Y0-DKM-134

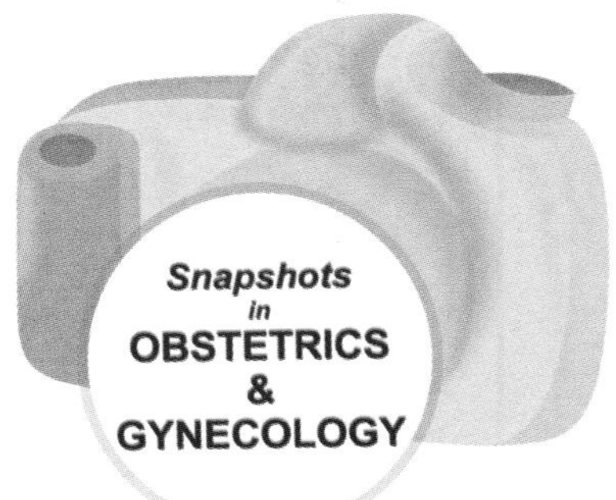
Snapshots
in
OBSTETRICS
&
GYNECOLOGY

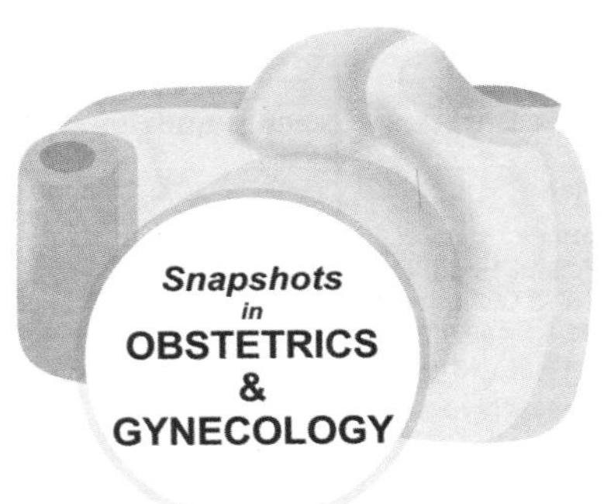

Richa Saxena MBBS MD

Obstetrician and Gynecologist

New Delhi, India

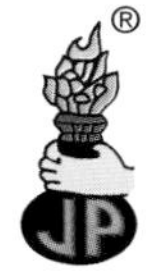

JAYPEE BROTHERS MEDICAL PUBLISHERS (P) LTD.

New Delhi • Panama City • London

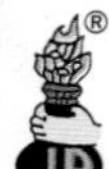

Jaypee Brothers Medical Publishers (P) Ltd.

Headquarter

Jaypee Brothers Medical Publishers (P) Ltd.
4838/24, Ansari Road, Daryaganj
New Delhi 110 002, India
Phone: +91-11-43574357
Fax: +91-11-43574314
Email: jaypee@jaypeebrothers.com

Overseas Offices

J.P. Medical Ltd.
83 Victoria Street, London
SW1H 0HW (UK)
Phone: +44-2031708910
Fax: +02-03-0086180
Email: info@jpmedpub.com

Jaypee-Highlights Medical Publishers Inc.
City of Knowledge, Bld. 237, Clayton
Panama City, Panama
Phone: +507-317-0496
Fax: +507-301-0499
Email: cservice@jphmedical.com

Website: www.jaypeebrothers.com
Website: www.jaypeedigital.com

Inquiries for bulk sales may be solicited at:
jaypee@jaypeebrothers.com

Snapshots in Obstetrics and Gynecology

First Edition: **2012**

ISBN 978-93-5025-802-6

Printed at Ajanta Offset & Packagings Ltd., New Delhi

Preface

Prayer does not fit us for the greater work; prayer is the greater work.

— Oswald Chanbers

Snapshots in Obstetrics and Gynecology is a small handbook which would serve as a ready reckoner and a pocket-sized reference source for both the general practitioners and the trainee students (especially the undergraduates). This book would prove to be useful in the day-to-day clinical practice of obstetrics and gynecology. Although it is a small handbook, the task of arranging the entire subject of obstetrics and gynecology into mere 500 small pages was a mammoth one, which could not have been made possible without the divine intervention and support of the almighty. So, I consider this book as a prayer which I offer and dedicate it to the almighty.

Everything should be made as simple as possible, but not simpler.

— Albert Einstein

This book aims at simplifying the subject of obstetrics and gynecology as much as possible. The idea behind "snapshots" is to present all important topics in obstetrics and gynecology, which are encountered in the clinical practice in form of brief snippets and snapshots. The book would also serve as a ready source of reference for a busy intern or an undergraduate student who does not have enough time to go through extensive literature.

The book has been broadly divided into two sections—obstetrics and gynecology. The section on obstetrics has 5 Chapters, while the section on gynecology has 10 Chapters. Various topics in each chapter have been termed as a "fragment". Each fragment has been arranged in the form of a predesignated template which has headings such as introduction, etiology, diagnosis, differential diagnosis, management, complications and clinical pearls. All these headings have been accompanied by relevant symbols.

Although utmost care has been taken while writing this text, I sincerely apologize for inadvertent errors, if any. Kindly email me your comments at: *richasaxena@womanhealthsimplified.com*

I would like to extend my thanks and appreciation to all the related authors and publishers whose references have been used in this book. Book creation is teamwork, and I acknowledge the way the entire staff of M/s Jaypee Brothers Medical Publishers (P) Ltd., New Delhi, India, worked hard on this manuscript to give it a final shape. Last but not the least, I would like to thank Shri Jitendar P Vij, the Chairman and Managing Director, Jaypee Brothers Medical Publishers, for being the guiding beacon and source of inspiration and motivation behind this book.

Richa Saxena

Contents

SECTION I: OBSTETRICS

1. General Obstetrics 3

1. Diagnosis of Pregnancy 3
2. Embryology and Early Fetal Development 10
   - 2.1 Gametogenesis 10
   - 2.2 Fertilization and Implantation 13
   - 2.3 Development of Human Placenta 17
   - 2.4 The Fetus 19
   - 2.5 The Fetal Circulation 22
   - 2.6 Development of Genitourinary System 25
3. Physiological Changes During Pregnancy 28
   - 3.1 Changes in Genital Organs and Breast 28
   - 3.2 Hematological Changes 32
   - 3.3 Cardiovascular Changes 34
   - 3.4 Changes in the Respiratory System 34
   - 3.5 Changes in Kidneys 34
   - 3.6 Changes in the Gastrointestinal Tract 35
   - 3.7 Carbohydrate Metabolism 36
   - 3.8 Changes in the Thyroid Glands 36
4. Lactation 37

2. Antenatal Assessment 39

1. Antenatal Care and Examination 39
2. Antepartum Fetal Surveillance 44
3. Pelvimetry 49
4. Different Pelvic Types 53
5. Fetal Skull 55

3. Labor and Delivery 58

1. Normal Labor and Delivery 58
2. Induction and Augmentation of Labor 70
3. Prolonged Labor 73
4. Obstructed Labor 77
5. Analgesia for Labor 80
6. Delivery by Forceps 82
7. Delivery by Vacuum 87
8. Cesarean Delivery 90
9. Breech Presentation 93
10. Transverse Lie 100
11. Occipitoposterior Position 104

12. Cord Prolapse 108
13. Compound Presentation 111
14. Face Presentation 112
15. Brow Presentation 115
16. Multifetal Gestation 117
17. Preterm Labor 122
18. Premature Rupture of Membranes 126
19. Post-term Pregnancy 130
20. Precipitate Labor 133
21. Version 134

4. Management of Special Cases in Obstetrics 138

1. Hypertensive Disorders in Pregnancy 138
   1.1 Preeclampsia 138
   1.2 Eclampsia 143
   1.3 Chronic Renal Disease During Pregnancy 145
2. Anemia During Pregnancy 147
   2.1 Iron Deficiency Anemia 147
   2.2 Megaloblastic Anemia 153
3. Gestational Diabetes 155
4. Cardiac Disease in Pregnancy 159
5. Spontaneous Abortion or Miscarriage 163
6. Medical Termination of Pregnancy 166
7. Gestational Trophoblastic Diseases 170
   7.1 Complete Hydatidiform Mole 170
   7.2 Partial Mole 174
   7.3 Gestational Trophoblastic Neoplasia 175
8. Antepartum Hemorrhage 177
   8.1 Placenta Previa 177
   8.2 Abruption Placenta 181
9. Abnormalities of Amniotic Fluid 185
   9.1 Oligohydramnios 185
   9.2 Polyhydramnios 188
10. Rh Negative Pregnancy 190
11. Vomiting in Pregnancy 194
12. Intrauterine Growth Retardation 198
13. Thyroid Disorders During Pregnancy 202
14. Connective Tissue Diseases During Pregnancy 204
15. Previous Cesarean Delivery 207
16. Bad Obstetric History 210
17. Liver Disease During Pregnancy 212
18. Obstetric Hysterectomy 213
19. Intrauterine Death 217

5. Postnatal Period 220

1. Puerperium 220
2. Complications in the Puerperium 223
   2.1 Puerperal Pyrexia 223
   2.2 Mastitis 225

2.3 Deep Vein Thrombosis (DVT) 226
2.4 Pulmonary Embolism 228
2.5 Amniotic Fluid Embolism 230
3. Episiotomy and its Repair 233
4. Perineal Injuries 236
5. Manual Removal of Placenta 239
6. The Newborn Infant 244
6.1 Care of a Newborn 244
6.2 Asphyxia Neonatorum 248
7. Postpartum Hemorrhage 253
8. Uterine Rupture 259
9. Uterine Inversion 261

SECTION II: GYNECOLOGY

6. General Gynecology 267

1. Gynecological Examination 267
2. Normal Gynecological Anatomy 270
3. Menstrual Cycle 277
4. Adolescent and Pediatric Gynecology 283
4.1 Puberty 283
4.2 Precocious Puberty 286
4.3 Delayed Puberty 288
5. Sex and Intersexuality 290
6. Ambiguous Genitalia 292
7. Hirsutism 295
8. Menopause and Hormone Replacement Therapy 297
9. Injuries of the Female Genital Tract 302
10. Tuberculosis of the Genital Tract 305

7. Abnormalities of Menstruation 309

1. Dysfunctional Uterine Bleeding 309
2. Menorrhagia 314
3. Leiomyoma 317
4. Dysmenorrhea 324
5. Premenstrual Syndrome 326
6. Postmenopausal Bleeding 330

8. Gynecological Oncology 334

1. Endometrial Cancer 334
2. Ovarian Cancer 338
3. Cancer of the Cervix 342
3.1 Cervical Intraepithelial Neoplasia 342
3.2 Invasive Cancer of the Cervix 347
4. Vaginal Cancer 352
5. Vulvar Cancer 355
6. Cancer of the Fallopian Tubes 358

9. Gynecological Surgery 361

1. Principles of Gynecological Surgery 361
2. Abdominal Hysterectomy 369
3. Vaginal Hysterectomy 376
4. Laparoscopic Assisted Vaginal Hysterectomy 379
5. Diagnostic and Operative Laparoscopy 382
6. Diagnostic and Operative Hysteroscopy 386

10. Disorders of the Uterus 391

1. Pelvic Prolapse 391
2. Uterine Retroversion 402
3. Chronic Pelvic Pain 405
4. Endometriosis 407
5. Adenomyosis 413
6. Uterine malformations 416

11. Gynecological Infections 424

1. Sexually Transmitted Diseases 424
   - 1.1 Chlamydial Infection 424
   - 1.2 Genital Herpes 426
   - 1.3 Gonorrhea 428
   - 1.4 Syphilis 430
2. Vaginal Discharge 431
3. Pelvic Inflammatory Diseases 437

12. Infertility 444

1. Amenorrhea 444
2. Male Infertility 451
3. Female Infertility 454
4. Assisted Reproductive Techniques 457

13. Disorders of Ovaries and Fallopian Tubes 460

1. Benign Ovarian Tumors 460
2. Polycystic Ovarian Disease 466
3. Disorders of Fallopian Tubes 469
   - 3.1 Salpingitis 469
   - 3.2 Ectopic Pregnancy 471
4. Disorders of Broad Ligament and Parametrium 477
   - 4.1 Parametritis 477
   - 4.2 Broad Ligament Leiomyoma 478
   - 4.3 Broad Ligament Hematoma 479

14. Urogynecology 482

1. Genitourinary Fistulae 482
2. Urinary Incontinence 488
   - 2.1 Stress Urinary Incontinence 490
   - 2.2 Urge Incontinence 495

15. Contraception **497**

1. Hormonal Method of Contraception 499
   1.1 Combined Hormonal Contraception (Oral Contraceptive Pills) 499
   1.2 Progestogen Only Contraception (Progestogen Only Pill) 501
   1.3 Injectable Contraceptives 502
   1.4 Subdermal Implants 504
2. Intrauterine Devices 506
3. Natural Family Planning Methods 511
4. Barrier Method of Contraception 512
5. Emergency Contraception 515
6. Permanent Method of Contraception 517
   6.1 Tubal Sterilization 517
   6.2 Vasectomy 521

Abbreviations *525*

Index *527*

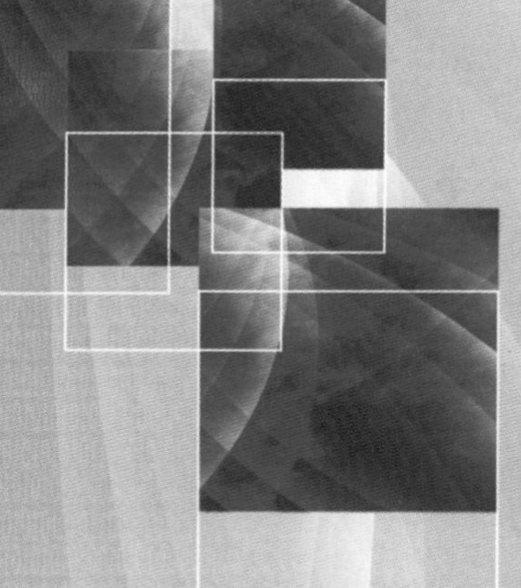

Section I

OBSTETRICS

- General Obstetrics
- Antenatal Assessment
- Labor and Delivery
- Management of Special Cases in Obstetrics
- Postnatal Period

CHAPTER 1

General Obstetrics

1. DIAGNOSIS OF PREGNANCY

INTRODUCTION

Reproductive activities in humans are likely to result in pregnancy, which can be defined as conception of one or more fetuses (embryos) in the uterine cavity of the women. Menstrual age or gestational age of pregnancy is the duration of pregnancy calculated from the first day of the last menstrual period. Gestational age is typically taken to be equal to 10 lunar months or 9 calendar months and 7 days or 280 days or 40 weeks. Fertilization occurs 14 days prior to the expected missed period. Thus, true gestational age is equal to 280 days minus 14 days, which is equal to 266 days. This is known as fertilization or ovulatory age. The whole period of pregnancy can be divided into three phases: the first trimester: 1–12 weeks; second trimester: 3–27 weeks and the third trimester: 28–40 weeks.

ETIOLOGY

Endocrinological Changes during Pregnancy

Various physical and physiological changes during pregnancy are related to the interplay between various hormones (**Fig. 1.1**). If pregnancy does not occur, the corpus luteum regresses. However, if the pregnancy does occur, the function of corpus luteum needs to be maintained in order to ensure sustained progesterone production. Following implantation, human chorionic gonadotropin (hCG) and possibly human placental lactogen (hPL) help in maintaining the growth and function of corpus luteum. Between 6–8 weeks of gestation, the functions of corpus luteum get transferred to placenta and it becomes responsible for production of protein and steroid hormones, which are responsible for various physical and physiological changes. Various hormones produced by placenta are:

- *Hypothalamic-like hormones*: Corticotropin releasing hormone (CRH), gonadotropin releasing hormone (GnRH), thyrotropin releasing hormone (TRH), growth hormone releasing hormone (GHRH)

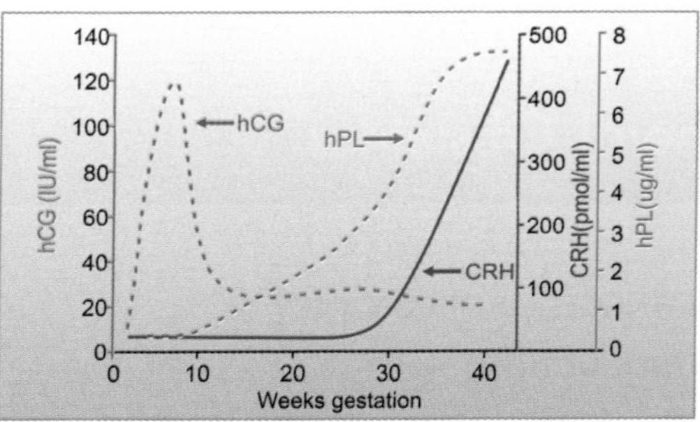

Figure 1.1: Endocrinological changes during pregnancy

- *Pituitary-like hormones*: Adrenocorticotropic hormone (ACTH), hCG, human chorionic thyrotropin (hCT), hPL
- *Other pregnancy proteins*: These include pregnancy associated plasma proteins (PAPP-A), relaxin, prolactin, atrial natriuretic peptide, etc.
- *Growth factors*: These include inhibin, activin, transforming growth factor-β (TGF-β), IGF I and II, epidermal growth factor (EGF)
- *Steroid hormones*: These include estrogen, progesterone and cortisol.

Some important hormones produced by placenta are hereunder described in details:

- *Human chorionic gonadotropin*: hCG is a glycoprotein with high carbohydrate content, which is produced from the trophoblastic cells following implantation. Hyperglycosylated hCG is a form of hCG produced by invasive cytotrophoblast cells in early pregnancy and implantation. This hormone can be detected in maternal plasma or urine by 8–9 days following ovulation. The doubling time of hCG varies from 1.4 to 2.0 days. Serum hCG levels increase from the day 1 of implantation and reach peak levels at 60–70 days, with the concentration ranging between 100–200 IU/mL. Soon thereafter, the concentration of hCG falls, reaching a value of 10–20 IU/mL between 100–130 days. Thereafter the levels of hCG remain constant throughout pregnancy with a slight secondary peak at 32 weeks. hCG disappears from circulation within 2 weeks following the delivery. The α subunit of hCG is biochemically similar to LH, FSH and TSH, whereas β subunit is relatively unique to hCG. The functions of hCG are as follows:
  - The function of hCG before 6 weeks of gestation is rescue and maintenance of corpus luteum and acting as a stimulus for secretion of progesterone by the corpus luteum.

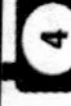

- It has immunosuppressive activity which inhibits the maternal process of fetal immunorejection
- It stimulates steroidogenesis from both adrenals and placenta

- *Human placental lactogen*: hPL, also known as the human chorionic somatomammotropin, is synthesized by the syncytiotrophoblastic cells of the placenta. It antagonizes the action of insulin and causes lipolysis, proteolysis and promotes the transfer of glucose and amino acids to the fetus.

Maternal-Fetal-Placental Unit

Placenta is not capable of independent steroidogenesis like the ovary. For steroidogenesis, it depends upon the precursors derived from the fetal and partly from the maternal sources. This concept is known as maternal-fetal-placental unit (**Fig. 1.2**). Precursors from fetal origin are not required for progesterone synthesis as in estrogen production. LDL cholesterol, derived from the mother, is used for progesterone synthesis (via pregnenolone).

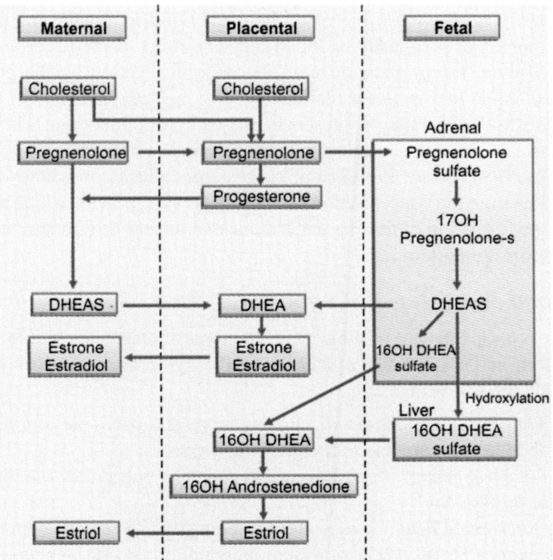

Figure 1.2: Maternal-fetal-placental unit

DHEA: Dehydroepiandrosterone; DHEAS: Dehydroepiandrosterone sulfate; OH: Hydroxy

DIAGNOSIS

History and Physical Examination

First Trimester of Pregnancy

- *Cessation of menstruation*: Cessation of menstrual cycles in a woman belonging to the reproductive age group, who had previously experienced spontaneous, cyclical, predictable periods, is the first most frequent symptom of pregnancy. Since there may be considerable variation in the length of ovarian and thus menstrual cycle among women, amenorrhea is not a reliable indicator of pregnancy, until 10 days or more after the onset of expected menses
- *Nausea and vomiting*: Also known as morning sickness, these symptoms appear 1 or 2 weeks after the period is missed and last until 10–12th week. Its severity may vary from mild nausea to persistent vomiting, e.g. hyperemesis gravidarum (refer to Chapter 4 for details)
- *Urinary symptoms*: Increased frequency of urination during the early months of pregnancy is due to relaxant effect of progesterone on the bladder, in combination with the pressure exerted by the gradually enlarged uterus on the bladder
- *Mastodynia*: It may be present in early pregnancy and ranges in severity from a tingling sensation to frank pain in the breasts
- *Cervical mucus*: Presence of progesterone during pregnancy helps in lowering the concentration of NaCl in cervical mucus, which prevents the formation of ferning pattern; instead the cervical mucus shows an ellipsoid pattern.

Second Trimester of Pregnancy

There is disappearance of subjective symptoms of pregnancy such as nausea, vomiting and frequency of micturition. Other symptoms, which may appear include the followings:

- *Abdominal enlargement*: Progressive enlargement of the lower abdomen occurs due to the growing uterus
- *Fetal movements*: Fetal movements generally occur after 18–20th week of gestation
- *Quickening*: Fetal movement (quickening) can usually be seen or heard between 16–18 weeks of gestation in a multigravida. A primigravida, on the other hand, is capable of appreciating fetal movements after approximately 2 weeks (i.e. 18–20 weeks)

- *Fetal heart sounds*: This is the most definitive clinical sign of pregnancy and can be detected between 18–20 weeks of gestation. The rate usually varies from 120 to 160 beats per minute
- *Palpation of fetal body parts*: The fetal body can usually be palpated by the 18–20 week of gestation unless the patient is obese; there is abdominal tenderness or there is an excessive amount of amniotic fluid
- *External ballottement*: This can be elicited as early as 20th week of gestation because the size of fetus is relatively smaller in comparison to the amniotic fluid **(Fig. 1.3)**
- *Internal ballottement*: This can be elicited between 16–28 weeks of gestation **(Fig. 1.4)**
- *Skin changes*: There is appearance of pigmentation over the forehead and cheeks by 24th week of gestation. There is appearance of linea nigra **(Fig. 1.5)** and stria gravidarum **(Fig. 1.6)** over the abdomen
- *Breast changes*: Refer to the successive fragments
- *Uterine changes*: Refer to the successive fragments.

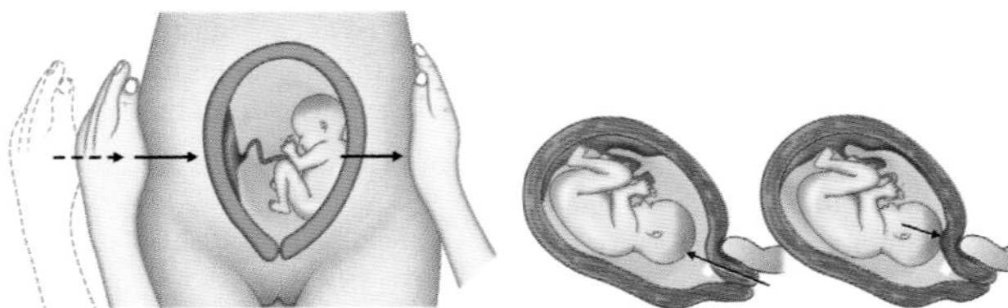

Figure 1.3: External ballottement

Figure 1.4: Internal ballottement

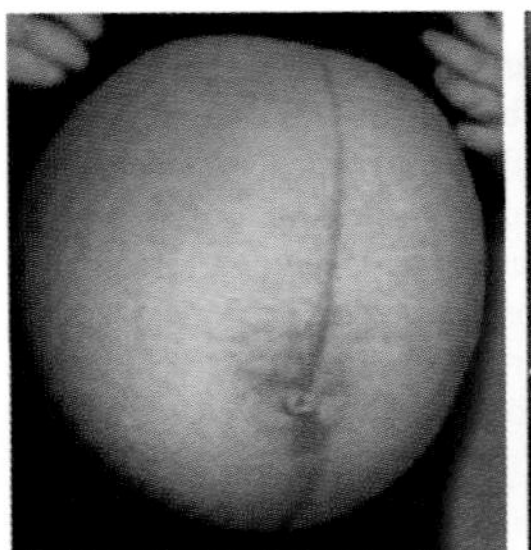

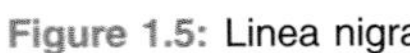

Figure 1.5: Linea nigra

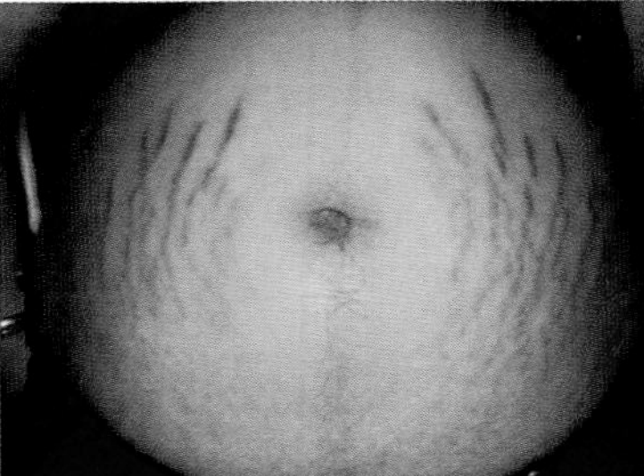

Figure 1.6: Stria gravidarum

Changes in the Third Trimester

- *Abdominal enlargement*: There occurs progressive enlargement of the abdomen, which can result in development of symptoms of mechanical discomfort such as palpitations and dyspnea. Lightening is another phenomenon, which occurs at approximately 38 weeks of gestation especially in the primigravida. This results in a slight reduction in fundal height, which provides relief against pressure symptoms
- *Frequency of micturition*: There is an increased frequency of micturition, which had previously disappeared in the second trimester
- *Fetal movements become more pronounced*: The fetal movements become more pronounced and palpation of fetal parts becomes easier
- Braxton Hicks contractions become more evident
- Fetal lie, presentation and period of gestation can be determined.

Investigation

- *Pregnancy test*: The laboratory test for pregnancy is based on the identification of hCG, which can be detected as early as 7–9 days after fertilization by highly sensitive techniques. The samples may be blood or urine. hCG has been described in the previous parts of this fragment.

Currently, the following four main types of hCG assays are used:

- Radioimmunoassay
- Immunoradiometric assay
- Enzyme-linked immunosorbent assay (ELISA)
- Fluoroimmunoassay.

Most current pregnancy tests have sensitivity to detect hCG levels of approximately 25 mIU/mL and involve the use of antibodies which are highly specific for β-subunit of hCG.

The most commonly employed technique is sandwich type immunoassay. In this test, a monoclonal antibody against β subunit is bound to a solid-phase support. The attached antibody is exposed to and binds with hCG in the serum or urine. A second antibody is then added to sandwich the bound hCG. In some assays, the second antibody is linked to an enzyme such as alkaline phosphatase. When the substrate for the enzyme is added, a color develops, intensity of which is proportional to the amount of enzyme and, therefore, to the amount of second antibody bound. The sensitivity for detection of hCG in serum is as low as 1.0 mIU/mL with this technique.

- *Basal body temperature (BBT)*: A persistent elevation of BBT for longer than 18 days may be presumptive evidence of pregnancy

- *Progesterone test*: If administration of progesterone to a woman with amenorrhea does not result in bleeding, she is most likely pregnant. If the woman is not pregnant, bleeding should occur within 7–10 days of progesterone administration
- *Ultrasonography*: Transvaginal ultrasonography (TVS) may demonstrate the gestational sac (GS) by 4–5 weeks of gestation **(Fig. 1.7)**, while transabdominal ultrasonography (TAS) is able to detect GS by 5–6 weeks of gestation. By 35 days of gestation, a normal sac is visible in all women and by 6 weeks, fetal cardiac activity can be visualized. Up to 12 weeks, the crown-rump length is predictive of gestational age within 4 days. With the advent of TVS, the diagnosis of pregnancy can be made even earlier than is possible with TAS
- The yolk sac can normally be recognized by 5–6 weeks gestation and is seen until approximately 10 weeks' gestation **(Fig. 1.8)**. When the GS is larger than 10 mm and no yolk sac is identified, an abnormal pregnancy is likely. This situation may be referred to as a blighted ovum or anembryonic pregnancy. Similarly, a yolk sac larger than 7 mm without evidence of a developing fetal pole suggests a nonviable pregnancy. The diagnosis of intrauterine pregnancy can be made once the yolk sac is present.

DIFFERENTIAL DIAGNOSIS

- *Pseudocyesis (spurious or false pregnancy)*: This is a psychological disorder where the woman feels that she is pregnant, but there is no pregnancy

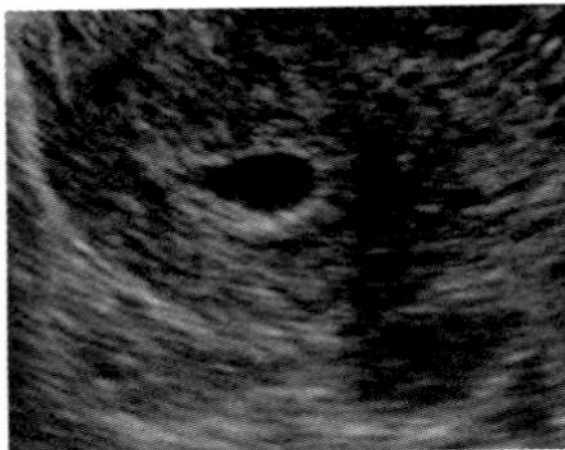

Figure 1.7: Gestational sac of size 4 mm observed on a transvaginal scan

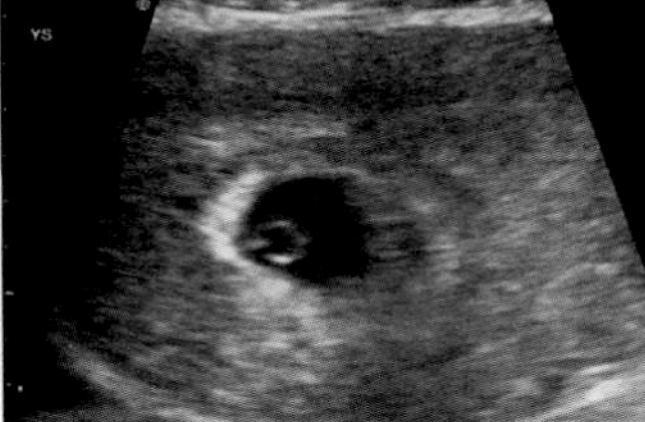

Figure 1.8: Yolk sac observed in a gestational sac at 6 weeks of gestation

- *Tumors*: Cystic ovarian tumors or fibroids
- *Encysted peritonitis*: This could be related to previous tubercular infection
- *Distended urinary bladder*.

MANAGEMENT

Management of pregnancy has been described in the successive chapters of this book.

CLINICAL PEARLS

- TVS is the most accurate means of confirming intrauterine pregnancy and gestational age during the early first trimester and can help to detect signs of intrauterine pregnancy approximately 1 week earlier than TAS
- The clinician must remain vigilant for presence of signs, such as rising hCG levels, an empty uterus (observed on sonogram), abdominal pain and vaginal bleeding, because these may signal an ectopic pregnancy
- The most important estrogen during late pregnancy is estriol, which is produced by the syncytiotrophoblasts. Low estriol levels may be related to fetal death, fetal anomalies (adrenal atrophy, anencephaly, Down's syndrome), hydatidiform mole, etc.
- Low progesterone levels are observed in cases of ectopic pregnancy and abortion, whereas high progesterone values are observed in cases of hydatidiform mole, Rh isoimmunization, etc.

2. EMBRYOLOGY AND EARLY FETAL DEVELOPMENT

2.1. GAMETOGENESIS

This comprises of spermatogenesis **(Box 1.1)** and oogenesis **(Box 1.2)**.

Box 1.1: Spermatogenesis

Spermatogenesis: The process in which spermatogonia gets transformed into spermatozoon is known as spermatogenesis. The testes are responsible for producing sperms and male hormone, mainly testosterone. Spermatogenesis is primarily under the control of follicle-stimulating hormone (FSH) and testosterone. Testosterone is synthesized in the interstitial leydig cells from where it diffuses into the seminiferous tubules and plays an important role in the facilitation of the process of spermatogenesis, which involves the production of sperms.

Contd...

Contd...

Initial process of spermatogenesis involves mitotic division, which is responsible for converting spermatogonia to primary spermatocytes. The spermatozoa then develop through a process of meiosis so that eventually diploid spermatocytes get converted into four haploid spermatids. Stages of spermatogenesis are described in **Figure 1.9**. The spermatids transform into spermatozoa, by a process known as spermiogenesis.

Box 1.2: Oogenesis

Oogenesis: The various stages of oogenesis have been described in **Figure 1.10**. The primordial germ cells, after arriving in the female gonad, differentiate into oogonia around 9th week of gestation. These enter the first meiotic division and are converted into oocytes. Progression of meiosis to the diplotene stage is accomplished throughout the pregnancy and is completed by birth. In the last week before birth, all the primary oocytes complete the diplotene stage, but do not progress further. Instead, they get arrested in the diplotene stage of prophase. The primary oocytes remain arrested at this stage and do not undergo the completion of first meiotic division till the age of puberty, when the completion of first meiotic division occurs at the time of ovulation. Second meiotic division starts, but gets arrested in the metaphase, which is completed only at the time of fertilization.

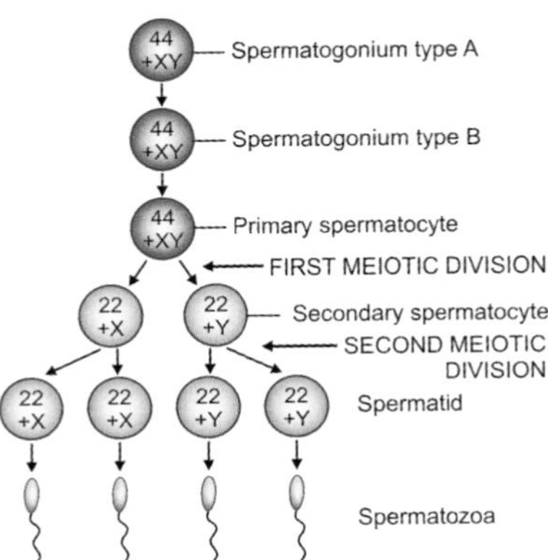

Figure 1.9: Stages of spermatogenesis

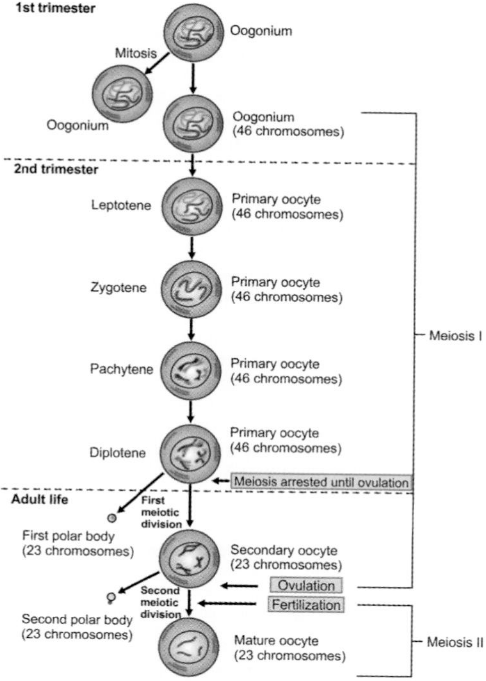

Figure 1.10: Stages of oogenesis

CLINICAL PEARLS

- The time required for the completion of the entire process of development of spermatozoon from the spermatogonium is about 70–75 days
- In males, testosterone gets converted into dihydrotestosterone in the peripheral tissues with the help of an enzyme 5-α reductase. Dihydrotestosterone is more potent than testosterone.

2.2. FERTILIZATION AND IMPLANTATION

Fertilization and implantation have been discussed in **Box 1.3**.

Box 1.3: Fertilization and implantation

Ovulation-Fertilization: Ovulation takes place as the ovarian follicle ruptures and the discharged oocyte is carried into the peritoneal cavity via the uterine tube. Once the oocyte has been extruded out, the cells of the empty ovarian follicle get converted into the corpus luteum which produces progesterone for about 14 days, in absence of fertilization and for 3–4 months if fertilization has taken place, after which it eventually dies off. The oocyte moves from the ovary to the uterine tube and may get fertilized by the male gamete in the ampulla of the uterine tube. Even though many spermatozoa may approach the oocyte, only one spermatozoon is allowed to enter the oocyte. It passes the zona pellucida by capacitation and acrosome reaction. The process of fertilization between two haploid gametes results in the formation of a diploid zygote, thereby restoring the number of chromosomes to that of the normal somatic cell. On fertilization, the chromosomal configuration can be of two types, either 44 (XY), i.e. a male child or 44(XX), i.e. a female child. The process of ovulation and fertilization has been summarized in **Figure 1.11**.

Cleavage Division and Formation of Morula

The zygote, a diploid cell with 46 chromosomes, formed as a result of fertilization of mature egg with a sperm undergoes numerous cleavage divisions to produce cells known as blastomeres **(Fig. 1.11)**. At this stage the zygote is present inside the fallopian tube and is surrounded by a thick zona pellucida. For 3 days as the blastomeres continue to divide, they produce a solid, mulberry-like ball of cells. This 16-celled ball is called morula. The morula enters the uterine cavity approximately 3 days after fertilization, and floats around in the cavity for a few more days. During this time, fluid gradually accumulates between the morula's cells, transforming the morula into a blastocyst.

Formation of Blastocyst

When the blastocyst reaches 58-celled stage at about 4–5th day of fertilization, it gets transformed into two types of cells: (1) trophoblast cells and (2) an inner cell mass **(Fig. 1.12)**. The inner cell mass (consisting of blastomeres) is destined to form the various tissues of the embryo. The trophoblast comprises of outer single layer of flattened cells, which later get converted into the future placenta. The cavity of the blastocyst is called the blastocoele.

Implantation begins with the burrowing of the blastocyst into the endometrium, which occurs by about 6–7 days after fertilization. The most

Contd...

Contd...

common site of implantation is upper posterior wall of the uterine cavity. By 8 day postfertilization, the trophoblast gets differentiated into an outer multinucleated syncytium known as syncytiotrophoblast and an inner layer of cytotrophoblasts.

As the trophoblastic cells invade deeper into the endometrium, by 10th day postfertilisation the blastocyst gets totally embedded within the endometrium **(Fig. 1.13A)**. As the blastocyst implants into the uterine wall, simultaneously it also prepares its cells and surrounding endometrium to develop into a placenta. As early as 7–8 days after fertilization, the inner cell mass or the embryonic disc gets differentiated into a top layer: ectoderm (epiblast) and an underlying layer of endoderm (hypoblast). Later, there is appearance of mesodermal cells between the ectoderm and endoderm. Small cells appear between the embryonic disc and trophoblast enclosing a space that later gets transformed into amniotic cavity. The ectoderm forms the floor of the amniotic cavity while the roof is formed by aminogenic cells. The endodermal germ layer produces additional cells which form a new cavity, known as the definitive yolk sac. As the amniotic fluid accumulates in the amniotic cavity, it enlarges. Small embryonic mesenchymal cells appear as isolated cells within the cavity of blastocyst. They soon line the cavity of blastocyst. When the blastocyst is completely lined with mesoderm, it is termed as chorionic vesicle. This is surrounded by a membrane called chorion which is composed of trophoblasts and mesenchyme. Soon numerous small cavities appear within the extraembryonic mesoderm. These cavities soon become confluent and form the extraembryonic coelom **(Fig. 1.13B)**. The extraembryonic coelom splits the extraembryonic mesoderm into two layers: (1) the extraembryonic somatopleuric mesoderm, lining the trophoblast and amnion and (2) the extraembryonic splanchnopleuric mesoderm, covering the yolk sac. With the development of extraembryonic coelom, the yolk sac becomes much smaller and is known as the secondary yolk sac. The membrane called amnion is composed of amniogenic cells along with somatopleuric extraembryonic mesoderm. As the folding of the embryo takes place, amniotic cavity completely surrounds the embryo **(Figs 1.14A to C)**. As the fetus grows, there is enlargement of the amniotic cavity, resulting in progressive reduction in the size of extraembryonic coelom. Eventually the extraembryonic coelom completely disappears, causing the amnion to come in contact with chorion and fuse with it to form the chorioamniotic membrane. As previously described, in the early stages, the embryo acquires the form of a three-layered disc. These three layers are also called as germ layers, from outside to inwards are: ectoderm (outer layer), mesoderm (middle layer) and endoderm (inner layer). These three layers of embryo are responsible for the formation of different organ systems and tissues giving the embryo more "human-like" appearance **(Figs 1.15A and B)**. When the embryo becomes about 10 weeks old, it is known as a "fetus".

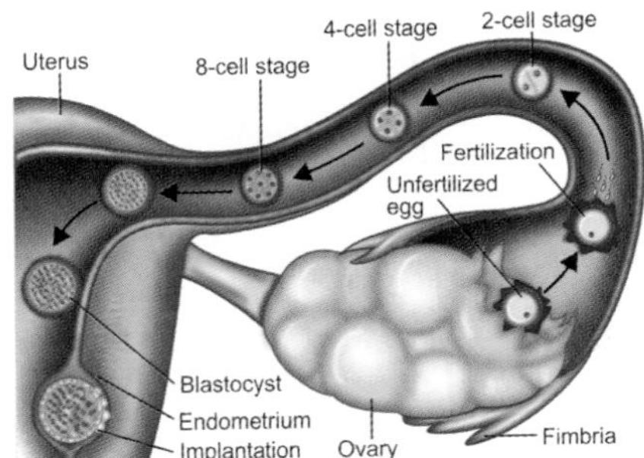

Figure 1.11: Ovulation-fertilization implantation

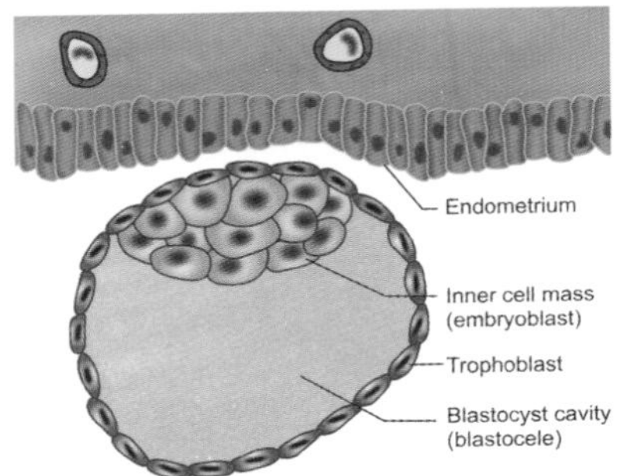

Figure 1.12: Blastocyst at a later stage with inner cell mass shifted to one side

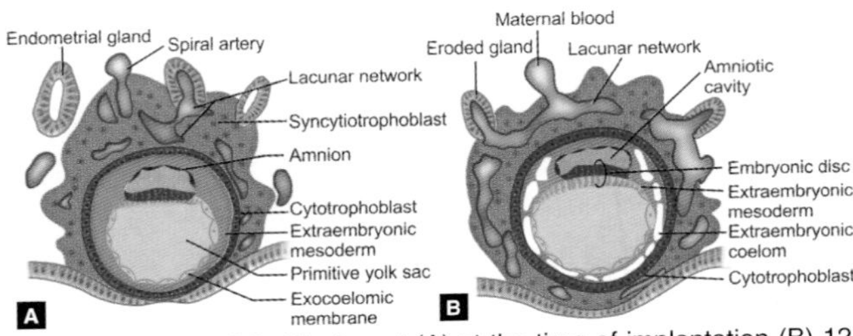

Figures 1.13A and B: Blastocyst (A) at the time of implantation (B) 12 days after fertilization

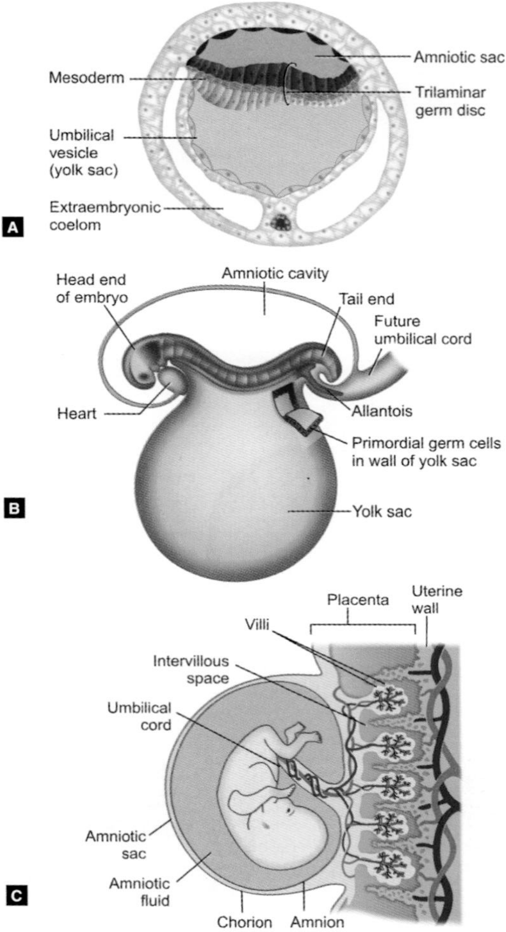

A

Mesoderm

Umbilical vesicle (yolk sac)

Extraembryonic coelom

Amniotic sac

Trilaminar germ disc

B

Head end of embryo

Amniotic cavity

Tail end

Future umbilical cord

Heart

Allantois

Primordial germ cells in wall of yolk sac

Yolk sac

C

Placenta

Uterine wall

Villi

Intervillous space

Umbilical cord

Amniotic sac

Amniotic fluid

Chorion

Amnion

Figures 1.14A to C: (A) Development of trilaminar germ disc; (B) development of early stage embryo; (C) development of fetus

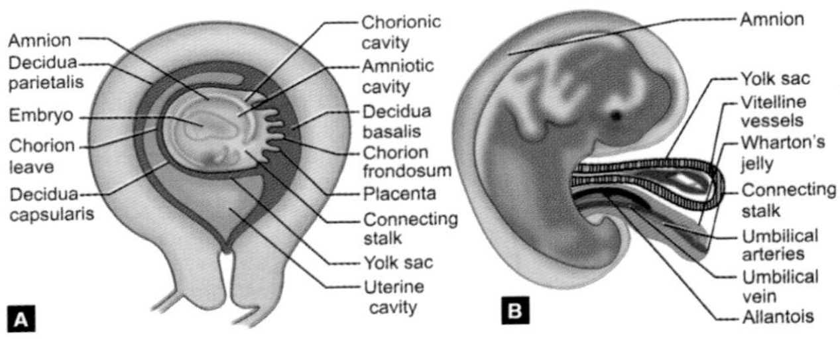

Figures 1.15A and B: (A) Uterus with embryo of 6 weeks size, (B) magnified view of a 6 weeks-sized embryo

2.3. DEVELOPMENT OF HUMAN PLACENTA

Development of human placenta has been discussed in **Box 1.4**.

Box 1.4: Development of human placenta

- The placenta is an organ with dual origin from both fetus and mother. A part of placenta develops from fetal chorion, and the rest develops from maternal endometrium. The fetal component consists of chorionic plate and chorionic villi, whereas the maternal component consists of decidua basalis. A structure known as cytotrophoblastic shell attaches the maternal and fetal component to one another
- After implantation, the syncytiotrophoblast starts secreting the hormone hCG. Under the influence of this hormone, the secretory changes taking place in the endometrial lining are further intensified resulting in conversion of endometrial lining into specialized cells, known as the decidua. This reaction is known as decidual reaction. By the 10th day of implantation, the blastocyst completely penetrates below the surface of decidua. The part of decidua at the site of the fetal portion gets transformed into chorion frondosum (the fetal precursor of mature placenta), whereas the maternal part is known as decidua basalis. The decidua at this stage can be classified into three portions. The side lying in contact with the blastocyst at the site of implantation is the decidua basalis; the decidua lying over the surface of the implanted blastocyst is the decidua capsularis; the remainder of the decidua lining the inside of the uterus is the decidua vera **(Fig. 1.15A)**. Initially, the decidua capsularis is separated from decidua parietalis by uterine cavity. With further enlargement of the uterine cavity, the decidua capsularis and decidua parietalis fuse with each other.

Contd...

Contd...

Stages of Chorionic Villi

- The chorionic villi are the finger-like projections arising from chorion and serve as precursors of human placenta. Chorionic villi of the placenta primarily function to transfer oxygen and other important nutrients between mother and fetus. In the early pregnancy, the villi are distributed over the entire periphery of the chorionic membrane. The chorionic villi in contact with decidua basalis, proliferate to form chorion frondosum, the fetal component of the placenta
- As the blastocyst with its surrounding trophoblasts grows and expands into the decidua, the outer pole of the mass expands outward toward the endometrial cavity. The opposite, inner most pole results in the formation of placenta comprising of villous trophoblasts and anchoring cytotrophoblasts. The development of chorionic villi passes through three stages: (1) primary villi [solid villi composed of cytotrophoblast core which is surrounded by syncytium **(Fig. 1.16)**]; (2) secondary villi [embryonic mesoderm has invaded the solid trophoblast columns **(Fig. 1.17)**]; (3) and finally tertiary villi [occurrence of angiogenesis in the mesenchymal core **(Fig. 1.18).**

Cytotrophoblastic Shell

- With increasing gestation, the cells of the cytotrophoblast in the tertiary villi proliferate and pass through the syncytiotrophoblast at the tip of the villi resulting in the formation of a continuous layer of cytotrophoblasts on the surface of decidua which is known as the cytotrophoblastic shell. This helps in fixing the chorionic villi to the decidua. Thus, the tertiary villi at one end are continuous with fetal component (chorion) and to the maternal component (decidua) at the other end.

Human Placenta

- The human placenta is rounded and discoidal in shape; the average diameter of the placenta being about 15–20 cm and weight about 500 grams. It is composed of multiple lobes called cotyledons, which are formed due to the presence of endometrial projections called septa. The placental cotyledons are visible on the maternal side of the placenta **(Fig. 1.19)**. On the other hand, the placenta shows a smooth surface from fetal side **(Fig. 1.20)** due to the presence of smooth chorion. At the center of the fetal surface the umbilical cord is attached. Despite the small size of a placenta, the surface area available for maternal-fetal exchange is greatly large due to the presence of villi. Each primary chorionic villus divides at least five times, forming villous trees. This leads to the formation of extremely large number of terminal villi, resulting in a large surface area, all of which is bathed in the uterine blood. Blood present in the intervillous spaces comes through the maternal endometrial arteries and is drained by maternal endometrial veins. The chorionic villi comprises of fetal blood as it contains branches of umbilical vein and umbilical arteries. The maternal blood in the intervillous space is separated from the fetal blood in placental villi through a membrane known as placental membrane or placenta barrier.

2.4. THE FETUS

The periods of fetal development **(Fig. 1.21)** are as follows:

- *Ovular period or germinal period*: This period lasts for first 2 weeks following ovulation
- *Embryonic period*: Begins from 3rd week following ovulation which extends up to 10 weeks of gestation
- *Fetal period*: Begins after 10 weeks of gestation and ends in delivery.

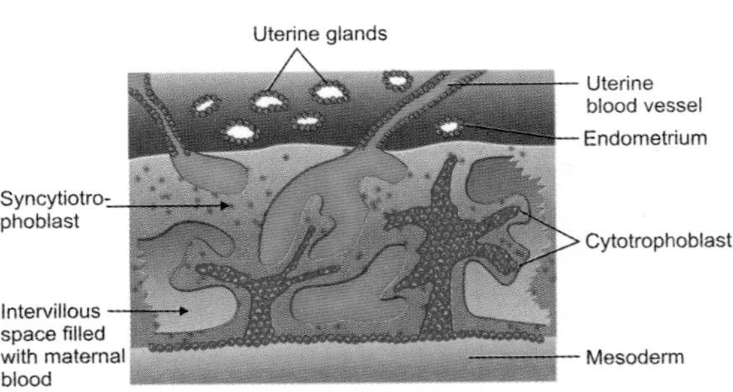

Figure 1.16: Primary villi

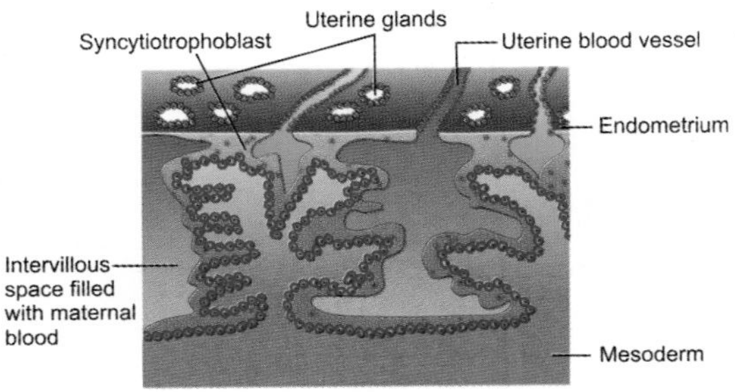

Figure 1.17: Secondary villi

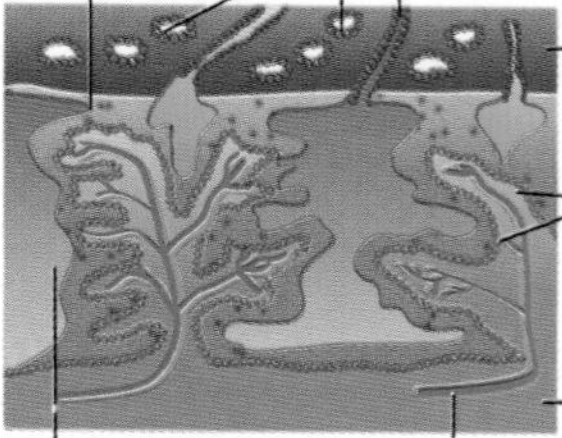

Figure 1.18: Tertiary villi

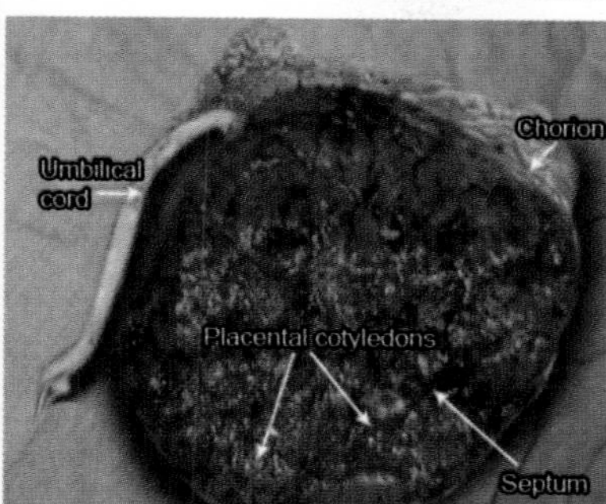

Figure 1.19: Maternal side of the placenta

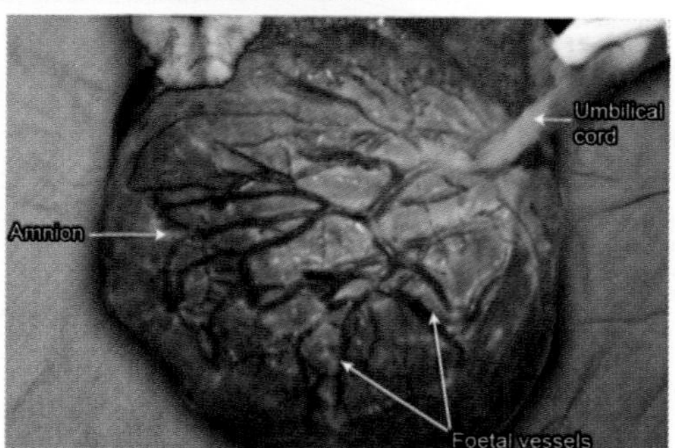

Figure 1.20: Fetal surface of the placenta

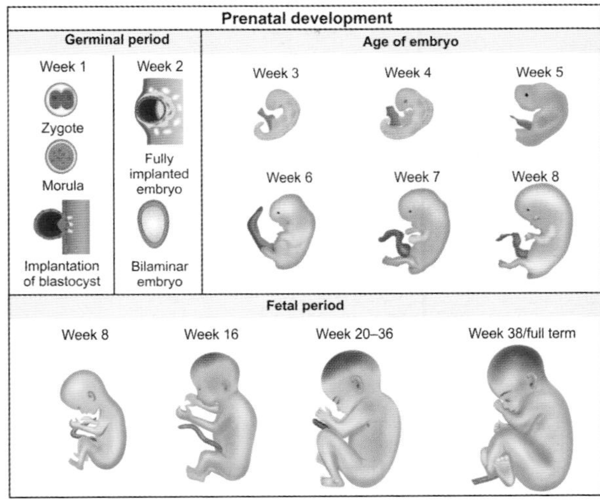

Figure 1.21: Various stages of fetal development

Embryo Development

Fate of development of different germ layers into various organ systems is described in **Table 1.1**.

Table 1.1: Fate of the germ layers

Layer	*Derivatives*
Endoderm	• Epithelial lining of respiratory and GI tract except part of the mouth, pharynx and the terminal part of the rectum (which are lined by the ectoderm) • Lining cells of all the glands which open into the digestive tube, including those of the liver and pancreas; the epithelium of the auditory tube and tympanic cavity; the trachea, bronchi and air cells of the lungs; the urinary bladder and part of the urethra; and the lining of the thyroid and parathyroid glands and the thymus • Various structures of digestive tract such as stomach, colon, liver, pancreas, urinary bladder

Contd...

Contd...

Layer	*Derivatives*
Mesoderm	• Cardiovascular system, reproductive/excretory organs, smooth and striated muscle, connective tissues, vessels, skeleton
Ectoderm	• Surface ectoderm—epidermis and other external structures • Neuroectoderm—central and peripheral nervous system, neural crest cells and derivatives

2.5. THE FETAL CIRCULATION

Adult circulation **(Box 1.5)** is described first followed by fetal circulation **(Box 1.6)**.

Box 1.5: Adult circulation

Adult Circulation: In normal adults, the deoxygenated blood from upper and lower parts of the body enters the right atrium via superior vena cava and inferior vena cava (IVC) respectively. The blood from right atrium enters the right ventricle via atrioventricular valves. The deoxygenated blood from right ventricle flows through the pulmonary artery to the lungs where it gets oxygenated. This oxygenated blood from lungs moves to the left atrium via the pulmonary veins. The oxygenated blood from left atrium moves to the left ventricle and is then distributed to the whole body via aorta and its branches **(Fig. 1.22)**.

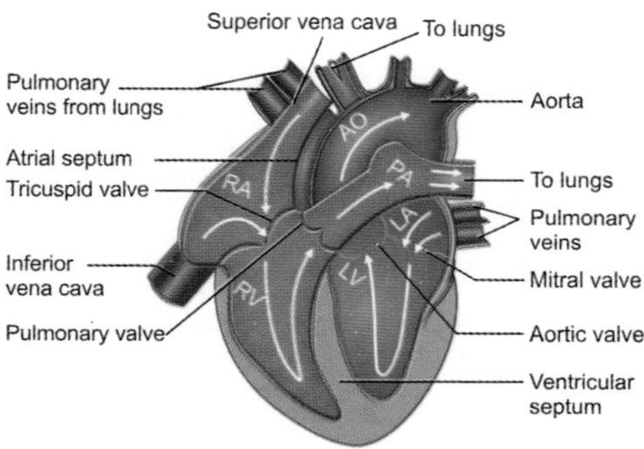

Figure 1.22: Adult circulation

Box 1.6: Fetal circulation

Fetal Circulation in Utero

Fetal circulation is characterized by presence of three shunts: (1) ductus venosus; (2) foramen ovale and (3) ductus arteriosus. These shunts permit the blood to bypass the liver and lungs, and shunt the most oxygenated blood from right to the left side of the heart **(Fig. 1.23)**.These shunts disappear following birth of the baby.

Also, in the fetus the lungs are not fully developed. Therefore exchange between the oxygenated and the deoxygenated blood does not take place in the lungs; rather it takes place in the placenta. Therefore, the fetal circulation differs from adult circulation in the following ways:

The deoxygenated blood from the hypogastric arteries, which are the direct continuations of the common iliac artery, moves into the two umbilical arteries. The umbilical arteries carry the deoxygenated blood from the fetus to the placenta. These arteries on reaching the placenta form numerous branches and enter the chorionic villi, where the exchange with oxygenated blood carried by maternal endometrial arteries takes place. The accompanying branches of umbilical veins in the chorionic villi, which carry the oxygenated blood, drain into umbilical vein, which carries the oxygenated blood to the fetus from placenta. As this oxygenated blood bypasses a shunt called ductus venosus, some of the oxygenated blood goes to the

Contd...

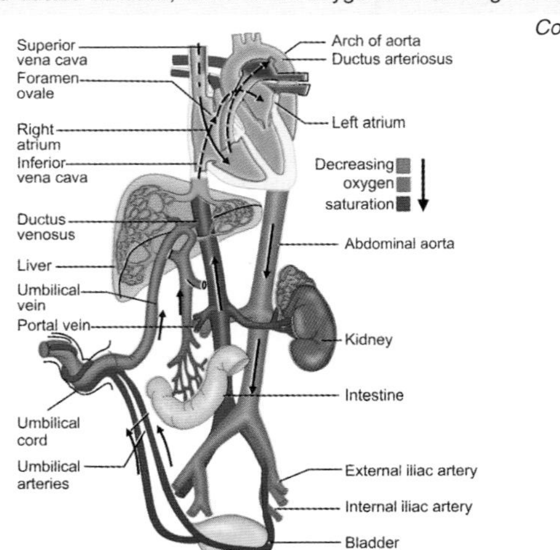

Figure 1.23: Fetal circulation just before birth

Contd...

liver, but most of it bypasses the liver and empties directly into the IVC. In IVC, there is oxygenated blood from umbilical veins along with deoxygenated blood returning from the lower extremities, pelvis and kidneys. While the deoxygenated blood from the lower parts of the body is drained into the right atrium via the IVC, the deoxygenated blood from the upper parts of the body is drained via the superior vena cava into the right atrium.

As the blood from the IVC enters the right atrium, a large proportion of it is shunted directly into the left atrium through an opening called the foramen ovale. A small valve called the septum primum, located at the atrial septum, prevents blood from moving in the reverse direction. The oxygenated blood in the left atrium mixes with a small amount of deoxygenated blood returning from the lungs (by means of pulmonary veins), and then enters the left ventricle and ascending aorta.

As the oxygenated blood from left atrium moves into the left ventricle and from there to the ascending aorta, the myocardium and brain are thereby supplied with the most oxygenated blood since the coronary and carotid arteries are the first to branch from the ascending aorta, before there is too much mixing with desaturated blood from other areas of the fetal heart. Although in the normal adult heart, all the blood from right atrium moves into the right ventricle and from there through pulmonary arteries to the lungs, in the fetal heart, a small amount of blood flows from the right atrium to the right ventricle and then through the pulmonary artery to the lungs. There is high resistance in the fetal pulmonary vessels that forces most of this blood to flow through the structure called ductus arteriosus into the descending aorta. Here it mixes with the blood from the proximal aorta to supply blood to the lower body.

Fetal Circulation Outside the Uterine Cavity

As the fetus is delivered out of the uterine cavity and the umbilical cord is clamped, the placental circulation ceases and the baby's lungs become functional. Thus, following the birth of the baby, two major changes take place:

- Decreased resistance of pulmonary vascular system following expansion of lungs
- Increased systematic vascular resistance due to breaking off from low resistance placental circulation. This causes blood to be shunted from left side of the heart to the right. Thus, heart starts working in series. This has two consequences:
    - The foramen ovale, which acts as a flap valve, closes due to increase in left atrial and decrease in right atrial pressure
    - The ductus arteriosus constricts due to exposure to increased PO_2. Although the functional closure occurs within 24–48 hours, permanent (anatomic) closure takes about 2–3 weeks for completion and results in the formation of a structure called ligamentum arteriosum. The hypogastric arteries on atropy becomes umbilical ligaments and the umbilical vein forms ligamentum teres. The ductus venosus closes and forms the ligamentum venosum.

2.6. DEVELOPMENT OF GENITOURINARY SYSTEM

Development of the genitourinary system has been discussed in **Box 1.7**.

Box 1.7: Development of the genitourinary system

Development of Gonads and Internal Genitalia

The sexual identity of individuals depends on their genetic, gonadal and phenotypic sex. Genetic or chromosomal sex is determined by the sex chromosomes, with XX karyotype being a genetic female and XY karyotype being a genetic male. Chromosomal sex is determined at the time of fertilization and is dependent on the presence of Y chromosome. In the absence of Y chromosome, the bipotential gonad differentiates into an ovary about 2 weeks later than when testicular development begins in the male. Gonadal sex, which is determined by the genetic sex, is established next. Gonadal sex is dependent on the presence of gonads: testes in males and ovaries in females. Gonadal sex controls the development of both internal and external genitalia. Internal genitalia in males comprise of testes, epididymis and vas deferens, while in females it comprises of fallopian tubes, uterus and cervix. Phenotypic sex is determined by the appearance of external genitalia and secondary sexual characteristics, which develop at the time of puberty.

The development of gonads begins during the 5th week of gestation in the human embryos with the development of a protuberance known as the genital or gonadal ridge. The primordial germ cells migrate into the developing gonad between 4–6th weeks of gestation, simultaneously proliferating at the same time. Initially the germ cells begin to divide by mitosis so that their number increases and they contain a diploid number of chromosomes. Soon thereafter, these cells undergo meiotic division, a process called gametogenesis, in which the number of chromosomes gets halved (haploid number).

The mesonephric ducts (Wolffian ducts) and paramesonephric ducts (Müllerian ducts) are two discreet duct systems, which coexist in all embryos during the ambisexual period of development (i.e. up to 8 weeks of gestation).

Under the influence of testosterone from the leydig cells of testes, the Wolffian ducts form the epididymis, vas deferens and seminal vesicles (male internal genitalia). The sertoli cells of testis produce a substance called MIS (Müllerian inhibiting substance), which suppresses the development of female internal genitalia from Müllerian ducts. In the absence of MIS, Müllerian ducts develop passively to form fallopian tubes, uterus and upper vagina **(Fig. 1.24)**. Development of vagina is described in **Figures 1.25A to D**. Differentiation of Müllerian ducts occurs in a cephalocaudal direction to form the female internal genital organs.

Contd...

Contd...

Development of External Genitalia

The external genitalia can be recognized as male or female by the 16th week of fetal life by ultrasound examination. External genitalia persists in the bipotential state until 9 weeks of gestation at which time it consists of a genital tubercle, urogenital sinus and lateral labioscrotal folds or swellings **(Fig. 1.26)**. Dihydrotestosterone, produced by the testes, determine the development of external genitalia. In the absence of masculinizing effect of dihydrotestosterone, the undifferentiated external genitalia develop along the female lines. The genital tubercle develops into the clitoris and genital folds into labia majora. Under the influence of testosterone, the genital tubercle forms the penis, the edges of the urogenital sinus fuse to form the penile urethra and the labioscrotal folds fuse to form the scrotum. This process is complete by 12–14 weeks of gestation. The urogenital sinus (UGS), which is of endodermal origin, is derived from the cloaca. It gives rise to caudal two-thirds of vagina in females; and forms prostate, bulbourethral glands, and urethra in males.

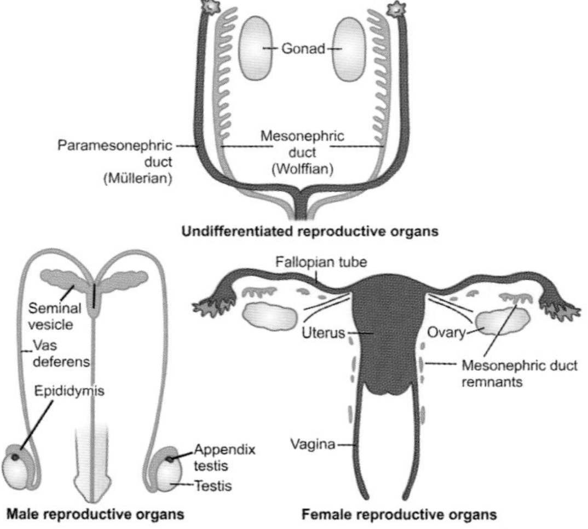

Figure 1.24: Formation of female internal genitalia from paramesonephric ducts and formation of male internal genitalia from Wolffian ducts

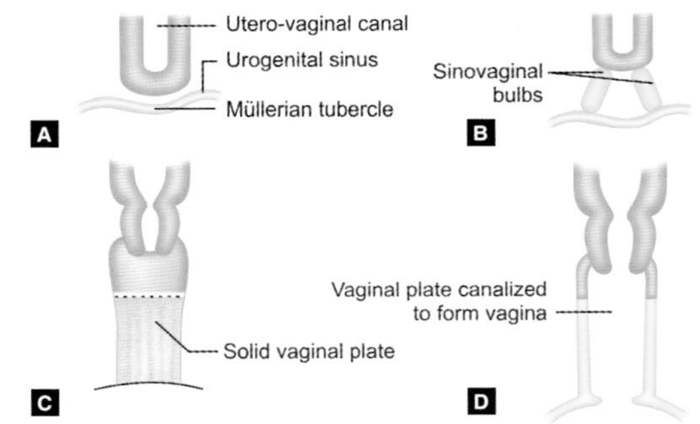

Figures 1.25A to D: Development of vagina: (A) mesoderm of uterovaginal canal pressing on the posterior wall of the endodermal urogenital sinus forming Müllerian tubercle; (B) proliferation of the endoderm of urogenital sinus results in the formation of sinovaginal bulbs; (C) solid vaginal plate formed due to fusion of mesoderm of uterovaginal canal and endoderm of sinovaginal bulbs; (D) vagina formed by canalization of vaginal plate (part derived from mesoderm is brown; part derived from endoderm is yellow)

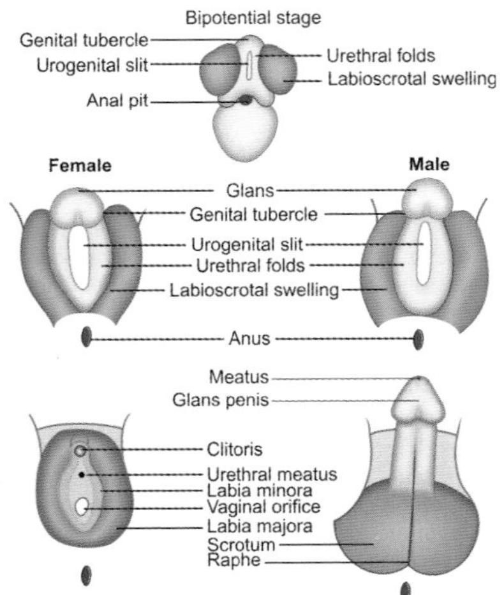

Figure 1.26: Development of external genitalia

CLINICAL PEARLS

- The uterus and upper one-third of the vagina develop from the paramesonephric ducts, while the lower two-thirds of the vagina develop from the urogenital sinus. By the 5th month the vagina is usually completely canalized
- The Wolffian duct degenerates in female fetus. It can sometimes still be traced in adult females, when it is known as Gartner's duct, which runs medially through the broad ligament and down the side of the vagina
- The pronephros and mesonephros develop to form the primitive kidney but disappear subsequently, and finally the metanephros appears to form the definitive kidney.

3. PHYSIOLOGICAL CHANGES DURING PREGNANCY

3.1. CHANGES IN GENITAL ORGANS AND BREAST

Changes, which take place during pregnancy in the genital organs, are described in **Box 1.8**, whereas those occurring in the breasts are described in **Box 1.9**.

Box 1.8: Changes in genital organs

Vagina

- *Chadwick's or Jacquemier's sign*: The vaginal walls show a bluish discoloration as the pelvic blood vessel becomes congested. This sign can be observed by 8–10 weeks of gestation
- *Osiander's sign*: There is increased pulsation in the vagina felt through the lateral fornix at 8 weeks of gestation.

Uterus

- Enlargement of the uterus occurs due to hypertrophy and hyperplasia of the individual muscle fibers under the influence of hormones such as estrogen and progestogens
- Uterine enlargement is more marked in the fundus. The uterine musculature during pregnancy is arranged in the form of three layers: (1) an outer hood-like layer arching over the fundus and extending into the various ligaments; (2) middle layer composed of dense network of muscle fibers perforated in all directions by the blood vessels and (3) an inner layer comprising of sphincter-like fibers around the orifices of fallopian tube and internal os of the cervix
- Muscle fibers in the middle layer are arranged in an interlacing, "figure of 8" manner with blood vessels lying between these fibers **(Fig. 1.27)**.

Contd...

Contd...

As a result, when the uterine musculature contracts following the delivery of the fetus and placenta, the penetrating blood vessels are constricted, thereby preventing excessive blood loss. The occlusion of arteries during uterine contractions also diminishes placental perfusion, resulting in fetal hypoxia and/or fetal bradycardia

- For the first few weeks of pregnancy, the uterus maintains its original pear shape, but becomes almost spherical by 12 weeks of gestation. Thereafter, it increases more rapidly in length, than in width becoming ovoid in shape. Until 12 weeks, the uterus remains a pelvic organ after which it can be palpated per abdominally
- The uterus increases in weight from prepregnant 70 grams to approximately 1,100 grams at term
- Due to uterine enlargement, the normal anteverted position gets exaggerated up to 8 weeks. Since the enlarged uterus lies on the bladder making it incapable of filling, the frequency of micturition increases. However, after 8 weeks the uterus more or less conforms to the axis of the inlet
- *Hegar's sign*: At 6–8 weeks of gestation, the cervix is firm in contrast to the soft isthmus and fundus. Due to the marked softness of uterine isthmus, cervix and body of uterus may appear as separate organs. As a result, the isthmus of the uterus can be compressed between the fingers palpating vagina and abdomen, which is known as Hegar's sign **(Fig. 1.28)**
- *Palmer's sign*: Regular rhythmic uterine contractions which can be elicited during the bimanual examination can be felt as early as 4–8 weeks of gestation
- *Braxton Hicks contractions*: In the early months of pregnancy, uterus undergoes contractions known as Braxton Hicks contractions, which may be irregular, infrequent and painless without any effect on the cervical dilatation and effacement. Toward the last weeks of pregnancy, these contractions increase in intensity, thereby resulting in pain and discomfort for the patient and may occur after every 10–20 minutes, thereby assuming some form of rhythmicity. Eventually, these contractions merge with the contractions of labor
- There is hypertrophy of the uterine isthmus to about three times its original size during the first trimester of pregnancy
- After 12 weeks of pregnancy, the uterine isthmus unfolds from above downward to get incorporated into the uterine cavity and also takes part in the formation of lower uterine segment
- There is an increase in the uteroplacental blood flow ranging between 450–650 mL/minute near term. This increase is principally due to vasodilatation

Contd...

Contd...

- *Uterine soufflé*: This is a soft blowing sound synchronous with the fetal pulse. It is caused by rush of blood through the umbilical arteries. On the other hand, fetal soufflé is a sharp whistling sound synchronous with the fetal pulse. It is caused by the rush of blood through umbilical arteries.

Cervix

- There occurs hypertrophy and hyperplasia of the elastic and connective tissue fibers and increase in vascularity within the cervical stroma. This is likely to result in cervical softening (known as Godell's sign), which becomes evident by 6 weeks of pregnancy. Increased vascularity is likely to result in bluish discoloration beneath the squamous epithelium of portio vaginalis resulting in a positive Chadwick's sign
- With the advancement of pregnancy, there is marked proliferation of endocervical mucosa with downward extension of the squamocolumnar junction. There is copious production of cervical secretions resulting in the formation of a thick mucus plug which seals the cervical canal. This mucus plug is rich in cytokines and immunoglobulins, and acts as an immunological barrier to protect the uterine contents against infection from the vagina
- When the cervical mucus (secreted during pregnancy) is spread over the glass slide and dried, it shows a characteristic crystallization or beading pattern due to presence of progesterone.

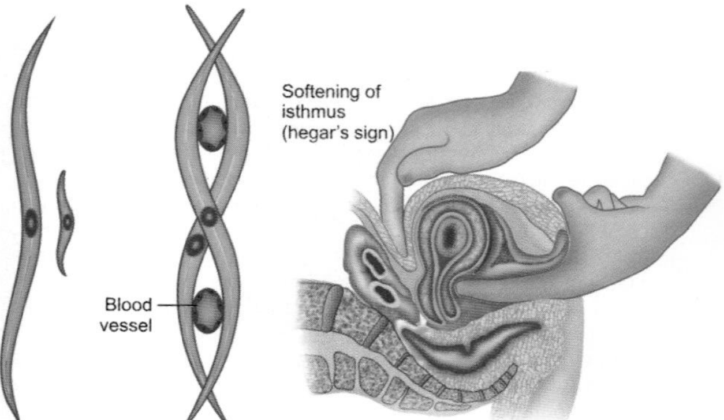

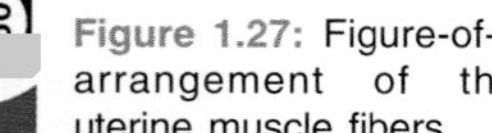

Figure 1.27: Figure-of-8 arrangement of the uterine muscle fibers

Figure 1.28: Hegar's sign

Box 1.9: Changes in the breast

Following changes are likely to take place in the breasts during pregnancy **(Fig. 1.29)**:

- Marked proliferation and hypertrophy of mammary ducts (under the effect of estrogen) and alveoli (under the effect of estrogen and progesterone)
- Hypertrophy of the connective tissue stroma and increased vascularity resulting in the appearance of bluish veins under the breast skin. The axillary tail of breasts becomes enlarged and painful
- The nipples become larger, erectile and pigmented. Hypertrophy of the sebaceous glands in the areola result in the formation of Montgomery's tubercles. Outer zone of irregular pigmented area appears around the areola in the second trimester, resulting in the formation of secondary areola. Sticky, thick, yellowish secretions can be squeezed from the breasts after about 12th week of pregnancy.

CLINICAL PEARLS

- Changes in the breasts are best evident in the primigravida in comparison to multigravida
- Presence of secretions from the breasts of a primigravida who has never lactated is an important sign of pregnancy.

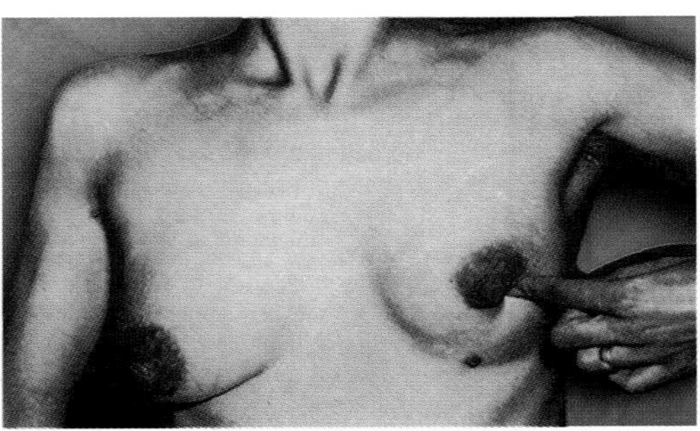

Figure 1.29: Breast changes during pregnancy

3.2. HEMATOLOGICAL CHANGES

Hematological changes which occur during pregnancy have been discussed in **Box 1.10**.

Box 1.10: Hematological changes during pregnancy

The following hematological changes occur during pregnancy **(Fig. 1.30)**:

- Increase in the blood volume starting from 6th week of pregnancy. By 30–32 weeks, the blood volume may have increased by 40–50% above the nonpregnant level
- The increase in the blood volume is due to an increase in the plasma volume (by 50%) and RBC volume (by 20–30%). The disproportionate increase in the plasma and RBC volume is likely to cause hemodilution, resulting in a physiological hemodilution of pregnancy
- Although more plasma than erythrocytes are added to the maternal circulation, the increase in erythrocyte volume averages to about 450 mL. Due to this, there is a slight decrease in the hemoglobin concentration, hematocrit and blood viscosity during pregnancy
- There is an increase in the concentration of total plasma proteins from a normal value of 180 grams in nonpregnant state to 230 grams at term. However, due to hemodilution there is an actual decrease in the concentration of plasma proteins from 7 gm% to 6 gm%. Moreover, there is a reduction in A:G ratio from 1.7:1 to 1:1
- There is neutrophil leucocytosis
- Average hemoglobin concentration at term is 12.5 gm/dL. A decline in hemoglobin value of less than 11 gm/dL especially late in pregnancy is abnormal and can be considered to be due to anemia (most likely iron deficiency anemia) rather than hypervolemia of pregnancy.

Coagulation Parameters

- Pregnancy is a hypercoagulable state. There is an increase in the fibrinogen levels from 200–400 mg% in the nonpregnant state to 300–600 mg% during pregnancy. There is also an increase in the activity of other clotting factors such as factors II, VII, VIII, IX and X. There is a slight decrease in the activity of other clotting factors such as factors XI and XIII.

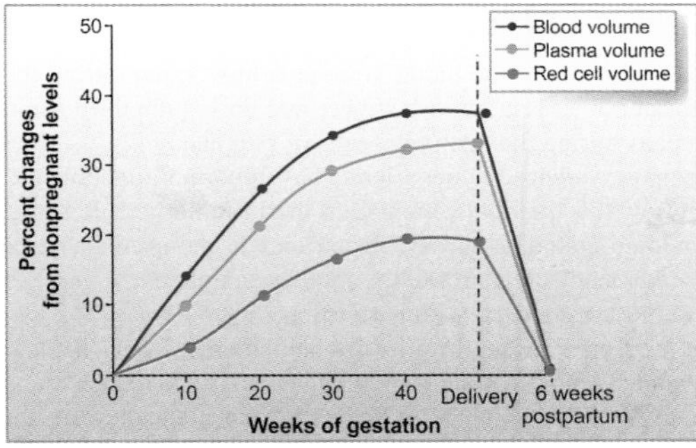

Figure 1.30: Hematological changes during pregnancy

Changes in iron requirements during pregnancy have been discussed in **Box 1.11**.

Box 1.11: Iron metabolism during pregnancy

Changes in Iron Requirements during Pregnancy

There is an increased iron requirement during pregnancy amounting to about 1,000 mg, which may occur due to the following reasons:

- 270 mg of iron is actively transferred to fetus. Fetus utilizes maternal iron for building up hemoglobin molecules
- 170 mg is lost through various routes of excretion, primarily the gastrointestinal tract
- Total amount of iron transferred to placenta and cord is 90 mg
- 450–500 mg of iron is utilized due to expansion in the total volume of circulating maternal erythrocytes.

Since pregnancy results in amenorrhea, this leads to a saving of nearly 240–300 mg of iron in form of menstrual blood. Thus total iron requirements during pregnancy are 600–700 mg (6–7 mg of daily requirement of elemental iron for about 100 days). Dietary iron along with that mobilized from the iron stores is usually insufficient to meet average demands imposed by pregnancy. Therefore, prescription of exogenous iron supplementation (an additional 20–30 mg of elemental iron per day) becomes a must during pregnancy.

CLINICAL PEARLS

- The expansion of the blood volume is most rapid during the second trimester. It rises at a much slower rate during the third trimester and plateaus during the last few weeks of pregnancy
- Pregnancy-induced hypervolemia has important functions: it helps in meeting the metabolic demands of the enlarged uterus; helps in providing abundant supply of nutrients to the growing placenta and the fetus and safeguarding the mother against the adverse effects of blood loss associated with parturition
- There is an average drop in the hematocrit of 5 U for a singleton pregnancy and 7 U for a twin pregnancy
- Changes in the coagulation factors during pregnancy ensure control of blood loss and hemostasis following the delivery of placenta.

3.3. CARDIOVASCULAR CHANGES

Changes in Cardiovascular system during pregnancy have been discussed in chapter 4 in the fragment of "cardiac disease in pregnancy".

3.4. CHANGES IN THE RESPIRATORY SYSTEM

During pregnancy, changes in the respiratory system have been discussed in **Box 1.12**.

Box 1.12: Changes in the respiratory system during pregnancy

- There occurs a state of hyperventilation, resulting in an increase in tidal volume and respiratory minute volume by 40%. This occurs due to the effect of progesterone on respiratory center and increase in the sensitivity of respiratory center to CO_2
- This hyperventilation causes changes in acid-base balance. There is fall in the arterial $PaCO_2$ from 38 to 32 mm Hg and a rise in PaO_2 from 95 to 105 mm Hg. These changes facilitate the transfer of CO_2 from fetus to the mother and O_2 from mother to the fetus. There is an overall rise in the pH and a base excess of 2 mEq/L. This results in respiratory alkalosis. Increased excretion of bicarbonates by the kidneys results in partial compensation.

3.5. CHANGES IN KIDNEYS

Changes occurring in the renal system during pregnancy have been discussed in **Box 1.13**.

Box 1.13: Changes occurring in the renal system during pregnancy

Glomerular Filtration Rate and Renal Plasma Flow

- There is an increase in GFR by 50% and RPF by 50–75% by 16 weeks of pregnancy and is maintained until 34 weeks. While the GFR remains elevated throughout pregnancy, RPF falls after 34 weeks of pregnancy
- As a result, there is reduction in maternal plasma levels of creatinine, blood urea, uric acid, etc.
- There is failure of complete absorption of substances, such as glucose, uric acid, amino acid, etc., from the renal tubules, resulting in an increased excretion of proteins, amino acids and glucose
- Serum creatinine levels decrease during normal gestation to greater than 0.8 mg/dL.

Acid-Base Balance

- There is decreased bicarbonate threshold, and progesterone stimulates the respiratory center. Therefore, serum bicarbonate decreases by 4–5 mEq/L.

Plasma Osmolality

- Serum osmolality decreases by 10 mOsm/L during normal gestation. Increased placental metabolism of vasopressin may cause transient diabetes insipidus during pregnancy.

CLINICAL PEARLS

- There is dilatation of ureters (above the pelvic brim), renal pelvis, calyces, etc., thereby resulting in stasis
- Stasis is particularly marked between 20–24 weeks of gestation.

3.6. CHANGES IN THE GASTROINTESTINAL TRACT

Changes occurring in the gastrointestinal tract during pregnancy have been discussed in **Box 1.14**.

Box 1.14: Changes occurring in the gastrointestinal tract during pregnancy

- There is increased congestion of the gums. Due to this, they may become spongy and thereby bleed to touch
- There is reduced muscle tone and motility of the entire gastrointestinal tract under the effect of progesterone. This may be responsible for producing constipation

Contd...

Contd...

- Relaxation of the cardiac sphincter may result in regurgitation of gastric acid into the esophagus, thereby producing chemical esophagitis and heart burns
- Gastric secretions are also reduced and the emptying time of the stomach is delayed. This results in a reduced risk for the development of peptic ulcer disease.

3.7 CARBOHYDRATE METABOLISM

Carbohydrate metabolism during pregnancy has been discussed in **Box 1.15**.

Box 1.15: Carbohydrate metabolism during pregnancy

Insulin Resistance

- Pregnancy is a diabetogenic state, resulting in development of insulin resistance. In the first half of pregnancy there is an increased sensitivity to insulin and therefore there is a tendency toward development of hypoglycemia. On the other hand, the second half of pregnancy (especially after 24 weeks of gestation) is related with development of insulin resistance.

Causes of insulin resistance during pregnancy include:

- There occurs hyperplasia and hypertrophy of the beta cells of pancreas.
- Steroid hormones (especially corticosteroids, estriol and progesterone), which are produced late in pregnancy, show an anti-insulin effect
- Some insulin may be destroyed by placenta and kidneys.

Changes Related with Carbohydrate Metabolism

- There is transfer of increased amount of glucose from the mother to the fetus throughout the pregnancy
- These changes help in ensuring continuous supply of glucose to the fetus
- There is mild fasting hypoglycemia, postprandial hyperglycemia and hyperinsulinemia as well as greater suppression of glucagon
- When fasting is prolonged in pregnant women, ketonemia rapidly results
- In the postprandial state, there is a switch from glucose to lipids as a source of principal fuel. Increasing levels of hPL with gestation is responsible for increased lipolysis and liberation of free fatty acids.

3.8. CHANGES IN THE THYROID GLANDS

Changes in thyroid glands during pregnancy have been discussed in **Box 1.16**.

Box 1.16: Changes in thyroid glands during pregnancy

- There is an increased production of thyroid hormones by 40–100% in order to meet the maternal and fetal requirements
- Moderate enlargement of thyroid glands is caused by glandular hyperplasia and increased vascularity
- There is a marked and early increase in hepatic production of thyroid binding globulins (TBG) and placental production of hCG. Levels of TBG start increasing from first trimester. They peak at 20 weeks of pregnancy and plateau during the remainder part of pregnancy. Increase in TBG increases serum thyroxine concentrations, whereas hCG has thyrotropin-like activity and stimulates maternal T4 production
- Levels of thyroid releasing hormone (TRH) are not increased during normal pregnancy. However, this hormone can cross the placenta and stimulates the fetal pituitary to secrete thyrotropin
- Normal suppression of TSH during pregnancy may result in misdiagnosis of subclinical hypothyroidism.

4. LACTATION

Lactation has been discussed in **Box 1.17**.

Box 1.17: Lactation

Lactation is the process of milk production, which occurs from the mammary glands. These are exocrine glands, whose function is to nourish the neonate. The endocrine control of lactation **(Fig. 1.31)** can be divided into the following stages:

- *Mammogenesis*: This stage is associated with preparation of the breast tissues. During pregnancy, there is growth of both ductal and lobuloalveolar systems
- *Lactogenesis*: There is synthesis and secretion of milk by breast alveoli during this phase. Although some amount of secretions are produced from the breasts throughout the pregnancy, actual milk secretion starts by 3rd or 4th postpartum days. With the decline in the levels of estrogen and progesterone following delivery, prolactin is able to produce its milk secretory activity in the previously fully developed mammary glands. Other hormones, which may enhance the secretory activity of mammary glands, include growth hormone, thyroxine, glucocorticoids and insulin
- *Galactokinesis*: During this phase, there is ejection of milk. Due to this, the milk is forced down the ampulla of lactiferous ducts from where it can be sucked by the infant
- *Galactopoiesis*: This phase is associated with maintenance of lactation. Prolactin is the most important hormone, which is responsible for galactopoiesis. Sucking is essential for maintenance of effective lactation. It helps in removal of milk produced by the glands as well as causes release of prolactin.

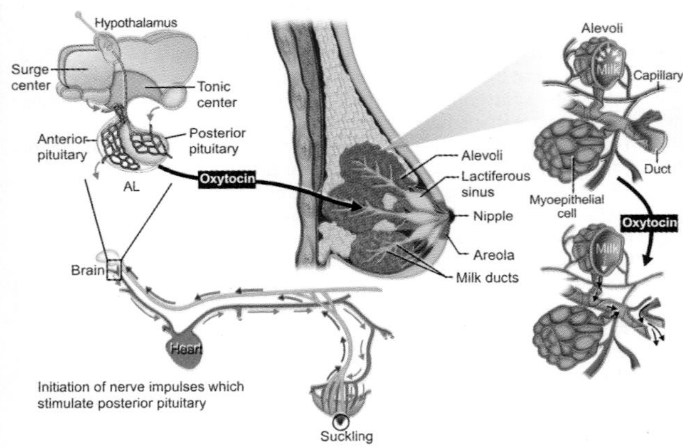

Figure 1.31: Endocrine mechanism of milk ejection: suckling of the breasts by the fetus causes the stimulation of paraventricular nucleus in the posterior lobe of pituitary gland, causing the release of oxytocin. This leads to the contraction of myoepithelial cells surrounding the alveolus, which causes the ejection of milk from alveoli into the ducts

CLINICAL PEARLS

- Milk ejection reflex can be inhibited by factors such as pain, breast engorgement, etc.
- The amount of milk produced in a healthy mother is about 500–800 mL/day.
- Drugs which help in improving milk production (galactogogues) include metoclopramide (10 mg, TDS), dopamine antagonists and intranasal oxytocin
- Drugs, which may cause milk suppression, include bromocriptine (dopamine agonists) and mechanical methods
- All babies, regardless of the type of delivery, must be given exclusive breast feeding up to 6 months of birth.

CHAPTER 2

Antenatal Assessment

1. ANTENATAL CARE AND EXAMINATION

Proper antenatal care **(Boxes 2.1 and 2.2)** helps in screening of high-risk cases (e.g. preeclampsia, anemia, diabetes, cardiac disease, etc.) and supervision of the present pregnancy.

Box 2.1: Antenatal assessment

A. *History Taking*

- *Past obstetric history*: The woman's past obstetric history must be denoted by the acronym GPAL, where G stands for gravid; P for parity; A for number of abortions and L for number of live births
- *Medical history*: The woman must be asked about the previous medical history of diabetes, epilepsy, hypertension, renal disease, rheumatic disease, heart valve disease, epilepsy, asthma, tuberculosis, psychiatric illness or any other significant illness she may have had in the past. History of any allergies (specifically allergy to penicillin) must also be enquired
- *Evaluation of exposure to medications*: Including exposure to over-the-counter and prescribed drugs, (including terato genic drugs such as isotretinoin, warfarin, etc.) must be enquired. Maternal use of alcohol, tobacco and other mood-altering substances must be enquired. History of receiving Rh immune globulins during her previous pregnancies must also be taken
- *Nutritional assessment*: The body mass index, defined as [weight in kilograms/(height in meters)^2] is the preferred indicator of nutritional status
- *Social assessment*: Identification of social, financial and psychological issues that could affect pregnancy planning must be done.

B. *Parameters to be Assessed at the Time of Each Antenatal Visit*

- Maternal weight
- Pallor, blood pressure, edema, jaundice, etc.
- Fetal well-being; fetal lie; position; presentation and number of fetuses; amniotic fluid volume; assessment of fetal growth

Contd...

Contd...

C. *Abdominal Examination*

- *Inspection*: Presence of previous scars over the abdomen, abdominal enlargement
- *Palpation*: Normally, the uterus cannot be palpated per abdomen during the first trimester; during the second trimester the fetus is identified by external ballottement; during the third trimester, palpation of the fetal parts and auscultation of fetal heart sounds can be done. Four Lepold's maneuvers for estimation of fetal lie, presentation, position and assessment of engagement need to be done. Measurement of abdominal girth, assessment of fetal growth pattern and liquor volume also needs to be done
- Fetal heart sounds can be heard with a stethoscope or a hand-held Doppler.

D. *Vaginal Examination*

This is usually done in the later months of pregnancy beyond 37 weeks. This involves assessment of cervical consistency, dilatation and effacement; fetal presentation and position; assessment of fetal membranes and amount of liquor; evaluation of the station of the presenting part; molding of fetal skull and pelvic assessment.

E. *Investigations*

- Determination of the patient's blood group (ABO and Rh)
- Hemoglobin estimation
- Urine test for protein and glucose (to be done at every visit)
- Serological screening test for syphilis
- Rapid HIV screening test (after pretest counseling and written consent)
- Microscopic examination of wet smear of any symptomatic vaginal discharge (i.e. itching, burning or offensive).

Box 2.2: Routine antenatal care

A. *Pregnancy Dating*

- The average duration of human pregnancy is 280 days from the first day of the last menstrual period (LMP) until delivery. Expected day of delivery is most commonly calculated using Naegele's rule

Naegele's rule: Using Naegele's rule, the estimated date of delivery is calculated by adding 9 calendar months and 7 days to the first day of the last menstrual (28-day cycle) period. For in vitro fertilization (IVF) pregnancies, date of LMP is 14 days prior to the date of embryo transfers.

Ultrasonographic dating: This is the most accurate from 7 to 11 weeks of pregnancy.

Contd...

Contd...

B. *Nutrition*

- Pregnant women require 15% more kilocalories than non-pregnant women, usually 100–300 kcal more per day, depending on the patient's weight and activity
- Consumption of iron-containing foods should be encouraged. Iron supplements containing 30 mg of elemental iron is prescribed daily starting from second trimester onward. For calcium, the prenatal daily requirement is 1,200 mg
- Pregnant women should avoid uncooked meat because of the risk of toxoplasmosis.

C. *Frequency of Antenatal Visits*

The antenatal visits should be at every 4-weekly up to 28 weeks; at every 2-weekly up to 36 weeks and thereafter weekly till the expected date of delivery. A minimum of four visits are mandatory: first at 16th weeks; second at 24–28 weeks; third at 32 weeks and fourth at 36 weeks.

D. *Weight Gain*

The total weight gain recommended for pregnancy based on the pre-pregnancy body mass index is described in **Table 2.1**. Gestational weight gain amounts to about 28–29 pounds. Distribution of weight gain during pregnancy is described in **Figure 2.1**.

The physiological average weight gain in healthy primigravid women eating without restriction is expected to be about 12.5 kg of which 1 kg is gained during the first trimester. Approximately 7 lbs (3.2 kg) is gained at 10–20 weeks and approximately 10 lbs (4.6 kg) at 20–30 weeks.

E. *Exercise and Employment*

In the absence of obstetric or medical complications, most patients are able to work throughout the entire pregnancy. Heavy lifting and excessive physical activity should be avoided.

F. *Immunizations*

- All women of childbearing age should be immune to measles, rubella, mumps, tetanus, diphtheria, poliomyelitis and varicella through natural or vaccine-conferred immunization
- All pregnant women should be screened for hepatitis B surface antigen. Pregnancy is not a contraindication to the administration of HBV vaccine for hepatitis B
- *Tetanus toxoid*: For unimmunized women, tetanus toxoid must be administered intramuscularly in the dosage of 0.5 mL at 6 weekly intervals, with the first dose being administered at 16–24 weeks. For women who have been immunized in the past, a booster dose of 0.5 mL may be administered in the third trimester

Contd...

Contd...

- Varicella zoster immune globulin should be administered to any newborn whose mother has developed chickenpox within 5 days before or 2 days after delivery.

G. *Sexual Intercourse*
No restriction of sexual activity is necessary for pregnant women. Avoidance of sexual activity must be recommended for women at risk of preterm labor, placenta previa or women with previous history of pregnancy loss.

H. *Genetic Counseling*
- *Noninvasive prenatal diagnostic tests*: These mainly include biochemical markers in the form of triple test or quadruple test. Addition of nuchal translucency to the biochemical markers helps in improving the accuracy of detection rate by 80%. The maternal serum triple screen is performed at 15–20 weeks of pregnancy and measures the following in maternal serum: maternal serum alpha-fetoprotein (MSAFP); hCG and unconjugated estriol levels. Low MSAFP levels, low levels of unconjugated estriol and high maternal serum hCG levels are associated with an increased risk of Down's syndrome.Quadruple test includes the same parameters as described with triple test along with high levels of inhibin A. If the woman is found to be at a high risk (> 1 in 250) for Down's syndrome based on the results of these tests, maternal age (> 35 years), they are then offered a diagnostic test—either amniocentesis or chorionic villus sampling (described in coming-up fragments).

Table 2.1: Recommended total weight gain for pregnant women based on their pre-pregnancy BMI for singleton gestation

Weight for height	*Body mass index (Kg/m^2)*	*Recommended total weight gain*	
		(Kg)	*(lb)*
Underweight	< 19.8	12.5–18	28–40
Normal weight	19.8–26.0	11.5–16	25–35
Overweight	26.0–29.0	7–11.5	15–25
Obesity	> 29	< 7	< 15
Twin gestation	—	15.5–20.4	35–45

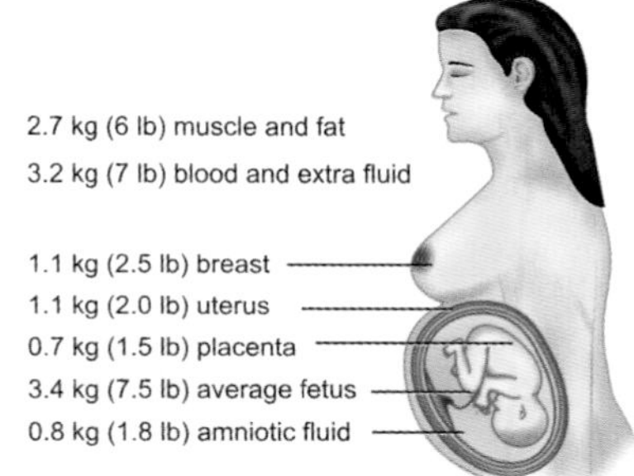

Figure 2.1: Distribution of weight gain during pregnancy

CLINICAL PEARLS

- Gravida refers to the number of pregnancies, including the present pregnancy the woman has ever had. This is irrespective of the fact whether the pregnancies were viable at the time of birth or not. Parity, on the other hand, refers to the number of previous viable pregnancies (including infants who were either stillborn or born alive)
- Pelvic assessment and assessment of cephalopelvic disproportion are best done with the onset of labor or just before induction
- Presence of or history of vaginal bleeding is a contraindication for vaginal examination
- Diminishing abdominal girth at term or earlier must arouse the suspicion of placental insufficiency
- The woman must be advised to report to the hospital immediately in case of presence of uterine contractions, passage of watery fluid per vagium, active vaginal bleeding, symptoms, such as intense headache, epigastric pain, vomiting, scanty urination, etc.
- Isotretinoin is highly teratogenic drug, which can cause craniofacial defects such as microtia, anotia, etc.Warfarin sodium, an anticoagulant, and its derivatives have also been associated with warfarin embryopathy
- Very overweight and very underweight women are at risk for poor pregnancy outcomes
- Periconceptual intake of folic acid reduces the risk of neural tube defects
- Down's syndrome is an autosomal chromosome abnormality in which an extra chromosome 21 material is present in the affected individual.

2. ANTEPARTUM FETAL SURVEILLANCE

The management protocol regarding antepartum fetal surveillance in all pregnant women is described in **Figure 2.2**.

METHODS OF FETAL ASSESSMENT

Daily fetal movement count using Cardiff count-to-10 method has been discussed in **Box 2.3**.

Box 2.3: Daily fetal movement count using Cardiff count-to-10 method

Method: While performing the kick count, the mother must lie on her left side in comfortable location. The mother is asked to report the time it takes for her to feel ten movements, no matter how small and is instructed to record them in the form of a chart. Whenever she feels a fetal movement, she is instructed to mark each movement on the chart until she has marked ten movements in all. Then she must note the time. If the women can feel about ten movements in an hour, it is considered as normal.

Nonstress Test (NST)

Box 2.4 describes the method of NST.

Box 2.4: Method of NST

The test involves attaching one belt of an external tocodynamometer to the mother's abdomen to measure fetal heart-rate and another belt to measure contractions. Fetal movement, heart-rate and "reactivity" of fetal heart are measured for 20–30 minutes **(Fig. 2.3)**. The classification of NST as reactive (normal or indicative of fetal well-being) or nonreactive (abnormal or may be indicative of fetal compromise is shown in **Table 2.2**.

Table 2.2: Classification of NST as either reactive or nonreactive

Test result	*Interpretation*
A reactive nonstress result	If there are accelerations of the fetal heart-rate of at least 15 beats per minute over the baseline, lasting at least 15 seconds, occurring within a 20 minute time block
Nonreactive nonstress test	If these accelerations don't occur, the test is said to be nonreactive. Additional testing may be required to determine whether the result is truly due to poor oxygenation

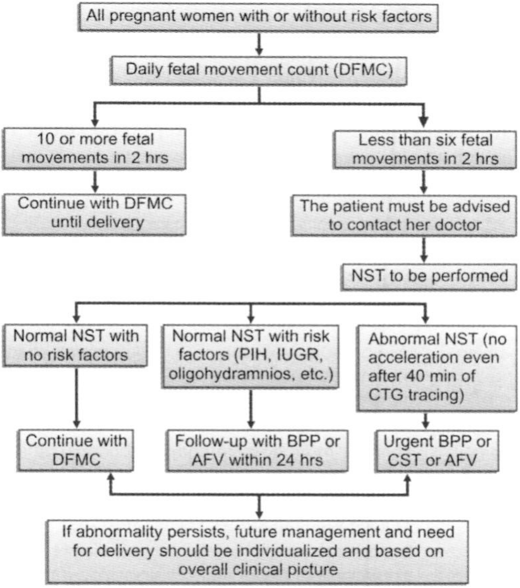

All pregnant women with or without risk factors
↓
Daily fetal movement count (DFMC)
↓

- 10 or more fetal movements in 2 hrs → Continue with DFMC until delivery
- Less than six fetal movements in 2 hrs → The patient must be advised to contact her doctor → NST to be performed
    - Normal NST with no risk factors → Continue with DFMC
    - Normal NST with risk factors (PIH, IUGR, oligohydramnios, etc.) → Follow-up with BPP or AFV within 24 hrs
    - Abnormal NST (no acceleration even after 40 min of CTG tracing) → Urgent BPP or CST or AFV

If abnormality persists, future management and need for delivery should be individualized and based on overall clinical picture

Figure 2.2: Management protocol regarding antepartum fetal surveillance

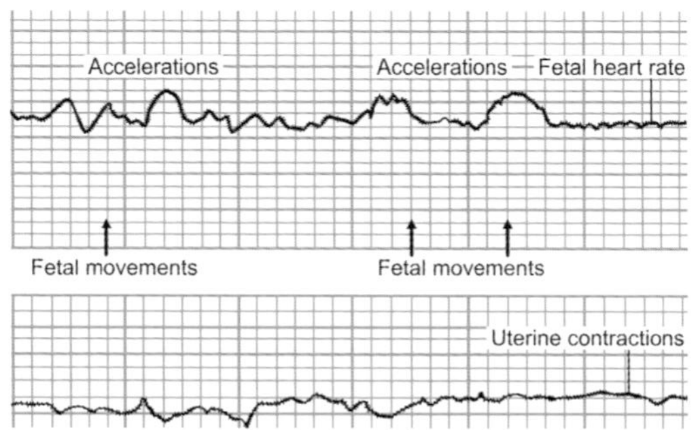

Figure 2.3: Reactive NST

Biophysical Profile (BPP)

The BPP has five components altogether, each scored 0 or 2 for a maximum score of 10; these are listed in **Table 2.3**. A BPP test score of at least 8 out of 10 is considered reassuring. A score of 6 or 7 out of 10 is equivocal, and must be repeated within 24 hours. A score of 4 or less out of 10 is non reassuring and strongly suggests preparing the patient for delivery.

Table 2.3: Biophysical profile criteria

Component	*Score of 2*	*Score of 0*
Amniotic fluid volume	Single vertical pocket of amniotic fluid is > 2 cm in two perpendicular planes	Largest vertical pocket of amniotic fluid is 2 cm or less
Fetal breathing movements	One or more episodes of rhythmic fetal breathing movements of 30 seconds or more within 30 minutes	Abnormal, absent or insufficient breathing movements
Fetal movement	Three or more discrete body or limb movements within 30 minutes	Abnormal, absent or insufficient movements
Fetal tone	At least one episode of flexion-extension of a fetal extremity with return to flexion, or opening or closing of a hand within 30 minutes	Abnormal, absent or insufficient fetal tone
Nonstress test	Reactive (normal)	Nonreactive (abnormal)

Contraction Stress Test (CST) or Oxytocin Challenge Test (OCT)

Box 2.5 describes the contraction stress test.

Box 2.5: Contraction stress test

Method: Mother is placed in dorsal supine position with a leftward tilt, and external monitors are applied. Contractions are induced either by nipple stimulation by the patient or by infusion of a dilute solution of oxytocin. An intravenous infusion of dilute oxytocin may be initiated at a rate of 0.5 mU/minute and doubled at every 20 minutes until an adequate contraction pattern is achieved (three contractions, within a 10-minute period, each lasting for 40 seconds or more). Interpretation of CST is described in **Table 2.4**.

Table 2.4: Interpretation of CST

Test result	*Interpretation*
Negative	No decelerations with the three contractions in the 10 minute window
Suspicious	Presence of intermittent late decelerations or severe variable deceleration
Unsatisfactory test	Less than three contractions or hyperstimulation (contractions lasting longer than 90 seconds and occurring every few minutes)
Positive	Late decelerations with 50% or more of the contractions

Doppler Ultrasonography

This is a noninvasive method of assessing fetal vascular impedance **(Fig. 2.4)**. This method helps in assessing fetal-placental unit by detecting the movement of blood flow through the maternal **(Fig. 2.5)** and fetal vessels **(Fig. 2.6)**. Some of important Doppler indices which help in evaluating the blood flow through uterine and umbilical blood vessels are shown in **Table 2.5**. In normal pregnancy, S/D ratio and pulsatility index (PI) decreases with an increase in the gestational age. Significant elevations in the S/D ratio have been associated with intrauterine growth retardation, fetal hypoxia or acidosis or both, and higher rates of perinatal morbidity and mortality. Absent and reversed end-diastolic flows are the more extreme examples of abnormal S/D ratio and may prompt delivery in some situations.

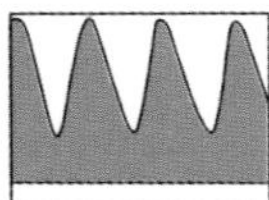

Normal pregnancy

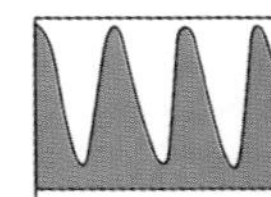

Reduced end diastolic velocity

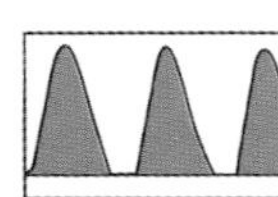

Absent end diastolic velocity

Reversed end diastolic velocity

Figure 2.4: Types of Doppler waveforms

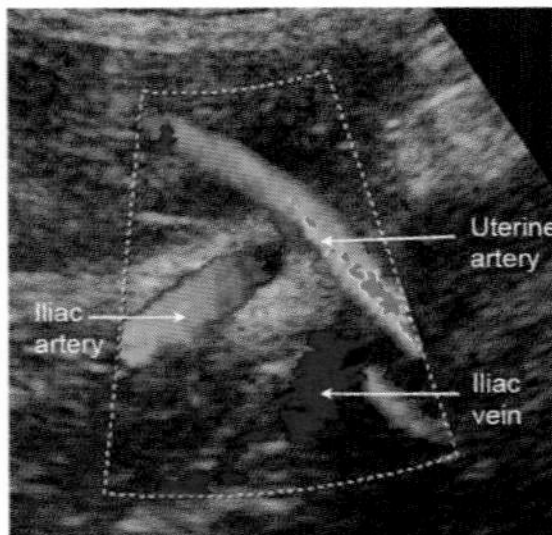

Figure 2.5: Uterine artery Doppler

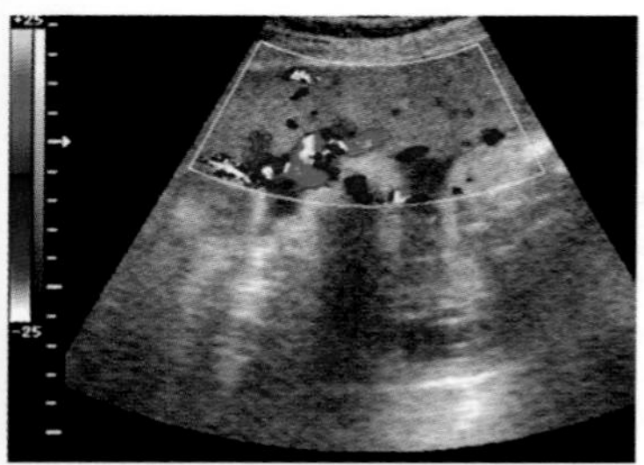

Figure 2.6: Umbilical artery circulation on color Doppler ultrasonography

Table 2.5: Types of Doppler indices

Doppler index	*Calculation of Doppler index*
S/D ratio	Peak systolic blood flow/End diastolic velocity
Pulsatility Index (PI)	$\frac{\text{Peak systolic velocity} - \text{End diastolic velocity}}{\text{Mean systolic velocity}}$
Resistance index (RI)	$\frac{\text{Peak systolic velocity} - \text{End diastolic velocity}}{\text{Peak systolic velocity}}$

Assessment of Pulmonary Maturity

This may especially be required in cases where premature fetal delivery is required (e.g. preeclampsia, IUGR, etc.). Some such tests of pulmonary maturity are described in **Box 2.6**.

Box 2.6: Assessment of pulmonary maturity

- Estimation of the pulmonary surfactant by lecithin/sphingomyelin (L/S ratio). L/S ratio of ≥ 2 is indicative of pulmonary maturity
- Clements shake bubble test: Increasing dilutions of amniotic fluid are mixed with 96% ethanol and shaken for 15 seconds. Formation of foam or bubbles which remain stable for about 15 minutes is a bedside test, which is indicative of pulmonary maturity
- Presence of phosphatidylglycerol or phosphatidylcholine ($\geq$ 500 ng/mL) in amniotic fluid is indicative of pulmonary maturity
- Presence of orange-colored cells on examination of desquamated fetal cells obtained from centrifuged amniotic fluid stained with 0.1% nile blue sulfate is noted. Presence of more than 50% orange colored cells is indicative of pulmonary maturity.

CLINICAL PEARLS

- NST is a noninvasive test which indicates whether the baby is receiving enough oxygen or not. Reduced oxygen supply to the fetus could be related to placental or umbilical cord problems. NSTs are usually performed after 28 weeks of gestation
- BPP is more accurate than a single test as it correlates five measurements to give a score. As a result, it is associated with much lower rates of false positives and false negatives.

3. PELVIMETRY

The anterior view of maternal pelvis is shown in **Figure 2.7**, and normal pelvic dimensions are described in **Table 2.6**.

Table 2.6: Normal pelvic dimensions

	Pelvic brim	*Pelvic cavity*	*Pelvic outlet*
Shape	Almost round, with anterior-posterior diameter being smaller than the transverse diameter **(Fig. 2.8)**	Round	Diamond-shaped
Boundaries	The pelvic inlet is bordered anteriorly by the posterior border of the symphysis pubis, posteriorly by the sacral promontory, and laterally by the linea terminalis	Pelvic cavity is bounded above by the pelvic brim and below by the plane of least-pelvic dimension, anteriorly by the symphysis pubis and posteriorly by sacrum	The pelvic outlet is bordered anteriorly by the lower margin of the symphysis, laterally by the ischial tuberosities, and posteriorly by tip of sacrum
Anterior-posterior diameter	Also known as true or anatomical conjugate, this is measured from the mid point of sacral promontory to the upper border of pubic symphysis and measures about 11 cm **(Fig. 2.9)**	It measures from the midpoint on the posterior surface of pubis symphysis to the junction of second and third sacral vertebra (12 cm)	It extends from the lower border of symphysis pubis to the tip of coccyx (as it moves backward during the second stage of labor) (13 cm)

Contd...

Contd...

	Pelvic brim	*Pelvic cavity*	*Pelvic outlet*
Oblique diameter	The right oblique diameter passes from right sacroiliac joint to the left iliopubic eminence, whereas the left diameter passes from left sacroiliac joint to the right iliopubic eminence (12 cm)	12 cm	—
Transverse diameter	It is the distance between the farthest two points on the ilio-pectineal line (13 cm)	It is the distance between two farthest points laterally. Since there are no bony landmarks, the diameter cannot be exactly measured and can be roughly estimated to be about 12 cm	It extends between the inner aspects of ischial tuberosities (11 cm)

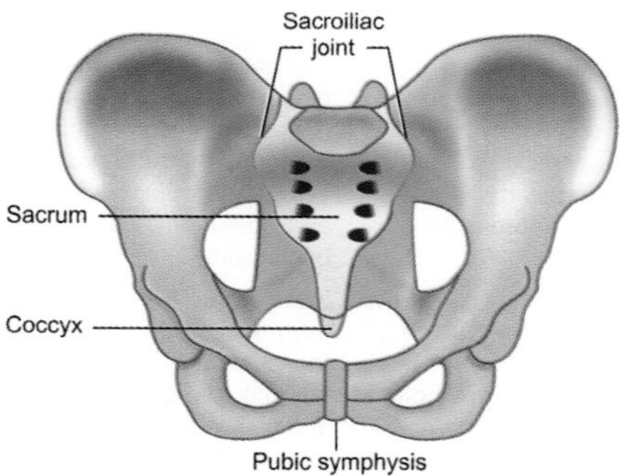

Figure 2.7: Anterior view of maternal pelvis

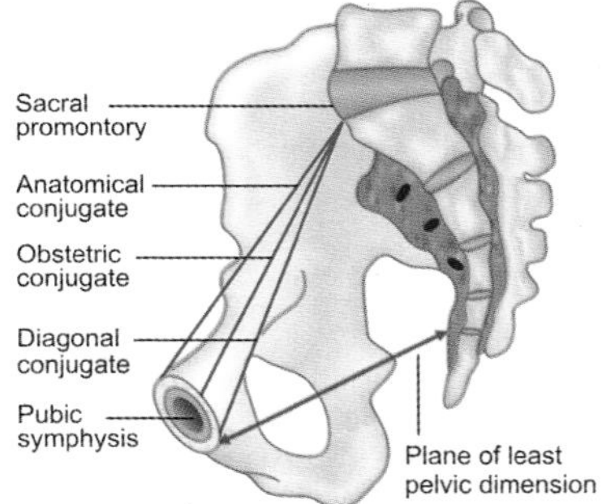

Figure 2.8: Medial view of maternal pelvis (from left)

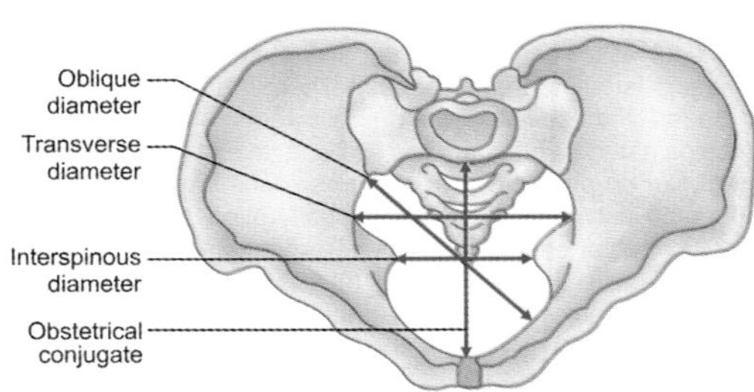

Figure 2.9: Superior view of pelvic inlet

CLINICAL PELVIMETRY

Clinical estimation of pelvic dimensions is described in **Box 2.7**.

Box 2.7: Clinical estimation of pelvic dimensions

Assessment of Pelvic Inlet

- For assessment of pelvic inlet, the sacral promontory and the retropubic area are palpated, and the diagnol conjugate is measured
- *Diagonal conjugate*: This is obtained by placing the tip of the middle finger at the sacral promontory and measuring to the point on the hand that contacts the symphysis. This is the closest clinical estimate of the obstetric conjugate and is 1.5–2.0 cm longer than the obstetric conjugate **(Fig. 2.10)**.

Contd...

Contd...

Assessment of Midpelvis

- For assessment of the midpelvis, the curve of the sacrum, the sacrospinous ligaments and the ischial spines are palpated.

Assessment of the Pelvic Outlet

- For assessment of the pelvic outlet, the subpubic angle, interischial, intertuberous diameter and mobility of the coccyx are determined
- *Bi-ischial diameter*: This is the distance between the ischial spines and measures about 10.5 cm
- *Bituberous diameter*: It extends between the inner aspects of ischial tuberosities and the measures about 11 cm
- The clinician must begin pelvic assessment by starting with the sacral promontory and then following the curve of the sacrum down the midline. In an adequate pelvis, the promontory cannot be easily palpated, the sacrum is well curved and the coccyx cannot be felt. In case of an inadequate pelvis, the sacral promontory is easily palpated and prominent, the sacrum is straight and the coccyx is prominent and/or fixed. After assessing the sacrum, the obstetrician must move his or her fingers lateral to the midsacrum where the sacrospinous ligaments can be felt. If these ligaments are followed laterally, the ischial spines can be palpated. In an adequate pelvis, at least two of the obstetrician's fingers can be placed over the sacrospinous ligaments. In case of an inadequate pelvis, the ligaments usually allow less than two fingers. Also, the ischial spines may appear sharp and prominent. Next the retropubic area is palpated. For this, the obstetrician must put two examining fingers with the palm of the hand facing upward, behind the symphysis pubis. The hand is then moved laterally to both sides
- In case of an adequate pelvis, the retropubic area is flat. In case of an inadequate pelvis, the retropubic area is angulated. To measure the subpubic angle, the examining fingers are turned so that the palm of the hand faces downward. At the same time, the third finger is also held out at the vaginal introitus, and the angle under the pubis is felt. If three fingers can be placed under the pubis, the subpubic angle is approximately 90°, which can be considered as adequate. If the subpubic angle allows only two fingers, the subpubic angle is about 60°, which is indicative of an inadequate pelvis. Finally, as the obstetrician's hand is withdrawn from the vaginal introitus, the intertuberous diameter is measured with the knuckles of the closed fist of the hand placed between the ischial tuberosities. If the pelvis is adequate, the intertuberous diameter allows four knuckles. In case of an inadequate pelvis the intertuberous diameter allows less than four knuckles.

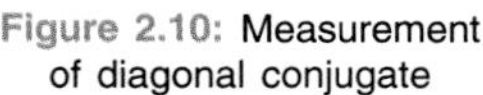
Figure 2.10: Measurement of diagonal conjugate

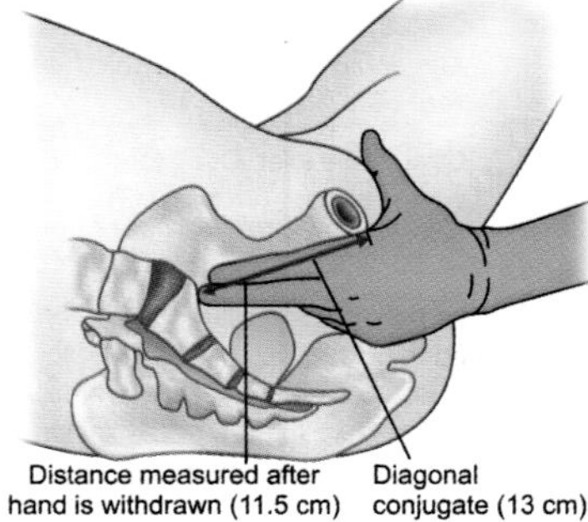

CLINICAL PEARLS

- The pelvic inlet separates the false pelvis from the true pelvis
- The plane of greatest diameter is bordered by the midpoint of the pubis anteriorly; the upper part of the obturator foramina laterally and the junction of the second and third vertebrae posteriorly
- The plane of least pelvic dimension extends from the lower border of pubic symphysis to the tip of ischial spines laterally and to the tip of 5th sacral vertebra posteriorly.

4. DIFFERENT PELVIC TYPES

Using the "Caldwell-Moloy" system, the pelvic shape can be classified into four basic types **(Fig. 2.11)**: (1) gynecoid; (2) android; (3) anthropoid and (4) platypelloid **(Table 2.7)**.

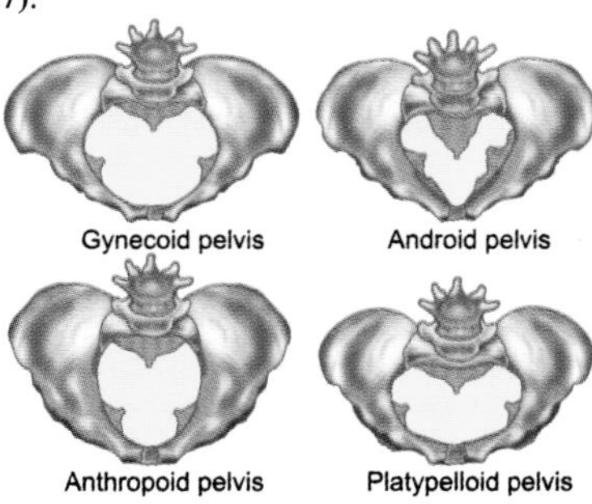

Figure 2.11: Different types of pelvises based on "Caldwell-Moloy" classification

Table 2.7: Pelvic types and characteristics

	Gynecoid (40–50%)	*Anthropoid (20%)*	*Android (30%)*	*Platypelloid (2–5%)*
Inlet	Oval at the inlet with anterior-posterior diameter being just slightly less than the transverse diameter	Oval, long and narrow. The anterior-posterior diameter of the inlet exceeds the transverse diameter giving it an oval shape	Heart shaped /triangular with the base toward the sacrum. As a result, posterior segment is short, and anterior segment is narrow	Pelvic brim is flat and transverse kidney shaped. diameter is much larger than the anterior-posterior diameter
Side walls	Straight	Straight	Convergent side walls (widest posteriorly)	The pelvic side walls diverge downward
Sub-pubic arch	Wide and curved subpubic arch (subpubic angle is not < 85°)	Subpubic arch is long and narrow; subpubic angle may be slightly narrowed	Long and straight subpubic arch; narrow subpubic angle	The subpubic arch is generally wide, and the subpubic angle is in the excess of 90°
Ischial spines	Ischial spines are not prominent	Ischial spines are not prominent	Prominent ischial spines	Ischial spines are not prominent
Sacrum	Sacrum is well-curved, and sacral angle exceeds 90%	Sacrum is long and narrow with usual curve; sacral angle is > 90°	Sacrum is inclined forward and straight; sacral angle is < 90°	The sacrum is prominent and the sacral promontory tends to encroach upon the area of the hind pelvis; sacral angle is > 90°
Bitu-berous diameter	Normal	Normal or short	Short	Wide
Sacro-sciatic notch	Wide and shallow	Wider and more shallow	Narrow and deep	Slightly narrow and small

CLINICAL PEARLS

- Gynecoid pelvis is the classical female pelvis, which is most favorable for delivery
- The platypelloid pelvis favors transverse presentations
- Anthropoid pelvis favors occiput posterior presentations
- Android pelvis is usually associated with difficult vaginal delivery, increased rate of perineal injuries and an increased rate of cesarean delivery.

5. FETAL SKULL

The important anterior-posterior diameters of the fetal skull which may engage are described in **Table 2.8** and **Figure 2.12**. Important transverse diameter of fetal skull includes biparietal diameter (which extends between the two parietal eminences and measures 9.5 cm). This diameter nearly always engages. Plane of engagement of fetal head depending upon its attitude is described in **Figure 2.13**.

Table 2.8: Anterior-posterior diameters of the fetal head which are likely to engage

Diameter	*Extent*	*Length*	*Attitude of head*	*Presentation*
Suboccipitobregmatic	Extends from the nape of the neck to the centre of bregma	9.4 cm	Complete flexion	Vertex
Suboccipitofrontal	Extends from the nape of the neck to the anterior end of anterior fontanel or center of sinciput	10 cm	Incomplete flexion	Vertex
Occipitofrontal	Extends from the occipital eminence to the root of the nose (glabella)	11.2 cm	Marked deflexion	Vertex

Contd...

Contd...

Diameter	*Extent*	*Length*	*Attitude of head*	*Presentation*
Mento-vertical	Extends from midpoint of the chin to the highest point on sagittal suture	13.9 cm	Partial extension	Brow
Submento-vertical	Extends from the junction of the floor of the mouth and neck to the highest point on sagittal suture	11.3 cm	Incomplete extension	Face
Submento-bregmatic	Extends from the junction of the floor of the mouth to the center of bregma	9.4 cm	Complete extension	Face

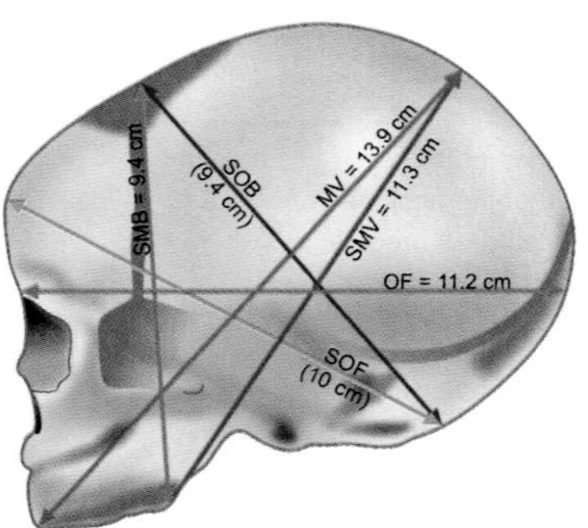

Figure 2.12: Diameters of fetal skull

(Abbreviations: SMB: Submentobregmatic; SOB: Suboccipitobregmatic; SOF: Suboccipitofrontal; OF: Occipitofrontal; SMV: Submentovertical; MV: Mentovertical)

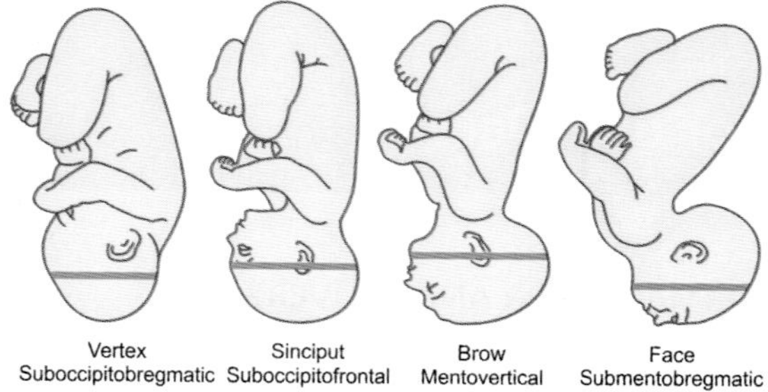

Figure 2.13: Engaging diameters of fetal head depending on the position of presenting part

CLINICAL PEARLS

- At the time of delivery of the baby, there is compression of the engaging diameter of head with the corresponding elongation of the diameter at right angles to it
- Wide gap in the suture lines of fetal skull is known as fontanel. There are a total of six fontanels in fetal skull, of which the anterior one is known as bregma and posterior one as lambda.

CHAPTER 3

Labor and Delivery

1. NORMAL LABOR AND DELIVERY

INTRODUCTION

Labor comprises of a series of events taking place in the genital organs which help to expel the fetus and other products of conception outside the uterine cavity into the outer world. It can be defined as the onset of painful uterine contractions accompanied by any one of the following: ROM; bloody show; cervical dilatation and/or effacement. It normally comprises of three stages: First stage, second stage and third stage. Since the most common fetal position is occipitolateral (transverse) position **(Fig. 3.1)**, the mechanism of labor in context to this position comprises of the following cardinal movements: engagement; flexion; descent; internal rotation; extension and external rotation of fetal head. Various stages of labor are described in **Table 3.1** and depicted in **Figures 3.2A and B**.

Table 3.1: Various stages of labor

Stages of labor	*Description*	*Characteristics*	*Duration in primigravida (in minutes)*	*Duration in multigravida (in minutes)*
Stage I	Starts from the onset of true labor pains and ends with complete dilatation of cervix	Can be divided into: **Latent phase:** slow and gradual cervical effacement and dilatation (up to 3 cm) **Active phase:** Active cervical dilatation (3 cm to 10 cm) and fetal descent. It comprises of: – Acceleration phase – Phase of maximum slope – Deceleration phase	—	—

Contd...

Contd...

Stages of labor	*Description*	*Characteristics*	*Duration in primigravida (in minutes)*	*Duration in multigravida (in minutes)*
Stage II	Starts from full dilatation of cervix and ends with expulsion of the fetus from birth canal	—	50	20
Stage III	It begins after expulsion of the fetus and is associated with expulsion of placenta and membranes	—	15	15
Stage IV	Stage of observation which lasts for at least 1 hour after the expulsion of afterbirths	—	60	60

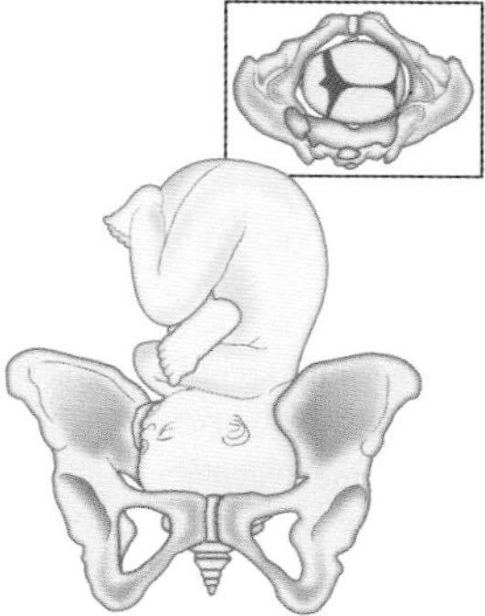

Figure 3.1: Occipitolateral (transverse) position of the fetal head

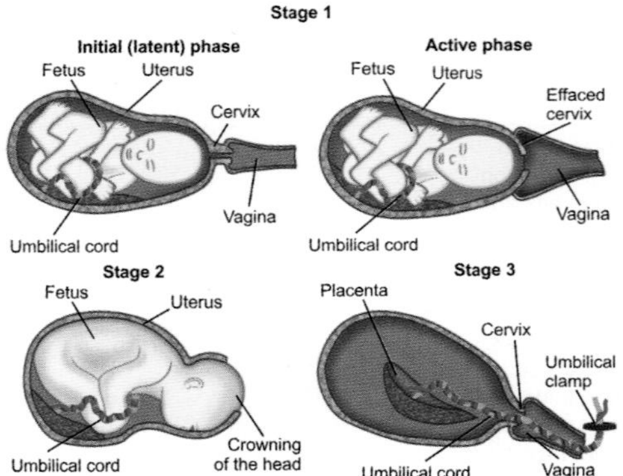

Figure 3.2A: Stages of normal labor

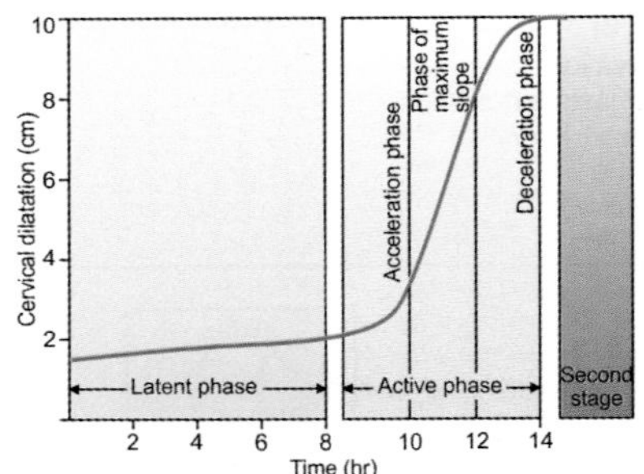

Figure 3.2B: Graphical representation of normal labor

ETIOLOGY

The exact mechanism for the initiation of labor is still unclear. However, the most likely mechanisms are as follows:

- *Mechanical factors*: Uterine distension
- *Endocrine factors*: There is increased cortisol secretion by fetal adrenals and increased production of estrogens and prostaglandins from the placenta. Together, these cause an increased release of oxytocin from the maternal pituitary and increased synthesis of contraction-associated proteins

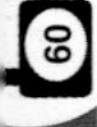

DIAGNOSIS

General Physical Examination

- Assessment of patient's vital signs
- Assessment of fetal heart rate
- Character of uterine contractions.

Abdominal Examination

The abdominal examination must comprise of the following:

- *Uterine height*: Estimation of height of uterine fundus **(Fig. 3.3)**
- *Fetal lie*: The fetal lie may be longitudinal, transverse or oblique **(Fig. 3.4)**
- *Fetal presentation*: This may be cephalic, podalic (breech) or shoulder **(Fig. 3.4)**
- Obstetric grips [Leopold's maneuvers **(Fig. 3.5)**]
- *Uterine contractions*: The uterus appears to be hard during the strong uterine contractions at the time of labor and it may be difficult to palpate the fetal parts
- Estimation of fetal descent
- Assessing the engagement of fetal presenting part by feeling how many fifths of the head are palpable above the brim of the pelvis **(Figs 3.6A and B)**
- Auscultation of fetal heart **(Fig. 3.7)**.

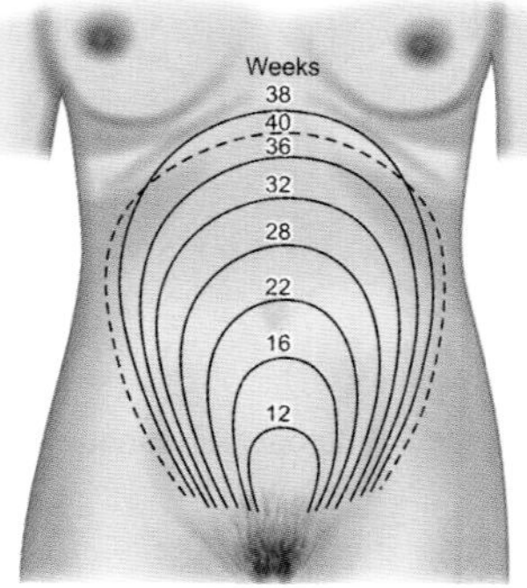

Figure 3.3: Estimation of the height of uterine fundus

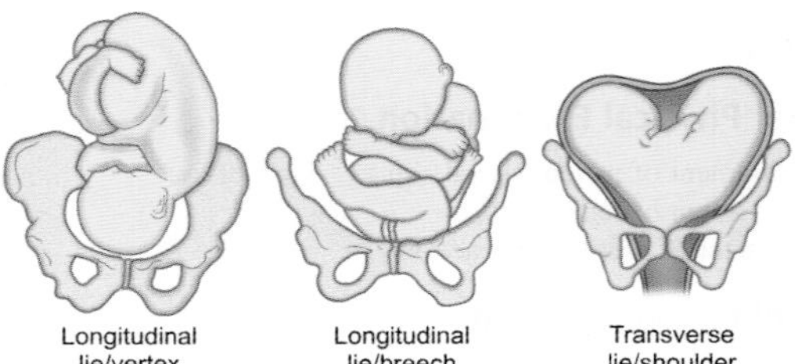

Figure 3.4: Different types of fetal lies and presentation

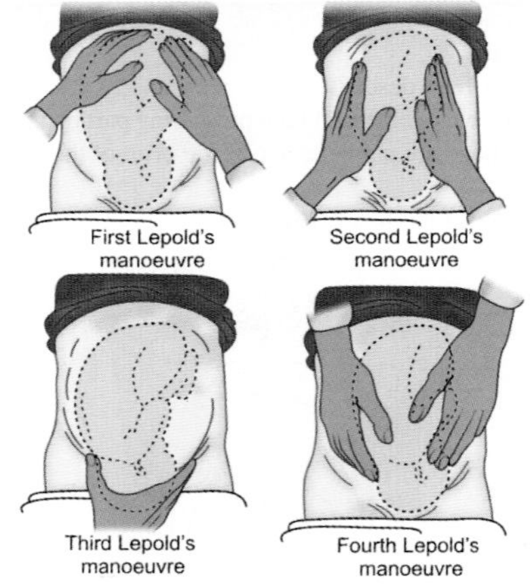

Figure 3.5: Leopold's maneuvers

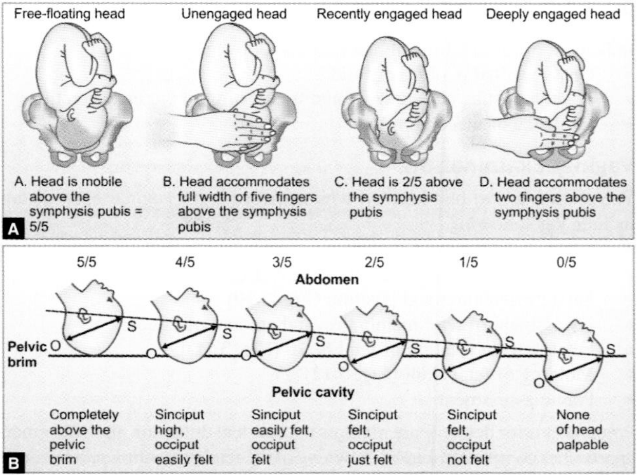

Free-floating head
Unengaged head
Recently engaged head
Deeply engaged head
A. Head is mobile above the symphysis pubis = 5/5
B. Head accommodates full width of five fingers above the symphysis pubis
C. Head is 2/5 above the symphysis pubis
D. Head accommodates two fingers above the symphysis pubis
A
5/5
4/5
3/5
2/5
1/5
0/5
Abdomen
Pelvic brim
Pelvic cavity
Completely above the pelvic brim
Sinciput high, occiput easily felt
Sinciput easily felt, occiput felt
Sinciput felt, occiput just felt
Sinciput felt, occiput not felt
None of head palpable
B

Figures 3.6A and B: Estimation of fetal descent through abdominal examination

Location of FHR in LOA position

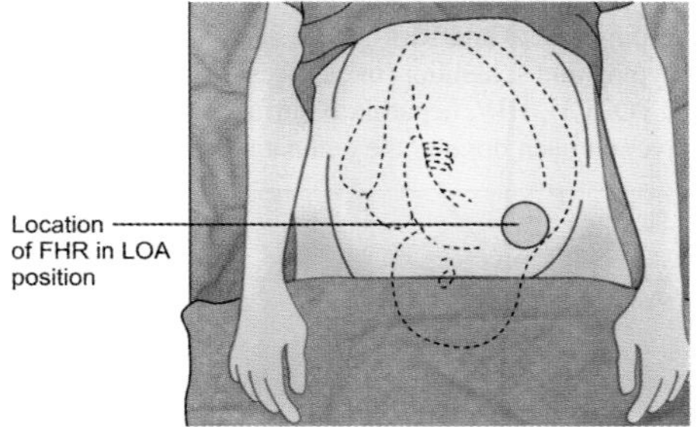

Figure 3.7: Auscultation of fetal heart rate

Per Speculum Examination

Indicators of ruptured membranes are as follows:

- Gross vaginal pooling of fluid
- Positive results on Nitrazine and fern testing of vaginal secretions
- Evidence of meconium.

Vaginal Examination

The parameters to be observed while performing a vaginal examination include the following:

- Cervical dilatation **(Fig. 3.8)**
- Cervical consistency and effacement **(Fig. 3.9)**
- Fetal presentation and position **(Fig. 3.10)**
- Assessment of fetal membranes and amount of liquor
- Fetal descent [Station of fetal head **(Fig. 3.11)**]
- Molding of fetal skull **(Fig. 3.12)**
- Pelvic assessment.

Preparations for delivery are made as the cervical dilatation and effacement approaches completion and/or crowning of the fetal presenting part becomes evident at the vaginal introitus.

Investigations

- Hematocrit with complete blood count
- Urine for proteins (dipstick examination)
- Blood typing (ABO and Rh)
- Blood typing and screening (in case cesarean section is anticipated)
- VDRL, TORCH, HIV, hepatitis B surface antigen (HBSAg) (in case they have not been done in the antenatal period).

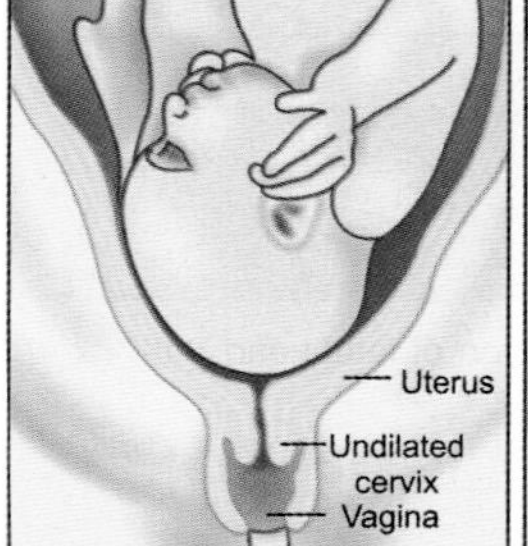

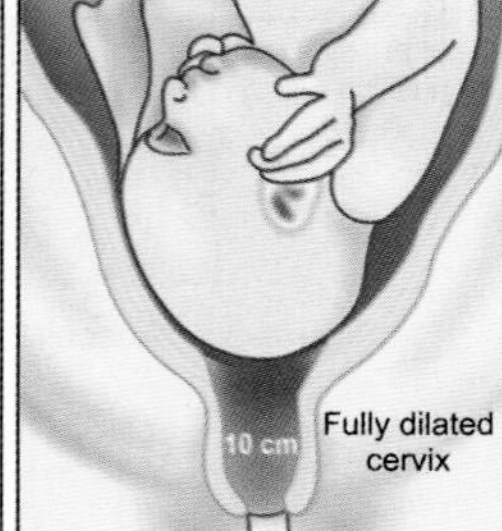

Figure 3.8: Dilation of cervix

Mucus
plug
Cervix
Vagina
Not effaced
Fully effaced cervix

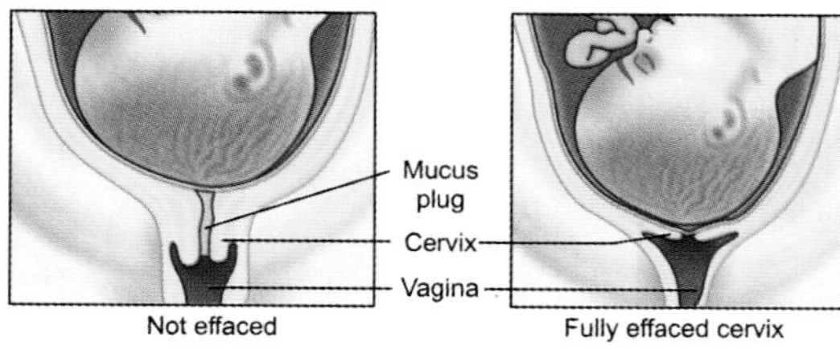

Figure 3.9: Effacement of cervix

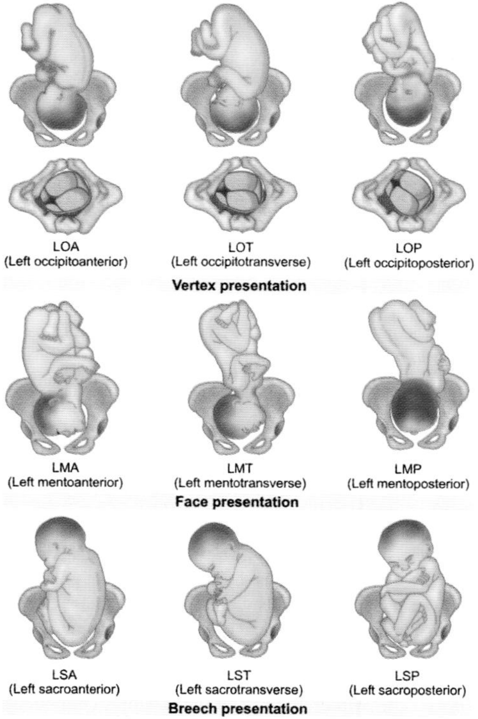

LOA
(Left occipitoanterior)
LOT
(Left occipitotransverse)
LOP
(Left occipitoposterior)
Vertex presentation
LMA
(Left mentoanterior)
LMT
(Left mentotransverse)
LMP
(Left mentoposterior)
Face presentation
LSA
(Left sacroanterior)
LST
(Left sacrotransverse)
LSP
(Left sacroposterior)
Breech presentation

Figure 3.10: Various positions possible with different presentations

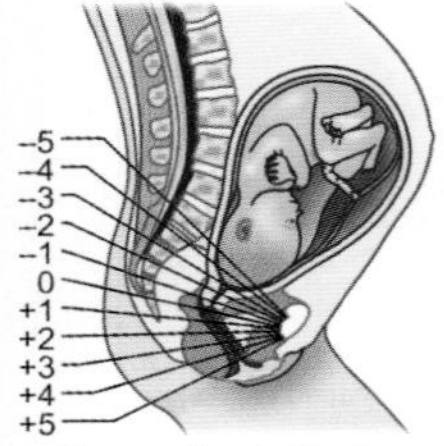

Figure 3.11: Station of fetal head

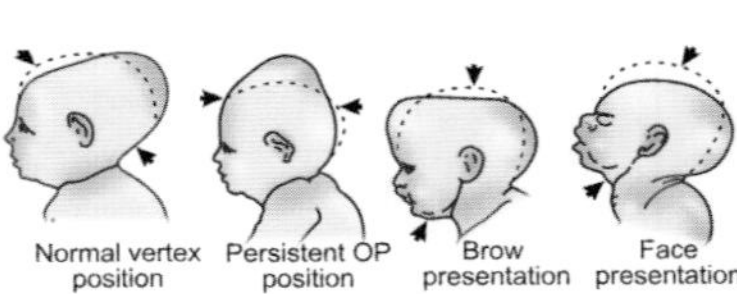

Figure 3.12: Molding of the fetal skull

MANAGEMENT OF NORMAL LABOR AND DELIVERY

Pre-Delivery Preparation

- *Patient position*: The patient is commonly placed in the dorsal lithotomy position with left lateral tilt
- Vulvar and perineal cleaning and draping with antiseptic solution must be done
- The sterile drapes must be placed in such a way that only the area immediately around the vulva and perineum is exposed
- If at any time during the abdominal examination, the bladder is palpable, the patient must be encouraged to void. If, despite of distended bladder, the patient is unable to void, catheterization is indicated
- *Patient monitoring*: Maternal BP and pulse should be recorded every hour during the first stage of labor and every 10 minutes during the second stage of labor. The fetal heart rate should be recorded immediately after a contraction at least every 30 minutes during the active phase of the first stage of labor and at least every 15 minutes during the second stage.
- *Induction of labor*: This has been described in a separate fragment
- *Fetal monitoring*: This has been discussed in Chapter 2
- *Partogram*: Normal labor should be plotted graphically on a partograph **(Fig. 3.13)**. The partograph is divided into a latent phase and an active phase. The latent phase ends while the active phase begins when the cervix is 3 cm dilated. Cervical dilation and descent of the presenting part are plotted in relation to an alert line and an action line. Alert line starts at the end of latent phase and ends with the full dilation of the cervix (10 cm) within 7 hours (at the rate of 1 cm/hour). The action

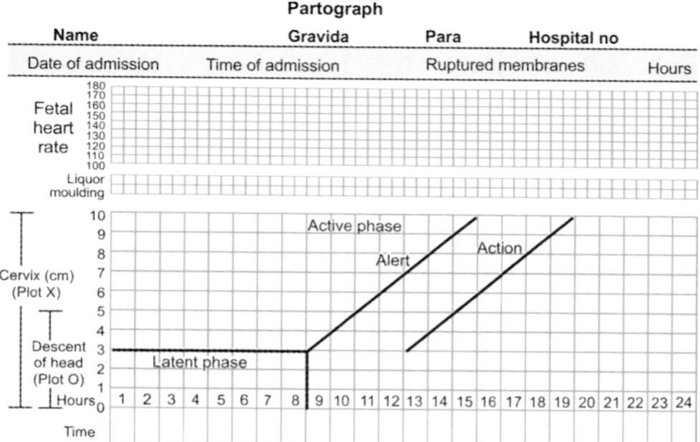

Figure 3.13: Partograph

line is drawn 4 hours to the right of the alert line. Labor is considered to be abnormal when the cervicograph crosses the alert line and falls on zone II, and intervention is required when it crosses the action line and falls in the zone III.

Delivery

Mechanism of normal labor has been described in **Figure 3.14** and comprises of the following steps:

- *Delivery of fetal head*: With the increasing descent of the head, the perineum bulges and thins out considerably. As the largest diameter of the fetal head distends the vaginal introitus, crowning is said to occur
- As the head distends the perineum and appears that tears may occur in the area of vaginal introitus, mediolateral surgical incision called episiotomy may be given
- As the fetal head progressively distends the vaginal introitus, the obstetrician in order to facilitate the controlled birth of the head must place the fingers of one hand against the baby's head to keep it flexed and apply perineal support with the other hand. Delivery of the fetal head can be achieved with the help of Ritgen maneuver. This helps in providing controlled delivery of the head and favors extension at the time of actual delivery so that the head is delivered with its smallest

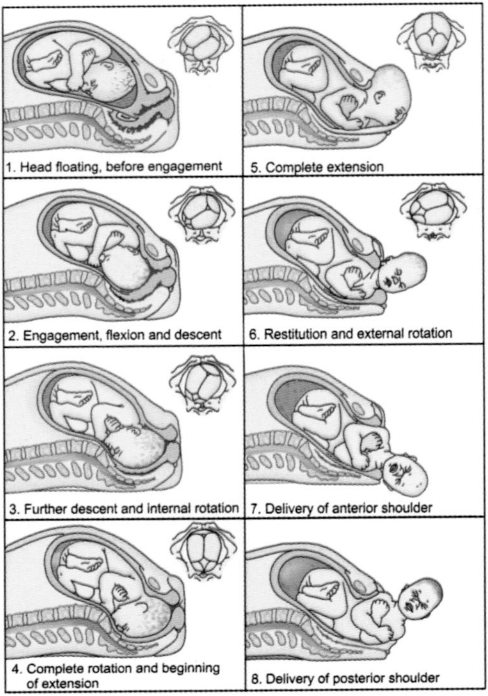

1. Head floating, before engagement

5. Complete extension

2. Engagement, flexion and descent

6. Restitution and external rotation

3. Further descent and internal rotation

7. Delivery of anterior shoulder

4. Complete rotation and beginning of extension

8. Delivery of posterior shoulder

Figure 3.14: Mechanism of normal labor

diameter passing through the introitus and minimal injury occurs to the pelvic musculature

- Once the baby's head is delivered, the woman must be encouraged not to push. The baby's mouth and nose must be suctioned
- The obstetrician must then feel around the baby's neck in order to rule out the presence of cord around the fetal neck
- *Delivery of the shoulders*: Following the delivery of fetal head, the fetal head falls posteriorly, while the face comes in contact with the

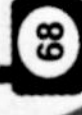

maternal anus. As the restitution or external rotation of the fetal head occurs, the occiput turns toward one of the maternal thighs, and the head assumes a transverse position. This movement implies that bisacromial diameter has rotated and has occupied the A-P diameter of the pelvis. Soon the anterior shoulder appears at the vaginal introitus. Following the delivery of the anterior shoulder, the posterior shoulder is born.

- *Delivery of the rest of the body*: This is followed by delivery of the rest of the body by lateral flexion
- *Clamping the cord*: The umbilical cord must be clamped and cut if not done earlier.

Post-Delivery Care

- The baby must be placed over the mother's abdomen and then handed over to the assisting nurse or the pediatrician
- The baby's body must be thoroughly dried, the eyes be wiped and breathing must be assessed
- In order to minimize the chances of aspiration of amniotic fluid, soon after the delivery of the thorax, the face must be wiped and the mouth and the nostrils must be aspirated
- The baby must be covered with a soft, dry cloth and then with a blanket to ensure that the baby remains warm and no heat loss occurs
- Following the delivery of baby, the placenta needs to be delivered. The obstetrician must look for signs of placental separation following the delivery of the baby
- The third stage of labor must actively be managed (as described in Chapter 5).

COMPLICATIONS

Important complications of pregnancy related to abnormal fetal presentation, medical disorders and complications specific to pregnancy have been discussed in this chapter as well as in the next chapter of this book.

CLINICAL PEARLS

- Episiotomy is no longer recommended as a routine procedure and is performed only if the obstetrician feels its requirement
- Commonest causes for abnormal hardness and tenderness of the uterus include abruption placenta or a ruptured uterus

- If PROM has occurred, digital examination may be deferred until the onset of active labor to reduce the risk of chorioamnionitis
- Intermittent auscultation of the fetal heart has been found to be equivalent to continuous electronic monitoring for the assessment of fetal well-being, provided that the nurse-to-patient ratio is 1:1.

2. INDUCTION AND AUGMENTATION OF LABOR

INTRODUCTION

Induction of labor can be defined as commencement of uterine contractions before the spontaneous onset of labor with or without ruptured membranes. It is indicated when the benefits of delivery to the mother or fetus outweigh the benefits of continuing the pregnancy. Induction of labor comprises of cervical ripening and labor augmentation. While cervical ripening aims at making the cervix soft and pliable, augmentation refers to stimulation of spontaneous contractions which may be considered inadequate due to failed cervical dilation or fetal descent.

INDICATIONS

Maternal

- Ruptured membranes with preeclampsia or eclampsia or non-reassuring fetal heart status
- Diabetes mellitus
- Renal disease
- Abruptio placenta
- Rh isoimmunization.

Indications Specific to Pregnancy

- Oligohydramnios
- Polyhydramnios.

Fetal

- Postmaturity
- Intrauterine growth restriction
- PROM
- Fetus with congenital anomalies
- Intrauterine death.

DIAGNOSIS

Clinical Presentation

Evaluation of state of cervix: This is done by calculation of the Bishop's score **(Table 3.2)**. A maximum score of 13 is possible with this scoring system. Labor is most likely to commence spontaneously with a score of 9 or more, whereas lower scores (especially those < 5) may require cervical ripening and/or augmentation with oxytocin.

Table 3.2: Bishop's score

Score	*Dilation (cm)*	*Effacement (%)*	*Station of the presenting part*	*Cervical consistency*	*Position of cervix*
0	Closed	0–30	– 3	Firm	Posterior
1	1–2	40–50	– 2	Medium	Mid position
2	3–4	60–70	– 1	Soft	Anterior
3	≥ 5	≥ 80	+ 1, + 2	—	—

Investigations

- *Ultrasound assessment of gestational age*: This would help to prevent induction in premature babies
- *Assessment of fetal lung maturity*: This may not be required in case where induction is medically indicated and the risk of continuing the pregnancy is greater than the risk of delivering a baby before lung maturity has been attained.

MEDICAL MANAGEMENT

Pharmacological methods for labor induction commonly comprise of prostaglandins [Dinoprostone (PGE_2), or misoprostol (PGE_1)] and/or oxytocin.

Dinoprostone helps in cervical ripening and is available in the form of gel (prepidil or cerviprime) or a vaginal insert (cervidil). Prepidil comprises of 0.5 mg of dinoprostone in a 2.5 mL syringe. The gel is injected intracervically every 6 hours for up to three doses in a 24-hour period. Cervidil, on the other hand is a vaginal insert containing 10 mg of dinoprostone. The main advantage of cervidil is that it can be immediately removed in case it causes hyperstimulation. Use of misoprostol for cervical ripening is an off-label use, which is still considered controversial by some clinicians. However, its use is recommended by the ACOG. A dose of 25 mg is placed transvaginally at every 3 hourly intervals for a maximum of 4 doses or it may be prescribed in the oral dosage of 50 mg orally at every 4 hourly intervals.

Oxytocin is a uterotonic agent which stimulates uterine contractions and is used for both induction and augmentation of labor. It can be started in low dosage regimens of 0.5–1.5 mU/minute or the high dosage regimen of 4.5–6.0 mU/minute, with incremental increases of 1.0–2.0 mU/minute at every 15–40 minutes. If an intrauterine pressure catheter is in place, measurement of intrauterine pressure ranging between 180–200 Montevideo units/period is an indicator of adequate oxytocin dosing.

SURGICAL MANAGEMENT

Various non-pharmacological methods for labor induction comprise of the following:

- Surgical methods such as low ROM and stripping of membranes
- Mechanical dilation (through use of dilators, osmotic dilation with laminaria tents, balloon catheters, etc.)

Surgical Procedure for ROM

- After placing the woman in lithotomy position, under all aseptic precautions, two fingers smeared with antiseptic ointment are introduced inside the vagina
- The index finger is passed through the cervical canal beyond the internal cervical os
- Using the index and the middle fingers, the fetal membranes are swept free from the lower uterine segment as far as can be reached with fingers
- While the fingers are still in the cervical canal, with the palmar surface upward, a long Kocher's forceps with closed blades is introduced along the palmer aspect of the fingers up to the membranes
- The blades of the Kocher's forceps are opened to grasp the membranes and tear it using twisting movements
- When the membranes rupture, there is a visible gush of amniotic fluid
- If the head is not engaged, an assistant must push the head to fix it to the brim in order to prevent cord prolapse.

Postoperative Care

- Color of liquor and cervical status following ROM is observed
- The clinician must detect cord prolapse, if present

- Quality of fetal heart rate must be assessed following ROM
- Fetal electrode may be applied in high-risk cases in order to assess the fetal heart status
- A sterile vulvar pad is applied
- Prophylactic antibiotics may be administered.

COMPLICATIONS

- Uterine hyperstimulation (with oxytocin and misoprostol), may result in uteroplacental hypoperfusion and fetal heart rate deceleration
- Prostaglandins may produce tachysystole, which may be controlled with terbutaline
- Maternal systemic effects, such as fever, vomiting and diarrhea, may be infrequently observed
- Failure of induction
- Uterine atony and postpartum hemorrhage
- Increased rate of cesarean delivery
- Chorioamnionitis
- Oxytocin may be responsible for producing water intoxication.

CLINICAL PEARLS

- Intracervical application of dinoprostone (PGE2, 0.5 mg gel) is the gold standard for cervical ripening
- 100 μg of oral or 25 μgms of vaginal misoprostol has been found to be similar in efficacy to intravenous oxytocin for labor induction.

3. PROLONGED LABOR

INTRODUCTION

Prolonged labor or dystocia of labor (dysfunctional labor) is defined as difficult labor or abnormally slow progress of labor.

Friedman's (1978) graphical representation of normal progress of labor using parameters, such as cervical dilatation and descent of fetal head, has been described in **Figure 3.2B** in the previous fragments. While the cervical dilatation follows a sigmoid curve, descent of the fetal head through the birth canal follows a hyperbolic shaped curve.

Abnormal progress of labor is defined as lack of change or minimal change in cervical dilatation or effacement during a 2-hour period (for each of the phase: latent and active phase) in a woman having regular uterine contractions before the beginning of active phase of labor or as a descent of less than or equal to 1.0 cm/hour in nullipara and less than or equal to 2.0 cm/hour in multipara during the second stage of labor (from complete cervical dilatation to delivery). Indicators for abnormal labor have been described in **Table 3.3**.

Table 3.3: Diagnostic criteria for abnormal labor

Indication	*Nullipara*	*Multipara*
Prolonged latent phase	> 20 hr	> 14 hr
Average second stage	50 min	20 min
Prolonged second stage without (with) epidural	> 2 hr (> 3 hr)	> 1 hr (> 2 hr)
	Protraction disorders	
Protracted active-phase dilation	< 1.2 cm/hr	< 1.5 cm/hr
Protracted descent	≤ 1 cm/hr	≤ 2 cm/hr
	Arrest disorders	
Prolonged deceleration	> 3 hr	> 1 hr
Secondary arrest of dilation*	> 2 hr	> 2 hr
Arrest of descent*	> 1 hr	> 1 hr
Failure of descent	No descent in the deceleration phase or the second stage of labor	
	Third stage disorders	
Prolonged third stage	> 30 min	> 30 min

* Adequate contractions > 200 Montevideo units per 10 minutes for 2 hours.

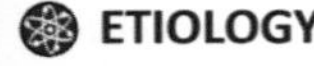

ETIOLOGY

Various causes for abnormal progress of labor are as follows:

Abnormalities in expulsive forces: These include:
- Hypotonic uterine dysfunction (uterine inertia)
- Hypertonic uterine dysfunction
- Poor maternal expulsive efforts (related to maternal fatigue or epidural analgesic use).

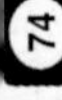

Fetal abnormalities: These include:

- Abnormalities in fetal size (e.g. fetal macrosomia, with fetal weight ≥ to 4000 gm)
- Abnormalities in fetal presentation (e.g. brow, shoulder, face)
- Abnormalities in fetal position (e.g. occiput posterior, occiput transverse, etc.)
- Abnormalities in fetal attitude (extension, asynclitism, etc.)
- Fetal congenital abnormalities (anencephaly, fetal ascites, fetal tumors, etc.).

Pelvic abnormalities: These include:

- Cephalopelvic disproportion
- Cervical dystocia.

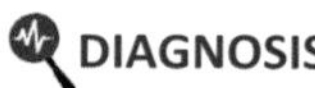

DIAGNOSIS

Clinical Presentation

Clinical presentation for abnormal progress of labor has already been described in the 'introduction' segment. Diagnosis involves understanding of the etiology of the problem and includes the following:

Evaluation of the fetal-pelvic relationship to determine if CPD is present: This involves the use of Müller Munro Kerr maneuver to assess for CPD, which has been described in details in the fragment of obstructed labor. Other findings suggestive of CPD on pelvic examination have also been described there.

Investigations

Insertion of an intrauterine pressure catheter: This helps in the evaluation of uterine activity. Diagnosis of uterine hypoactivity is made if uterine contractions occur more than 3 minutes apart, last for less than 40 seconds and produce a rise in intrauterine pressure of less than 50 mm Hg.

MANAGEMENT

Patients with prolonged latent phase can be managed in the following ways:

- *Therapeutic rest*: This involves administration of an intramuscular dose of 15 mg of morphine, following which the majority of patients would go to sleep within an hour. If the patient wakes up after 4–5 hours with no signs of active labor, this implies that she had false labor. In case the patient is in active labor on waking up, it implies that she was in the latent phase of labor

- *Stimulation with oxytocin*: In cases of uterine hypocontractility, oxytocin (30 units diluted in 500 mL of saline) must be started at a rate of 0.5–1.0 mU/minute and gradually increased by 1–2 mU/minute at every 20–30 minutes, until an adequate pattern of contractions is achieved. Amniotomy and oxygen infusion can also be tried in cases with reduced uterine activity. If there is no response even after 3 hours of augmentation with oxytocin, cesarean section may be required in most of the cases due to the possibility of an underlying CPD
- *Discontinuation of regional anesthesia*: If the cause of abnormal progress of labor is related to the administration of epidural analgesia, it must be discontinued
- *Assisted vaginal delivery*: Assisted vaginal delivery in the form of vacuum or forceps application can serve as a good option in cases of delayed second stage
- *Cesarean section*: This may appear to be treatment of choice when vaginal delivery appears to be unsafe.

COMPLICATIONS

Maternal

There is an increased incidence of the following:
- Traumatic injuries (cervical tears, uterine rupture, etc.)
- Increased incidence of operative deliveries
- Chorioamnionitis
- Postpartum hemorrhage
- Puerperal sepsis, subinvolution.

Fetal: These include:
- Fetal hypoxia, thick meconium
- Intracranial stress or hemorrhage
- Variable or delayed decelerations
- Fetal acidosis
- Five-minute APGAR score of less than 7
- Increased rate of admission to the NICU
- Increased perinatal morbidity and mortality.

CLINICAL PEARLS

- The evaluation of the descent of the fetal head may be complicated due to development of molding and caput formation

- In nulliparous patients, inadequate uterine activity is a common cause of primary dysfunctional labor, while in multiparous patients cephalopelvic disproportion is the common cause.

4. OBSTRUCTED LABOR

INTRODUCTION

This can be defined as a condition in which the progressive descent of the presenting part through the maternal genital tract is arrested despite of strong uterine contractions.

In primigravidas as a result of obstructed labor, features of maternal exhaustion and sepsis are apparent. However, the uterus becomes inert. On the other hand, in multigravidae, the uterus responds vigorously in face of obstruction, which may eventually lead to the rupture of uterus. Tonic contractions in the face of uterine obstruction result in formation of a circular groove between the upper and lower uterine segment, known as the pathological retraction ring or Bandl's ring. Eventually, there is rupture of uterus as the lower segment gives way due to marked thinning of the uterine wall.

ETIOLOGY

The most common cause of obstructed labor is mechanical obstruction, which results due to a mismatch between the size of fetal presenting part and the maternal pelvis. This could occur due to defects with the passage (bony pelvis) or the passenger (fetus).

Defects with the passage: These include:

- Cephalopelvic disproportion
- Cervical dystocia due to operative scarring of cervix, cervical or broad ligament fibroids, impacted ovarian tumors, etc.

Defects with the passenger: These include:

- Transverse lie
- Brow presentation
- Congenital malformations of the fetus (hydrocephalus)
- Compound presentation
- Occipitoposterior position
- Conjoint twins.

DIAGNOSIS

General Physical Examination

- Patient may be in severe pain
- Features of exhaustion and ketoacidosis may be present.

Abdominal Examination

- Upper uterine segment may be hard and tender
- Pathological retraction ring (Bandl's ring) may be placed obliquely between the umbilicus and the pubic symphysis and rises in the course of time
- Fetal parts may not be well-defined
- FHS is usually absent
- Assessment of fetopelvic disproportion: The following methods can be used for the assessment of fetopelvic disproportion:

Abdominal method: In this method, the patient is placed in dorsal position with thighs slightly flexed. The index and the middle fingers of the right hand are placed above the pubic symphysis over the abdomen in such a way that the inner surface of the fingers is line with the anterior surface of pubic symphysis **(Fig. 3.15A)**. The fetal head in grasped by clinician's left hand and pushed down towards the pelvis.

Abdominal vaginal (Müller Munro Kerr) method: This is a bimanual method **(Fig. 3.15B)** for assessing the pelvis and comprises of the following steps:

After taking all aseptic precautions, the obstetrician introduces two fingers of the right hand inside the vagina with tips of the fingers placed at the level of ischial spines and thumb above the symphysis pubis. The fetal head is then grasped by the left hand and pushed in a downward and backward direction into the pelvis. The conclusions which can be reached depending upon the findings on abdominal method as well as the abdominovaginal examination are:

- No disproportion: Fetal head can be pushed down up to the level of ischial spines without any overlapping of the parietal bones
- Slight or moderate disproportion: The head can be pushed down a little but not up to the level of ischial spines and there is only a slight overlapping of the parietal bones
- Severe disproportion: The fetal head cannot be pushed down and instead the parietal bone overhangs the symphysis pubis.

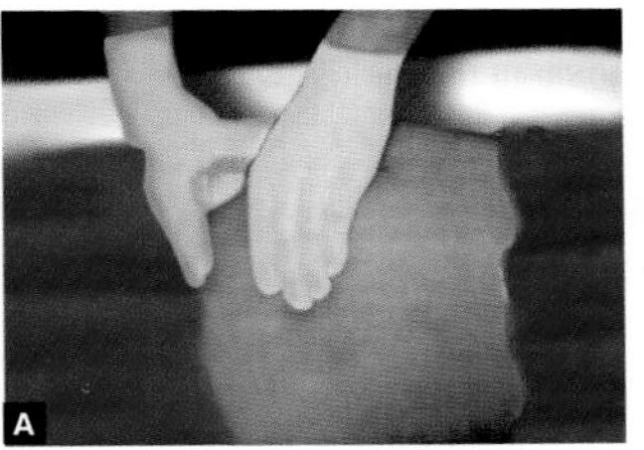

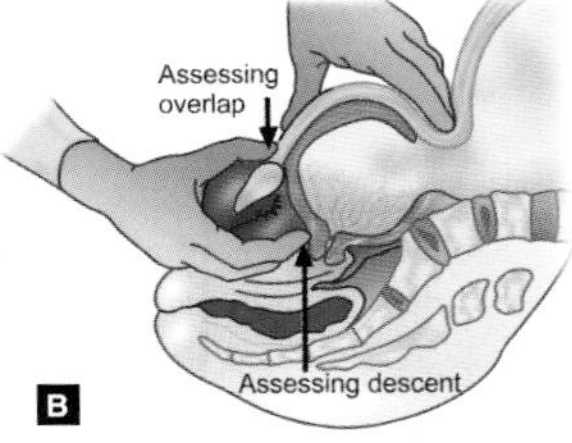

Figures 3.15A and B: (A) Abdominal method (B) Abdominal vaginal (Müller Munro Kerr) method

Vaginal Examination

- Vagina may be hot and dry
- Cervix may be fully dilated
- Offensive discharge may be present
- Membranes may be absent.

Investigations

- Blood samples for grouping and cross matching
- Vaginal swabs for culture and sensitivity.

MANAGEMENT

- Most important step in the prevention of obstructed labor is early recognition of prolonged labor or abnormal progress of labor by plotting the progress of labor on a partograph
- Taking steps for relieving the obstruction as soon as possible
- Checking against dehydration and ketoacidosis
- Controlling sepsis
- Correction of fluid and electrolyte balance
- Antibiotics: Usually a combination of third generation cephalosporin (e.g. ceftriaxone) and metronidazole is administered
- A timely cesarean section gives the best results.

COMPLICATIONS

Maternal: These include:

- Pressure necrosis of the bladder base and urethra resulting in the development of genitourinary fistulae (more common in the primigravida)

- Maternal exhaustion, dehydration and/or metabolic acidosis
- Rupture of the uterus (more common in the multigravida)
- Postpartum hemorrhage and shock
- Sepsis
- High maternal mortality and morbidity
- Secondary amenorrhea following hysterectomy due to rupture
- Sheehan's syndrome due to massive postpartum hemorrhage.

Fetal: These include:
- Asphyxia
- Acidosis
- Intracranial hemorrhage
- Infection.

CLINICAL PEARLS

- Oxytocin must not be used for stimulating uterine contractions in cases of suspected obstruction
- Obstructed labor must be urgently handled like an obstetric emergency
- Conscious efforts must be made to exclude rupture of the uterus in every case of obstructed labor.

5. ANALGESIA FOR LABOR

INTRODUCTION

Epidural analgesia has presently become a commonly employed technique for providing pain relief during labor. Epidural analgesia should be administered only once the diagnosis of labor has been established and the patient requests for pain relief. It should be provided by practitioners only in settings where facilities for resuscitation are immediately available. This technique involves injection of a local anesthetic agent into the epidural space (between the dura mater and the ligamentum flavum) in the space between the vertebra L3 and L4 **(Fig. 3.16)**. An indwelling catheter is usually kept in place for repeat injections or continuous infusion.

INDICATIONS

- Provision of pain relief during first and second stages of labor
- Facilitation of patient cooperation during labor and delivery
- Provision of anesthesia for episiotomy or forceps delivery or extension for cesarean delivery.

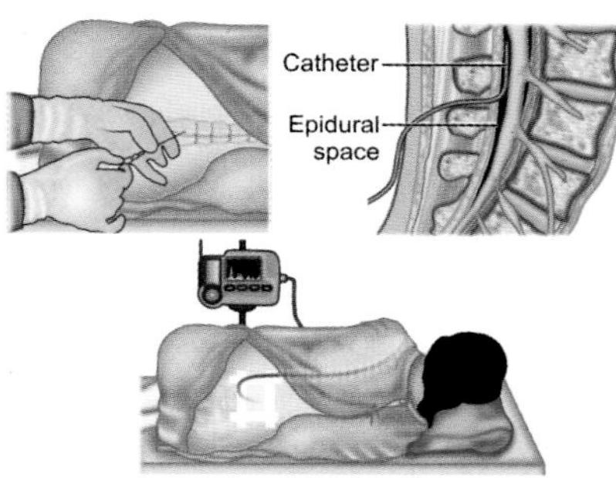

Figure 3.16: Administration of epidural analgesia

SURGICAL MANAGEMENT

Preoperative Preparation

- Informed consent must be obtained from the patient
- Prehydration with 500–1,000 mL of crystalloid solution in order to prevent the development of postprocedural hypotension
- Patient is placed in lateral decubitus or sitting position.

Steps of Surgery

- Under all aseptic precautions, the epidural needle is inserted in the epidural space between the vertebra L3 and L4. Epidural space can be identified by loss-of-resistance at the time of needle insertion
- An epidural catheter is threaded by 3–5 cm into the epidural space
- A test dose of 3 mL of 1.5% lidocaine with 1:200,000 epinephrine or 3 mL of 0.25% bupivacaine with 1:200,000 epinephrine is injected
- If the test dose is negative, approximately 10 mL of 0.25 % bupivacaine (Marcaine) or 0.25% of ropivacaine, with or without a small dose of a lipid-soluble opioid (e.g., fentanyl or sufentanil), are injected
- Following this, epidural analgesia may be maintained either with intermittent bolus injections or continuous epidural infusion. Patient-controlled epidural analgesia may also be used.

Postoperative Care

- Following the administration of epidural analgesia, the woman is placed in lateral or semilateral position in order to avoid aortocaval compression

- Blood pressure must be recorded at every 5 to 15 minutes interval for an hour following the procedure
- Continuous fetal heart rate monitoring at least for an hour following the procedure is required to detect any abnormalities in the fetal heart rate
- Hourly monitoring of the level of analgesia and intensity of motor blockade is required.

COMPLICATIONS

Immediate: These include:
- Maternal hypotension
- Rarely convulsions and/or cardiac arrest induced by local anesthetics
- Increase in the duration of labor (controversial)
- Increased requirement for instrumental vaginal delivery and cesarean section (controversial).

Delayed: These include:
- Postdural puncture headache
- Transient backache
- Rarely, epidural abscess, meningitis, or permanent neurologic deficit.

CLINICAL PEARLS

- Use of epidural analgesia helps in avoiding opioid-induced maternal and neonatal respiratory depression
- Epidural analgesia must not be administered in the presence of active maternal hemorrhage, coagulation disorders, maternal septicemia and/or infection at the insertion site
- During the second stage of labor, it is important to ensure that the segmental extent of epidural analgesia has spread to include the S2-4 nerve roots in order to maintain analgesia in the perineal region.

6. DELIVERY BY FORCEPS

INTRODUCTION

When the normal vaginal delivery is not possible, the obstetrician has to resort to operative delivery, which can be of two types:
1. Abdominal method (cesarean section) and
2. Vaginal assisted delivery (forceps delivery or vacuum extraction)

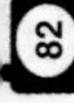

Delivery by forceps is a type of assisted vaginal delivery, which makes use of manual traction (forceps) to facilitate the delivery of fetus.

INDICATIONS

Maternal Indications

- *Termination of second stage of labor*: This may be required in case of maternal exhaustion, severe preeclampsia, severe bleeding, cardiac or pulmonary disease, etc.
- *Prolonged second stage*: Prolonged second stage of labor has been described by Friedman, as nulliparous woman, who fails to deliver after 3 hours with and 2 hours without regional anesthesia. It also includes multiparous woman, who fails to deliver even after 2 hours with or 1 hour without regional anesthesia

Fetal Indications

- *Suspicion of fetal compromise in the second stage of labor*: This may be related to conditions such as fetal umbilical cord prolapse, premature separation of placenta, etc.
- *Fetal malposition*: In the hands of an experienced surgeon, fetal malpositions, such as the after-coming head in breech vaginal delivery and occipitoposterior positions can be indications for forceps delivery.

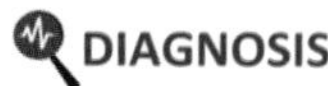

DIAGNOSIS

Clinical Presentation

Clinical classification of forceps application is based on ACOG Criteria **(Table 3.4)**, which is based on the station and rotation of fetal head.

Table 3.4: ACOG criteria for classification of instrumental delivery

Procedure	*Criteria*
Outlet forceps	The fetal scalp is visible at the introitus, without separating the labia. • The fetal skull has reached the pelvic floor • The sagittal suture is in anteroposterior diameter or right or left occiput anterior or posterior position • The fetal head is at or on the perineum • The rotation does not exceed 45°
Low forceps	Leading point of fetal skull is at station ≥ + 2 and not on the pelvic floor. • The degree of rotation does not matter. It could be either:

Contd...

Contd...

Procedure	*Criteria*
	○ Rotation is 45° or less (left or right occiput anterior to occiput anterior or left or right occiput posterior to occiput posterior)
	○ Rotation is 45° or more
Mid pelvic	Station is above +2 cm, but the head is engaged
High pelvic application	Not included in the classification system

Source: American Academy of Pediatrics and American College of Obstetricians and Gynecologists. Guidelines for Perinatal Care, 6th edition. Washington DC: AAP and ACOG; 2007. p. 158.

Investigations

Prerequisites for forceps application have been described later in the text. Besides this, no special investigations are required prior to forceps application.

DIFFERENTIAL DIAGNOSIS

The main differential diagnosis in this case would be to choose between the other options for assisted vaginal delivery (vacuum delivery) or to consider operative abdominal delivery (cesarean section).

SURGICAL MANAGEMENT

Preoperative Preparation

Prerequisites for forceps delivery include the following:

- Maternal verbal consent
- *Assessment of the maternal pelvis*: The forceps must only be applied in cases where there is no fetopelvic disproportion
- *Engagement of fetal head*: The fetal head must be engaged before application of forceps
- *The presentation, position and station of the presenting part*: These must be reconfirmed just before the procedure
- *Cervical dilatation and effacement*: The cervix must be fully dilated and effaced
- *Status of the membranes*: The fetal membranes must have ruptured
- *Bladder to be emptied*: The bladder should be emptied, preferably with help of a catheter

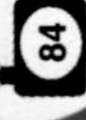

- *The woman's position*: The woman should be placed in the "lithotomy position" or the left lateral position. After placing in the proper position, she must be adequately cleaned and draped under all aseptic precautions
- *Adequate analgesia*: While some surgeons use only local infiltration of anesthesia to the perineal body prior to forceps application, others may prefer to use pudendal block anesthesia augmented with intravenous sedation
- *Facilities for operative delivery*: Adequate facilities for cesarean section should be available in case the delivery by forceps fails.

Steps of Surgery

The proper application of forceps is shown in **Figures 3.17A to F**.

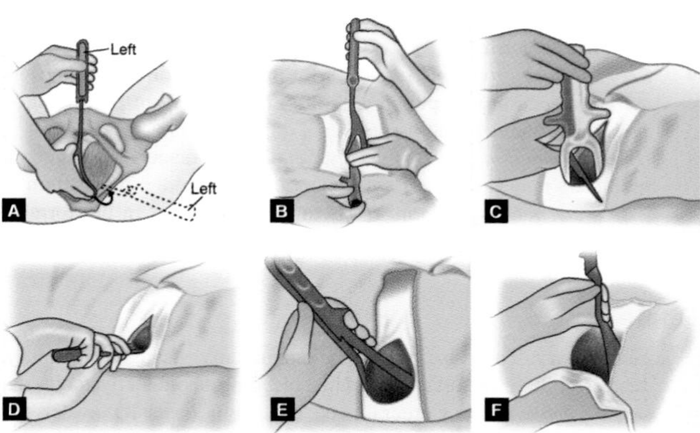

Figures 3.17A to F: (A) The left blade is introduced into the left side of the maternal pelvis; (B) the left blade is in place and the right blade is introduced by the right hand; a median or mediolateral episiotomy may be performed at this point; (C) the forceps have been locked; (D) application of horizontal traction with the operator seated (E) as the fetal occiput bulges out, the traction is applied in the upward direction; (F) following the distension of vulval outlet by the fetal head, the branches of forceps are disarticulated and delivery of rest of the head is completed by modified Ritgen's maneuver

Postoperative Care

- *Maternal examination*: The mother's external genitalia must be carefully examined, in order to rule out presence of any cervical, vaginal, perineal and paraurethral lacerations or tears
- *Neonatal examination*: The newborn must be examined for lacerations, bruising and other injuries over the scalp and face.

COMPLICATIONS

Maternal

- *Injury to the maternal tissues*: Increased risk of perineal tears and lacerations (both vaginal and cervical)
- *Hemorrhage*: Severe maternal tissue injury and lacerations due to forceps application can sometimes result in extensive bleeding and maternal hemorrhage
- *Febrile morbidity*: This could be the manifestation of postpartum uterine infection and pelvic cellulitis, resulting from the infection caused by trauma to the tissues
- *Urinary retention and bladder dysfunction*: Damage to the urethral sphincters may result in urinary retention and bladder dysfunction
- *Late maternal complications*: These could manifest in the form of genitorurinary fistulae, pelvic organ prolapse and/or fecal or urinary incontinence

Fetal

- *Fetal injury*: These include cephalohematoma, facial nerve injury, depressed skull fractures, intracranial bleeding, shoulder dystocia, etc.
- *Other complications*: Cerebral palsy and subtly lower IQ levels.

CLINICAL PEARLS

- American College of Obstetrics and Gynecology (2001) has recommended forceps delivery as an acceptable and safe option for delivery
- Failed forceps or an unsuccessful attempt at forceps delivery can occur due to causes such as unsuspected cephalopelvic disproportion, misdiagnosis of the position of the head and incomplete dilation of the cervix.

7. DELIVERY BY VACUUM

INTRODUCTION

Vacuum application (ventouse) is emerging as an important procedure for assisted vaginal delivery, which is presently being favored over forceps delivery. Malmström developed the prototype of the modern vacuum extractor in Sweden. This instrument assists in delivery by creating a vacuum between it and the fetal scalp. The newer types of vacuum devices available today are shown in **Figures 3.18A and B**.

INDICATIONS

The classifications, indications and contraindications for vacuum delivery are almost same as that utilized for forceps delivery (described in the previous fragment). However, unlike the forceps, vacuum extractors cannot be used in cases of face presentation or after-coming head of breech. The vacuum must never be applied to an unengaged head.

DIAGNOSIS

This is same as that described in the fragment of forceps delivery.

DIFFERENTIAL DIAGNOSIS

The main differential diagnosis in this case would be to choose between the other options for assisted vaginal delivery (forceps delivery) or to consider operative abdominal delivery (cesarean section).

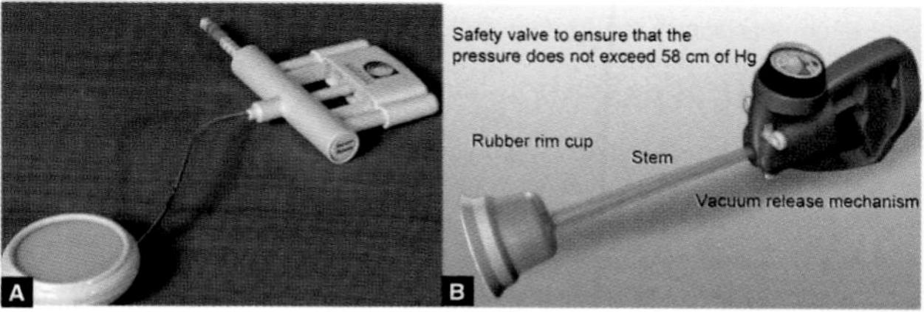

Figures 3.18A and B: Various types of vacuum extractor devices using hand-pump suction: (A) hand-held vacuum device with soft silastic cup and (B) Mity Soft Bell cup

SURGICAL MANAGEMENT

Preoperative Preparation

Prerequisites for vacuum application are similar to that of forceps application as described previously.

Steps of Surgery

Steps of vacuum application are shown in **Figures 3.19A to D**.

Postoperative Care

The postoperative care for vacuum delivery is same as that of forceps delivery and includes the followings:

- Inspection of maternal tissues (cervix, vagina, vulva and paraurethral tissues) for the presence of any tears, lacerations, injury, etc.
- Examination of the newly delivered infant for the presence of any injuries.

COMPLICATIONS

- *Neonatal injury*: Use of vacuum can result in development of injuries, such as scalp lacerations, bruising, subgaleal hematomas, cephalohematomas **(Figs 3.20A and B)**, intracranial hemorrhage, neonatal jaundice, subconjunctival hemorrhage, clavicular fracture, shoulder dystocia, injury of sixth and seventh cranial nerves, Erb's palsy, retinal hemorrhage, transient neonatal lateral rectus palsy and fetal death
- *Shoulder dystocia*: This occurs more commonly with vacuum delivery in comparison to the forceps delivery.

CLINICAL PEARLS

- The "ventouse" delivery is considered to be more physiological and similar to normal vaginal delivery, in comparison to the forceps delivery
- Similar to forceps delivery, the use of vacuum helps in avoiding the need of abdominal delivery
- While the use of vacuum is associated with minimal injury to maternal tissues in comparison to forceps delivery, it is associated with a higher incidence of injury to the fetal tissues
- The modern, soft, silastic vacuum cup, used nowadays can be safely applied to the fetal scalp without much chances of causing injury or fetal scalp trauma

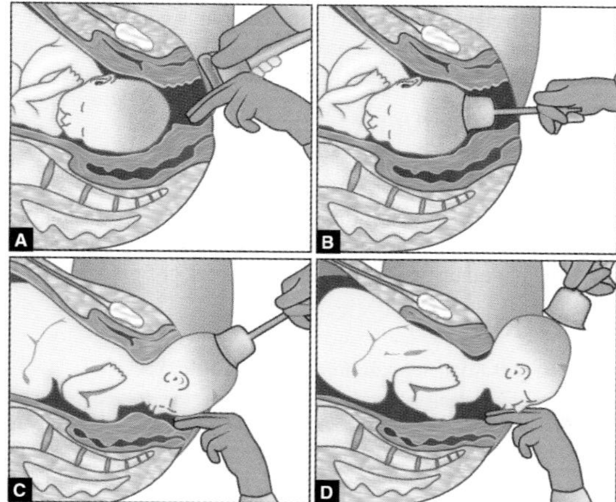

Figures 3.19A to D: (A) Insertion of the vacuum cup into the vagina following the separation of patient's labia by pressing the cup in inward and downward direction, so that the inferior edge of the cup lies close to the posterior fourchette; (B) application of the vacuum cup over the fetal head in such a way that the cup is placed as far posteriorly as possible (C) vacuum suction must be gradually created, by increasing suction by 0.2 kg/cm^2 at every 2 minutes. With the use of soft cups, it is possible to create negative pressure of 0.8 kg/cm^2 over as little as 1 minute; (D) application of traction at right angles to facilitate the delivery of fetal head. Traction should be repeated with each contraction, until crowning of the fetal head occurs. As the head clears the pubic symphysis, the delivery of head is completed by modified Ritgen's maneuver

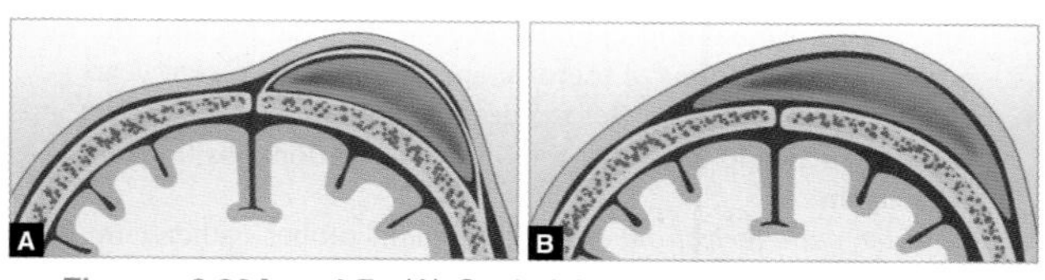

Figures 3.20A and B: (A) Cephalohematoma and (B) Subgleal hematoma

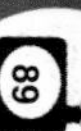

- The vacuum can be used, even if the occiput is not directly anterior or the head is in unrotated position or fetal head is deflexed or obstetrician is unsure about the exact fetal position.

8. CESAREAN DELIVERY

INTRODUCTION

Cesarean section is a surgical procedure commonly used in the obstetric practice. In this procedure the fetal delivery is attained through an incision made over the abdomen and uterus, after 28 weeks of pregnancy.

INDICATIONS

Indications for cesarean section are listed in **Table 3.5**.

Table 3.5: Indications for cesarean section

Indication for cesarean section	*Percentage of cases (%)*
Dystocia	37.5
Previous cesarean section	29
Abnormal presentations (Breech presentation or transverse lie)	14.5
Fetal distress	33.4
Preeclampsia	12

SURGICAL MANAGEMENT

Preoperative Preparation

- *Empty stomach*: In order to prevent the risk of aspiration at the time of administration of anesthesia, the patient should be nil per mouth for at least 12 hours before undertaking a cesarean section
- *Patient position*: The patient is placed with 15° lateral tilt on the operating table, in order to reduce the chances of hypotension
- *Anesthesia*: Spinal and epidural anesthesia have become the most commonly used forms of regional anesthesia in the recent years
- *Patient re-examination*: Before cleaning and draping the patient, it is a good practice to check the fetal lie, presentation, position and FHS once again
- *Bladder catheterization*: Foley's or plain rubber catheter must be inserted, following which the cleaning and draping of the abdomen is done

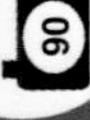

- *Preparation of the skin*: The area around the proposed incision site must be washed with antiseptic soap solution (e.g. savlon and/or betadine solution). The woman must be draped using sterile drapes immediately after the area of surgery has been adequately prepared in order to avoid contamination

Steps of Surgery

The essential steps in a cesarean delivery are summarized in **Figures 3.21A to H**.

Postoperative Care

- *Immediate postoperative care*: After the completion of surgery, monitoring of routine vital signs, urine output, vaginal bleeding and uterine tonicity needs to be done at hourly intervals for the first 4 hours
- *Analgesia*: Adequate analgesia needs to be provided, initially through the IV route and later with oral medications
- *Fluids and oral food after cesarean section*: As a general rule, about 3 liters of fluids must be replaced by intravenous infusion during the first postoperative day, provided that the woman's urine output remains greater than 30 mL/hour. In uncomplicated cases, the urinary catheter can be removed by 12 hours postoperatively, and the woman may be given a light liquid diet in the evening after the surgery
- *Ambulation after cesarean section*: The women must be encouraged to ambulate soon after 6–8 hours following the surgery in uncomplicated cases
- *Dressing and wound care*: The dressing must be kept on the wound for the first 2–3 days after surgery, so as to provide a protective barrier against infection.

COMPLICATIONS

- Abdominal pain
- Injury to bladder, ureters, etc.
- Increased risk of rupture uterus, antepartum or intrapartum intrauterine deaths and/or maternal deaths in future pregnancies
- Neonatal respiratory morbidity
- Requirement for hysterectomy during the surgery
- Increased duration of hospital stay
- Increased risk of complications, such as placenta previa and adherent placenta, during future pregnancies

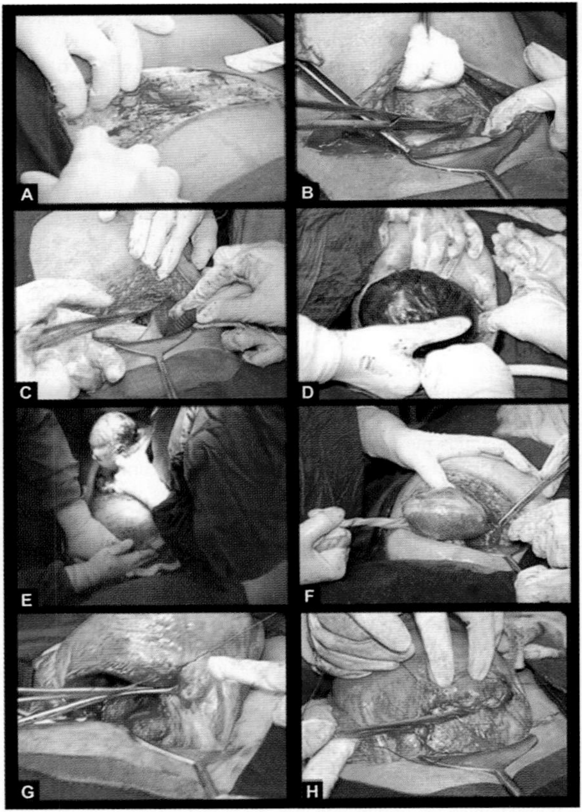

Figures 3.21A to H: Steps of cesarean delivery: (A) giving an incision over the abdomen and dissecting out different layers of skin; (B) application of Doyen's retractor after dissection of parietal peritoneum followed by Incision of visceral peritoneum; (C) giving a uterine incision; (D) delivery of fetal head; (E) delivery of the entire baby out of the uterine cavity; (F) delivery of the placenta; (G) clamping the uterine angles with green armytage clamps (H) stitching the uterine cavity

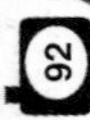

- *Infection*: This may occur in the form of endometritis or infection of the endometrial cavity and/or urinary tract infection
- *Thromboembolism*: Thromboembolism must be suspected, if the patient develops cough, swollen calf muscles or positive Homan's sign (passive dorsiflexion of the ankle by the examiner elicits sharp pain in the patient's calf).

CLINICAL PEARLS

- Pregnant women with a history of one previous lower segment transverse section may be offered either planned vaginal birth after cesarean (VBAC) or elective repeat cesarean section (ERCS) for future deliveries
- Although presently a large number of patients with previous cesarean delivery are being considered for VBAC, the risk of scar rupture, although small, still remains.

9. BREECH PRESENTATION

INTRODUCTION

Breech presentation is a type of abnormal presentation where the fetus lies longitudinally with the buttocks presenting in the lower pole of the uterus. The different types of breech presentations, like complete breech, footling breech and frank breech, are shown in **Figure 3.22**.

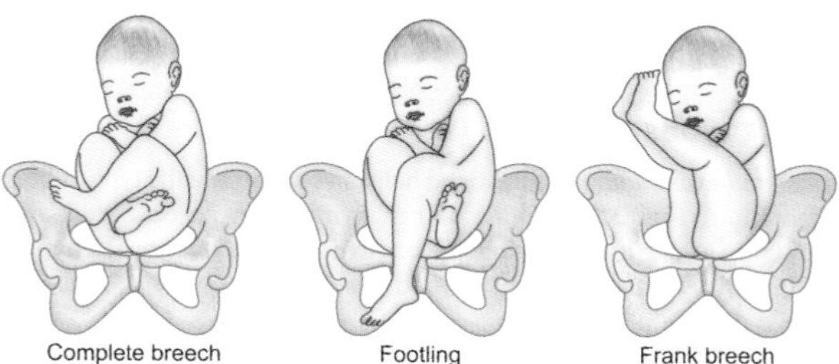

Figure 3.22: Different types of breech presentation

ETIOLOGY

- *Maternal factors*: Maternal risk factors for breech presentation include factors such as cephalopelvic disproportion; liquor abnormalities (polyhydramnios and oligohydramnios); uterine anomalies (bicornuate or septate uterus); space occupying lesions (e.g. fibroids in the lower uterine segment); placental abnormalities (placenta previa, cornuofundal attachment of placenta), multiparity (especially grand multiparas); cord abnormalities (very long or very short cord); previous history of breech delivery; etc.
- *Fetal factors*: These include factors such as prematurity; fetal anomalies (e.g. neurological abnormalities, hydrocephalus, anencephaly and meningomyelocele); intrauterine fetal death; etc.

DIAGNOSIS

Abdominal Examination

Fetal lie is longitudinal with fetal head on one side and breech on the other side. First Leopold's maneuver or fundal grip shows smooth, hard, ballotable structure suggestive of fetal head. On second Leopold's maneuver or lateral grip, there is a firm, smooth board-like fetal back on one side and knob-like structures suggestive of fetal limbs on other side. On pelvice grips, fetal head cannot be palpated. Instead there is soft broad irregular mass.

Pelvic Examination

Head is not felt in pelvis; instead an irregular, soft, non-ballotable structure suggestive of fetal buttocks, feet, anus, sacrum and/or external genitalia, etc. may be felt on the vaginal, examination. Very thick meconium may be present after ROM.

Investigations

Ultrasound examination: Ultrasound helps in confirming the type of breech presentation **(Fig. 3.23)**. Other things, which can be observed on the ultrasound, include the following: presence of uterine and/or fetal anomalies, fetal maturity, placental location and grading, adequacy of liquor and presence of multiple gestation.

The management options for breech presentation are basically of two types: first being external cephalic version (ECV) during pregnancy and the second being delivery by cesarean section or a breech vaginal delivery

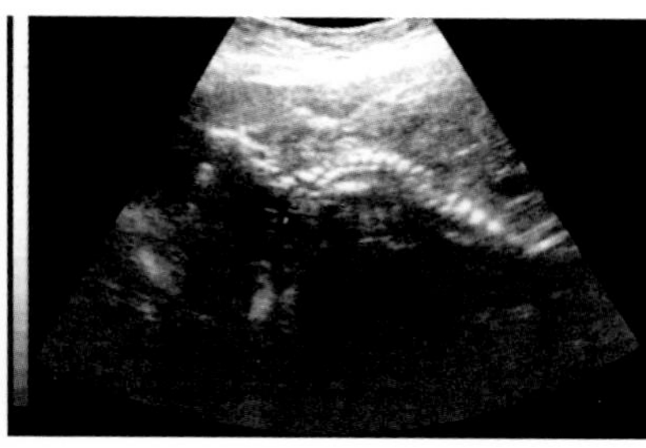

Figure 3.23: Ultrasound examination showing breech gestation

at term. The breech scoring system by Zatuchni and Andros (**Table 3.6**) can be used for deciding whether to perform a vaginal (score of > 3) or an abdominal delivery (score of 3 or less).

Table 3.6: Zatuchni and Andros score

Parameter	*0 point*	*1 point*	*2 point*
Parity	Primigravida	Multigravida	—
Gestational age	39 weeks or more	38 weeks	37 weeks
Estimated fetal weight	> 8 pounds (3690 gm)	7–8 pounds (3176–3690 gm)	< 7 pounds (< 3176 gm)
Previous breech (> 2500 gm)	None	One	Two or more
Cervical dilation by vaginal examination at the time of admission	2 cm or less	3 cm	4 cm or more
Station of the presenting part at the time of admission	– 3 or higher	– 2	–1 or lower

OBSTETRIC MANAGEMENT

External Cephalic Version

External cephalic version (ECV) can be defined as a procedure in which the clinician externally rotates the fetus from a breech presentation into a cephalic presentation. The detailed procedure of version has been described in a separate fragment of this chapter.

Elective Cesarean Delivery

Some of the absolute indications for cesarean section in cases of breech presentation are enumerated in **Box 3.1**. Details regarding cesarean delivery have been described in a separate fragment of this chapter.

Box 3.1: Absolute indications for cesarean section in breech presentation

- Cephalopelvic disproportion
- Placenta previa
- Estimated fetal weight > 4 kg
- Hyperextension of fetal head
- Footling breech (danger of entrapment of head in an incompletely dilated cervix)
- Severe IUGR
- Clinician not competent with the technique of breech vaginal delivery
- A viable preterm fetus in active labor

Trial of Breech (Vaginal Breech Delivery)

Although breech vaginal delivery is not routinely used, it may become unavoidable in certain circumstances **(Box 3.2)**. Obstetric steps for breech vaginal delivery are as follows:

- Once the buttocks have entered the vagina and the cervix is fully dilated, the woman must be advised to bear down with the contractions
- Episiotomy may be performed, if the perineum appears very tight
- A "no touch policy" by the clinician must be adopted until the buttocks and lower back deliver till the level of umbilicus
- Sometimes the clinician may have to make use of maneuvers like Pinard maneuver **(Figs 3.24 A to C)** and groin traction **(Fig. 3.25)**, if the legs have not delivered spontaneously
- The clinician should be extremely careful and gently hold the baby by wrapping it in a clean cloth in such a way that the baby's trunk is present anteriorly. In order to avoid compression on the umbilical cord, it should be moved to one side
- If the fetal arms are felt on the chest, the clinician must wait for them to deliver spontaneously. After spontaneous delivery of the first arm, the buttocks must be lifted toward the mother's abdomen to enable the second arm to deliver spontaneously. In case the fetal arms are extended, the clinician can use Lovset's maneuver **(Figs 3.26A to C)** to deliver the anterior shoulder or the maneuver, 'delivery of the posterior shoulders **(Fig. 3.27)**' in case the Lovset's maneuver, fails

- Once the shoulders are delivered, the baby's body with the face down must be supported on the clinician's forearm. One of the following maneuvers can be used for delivery of after-coming head of the fetus: Burns-Marshall Technique **(Figs 3.28A and B)**, Mauriceau Smellie Veit maneuver **(Fig. 3.29)** or delivery of after-coming head using forceps **(Fig. 3.30)**.

Box 3.2: Indications for breech vaginal delivery

- Estimated fetal weight 2,000-4,000 gm
- Frank or complete breech presentation
- Flexed fetal head, i.e. an extension angle of less than 90°
- No major fetal anomalies or placenta previa on ultrasound
- No obstetric contraindication for breech vaginal delivery (e.g. CPD, placenta previa, etc.)
- Delivery is imminent
- Presence of severe fetal anomaly or fetal death
- Mother's preference for vaginal birth.

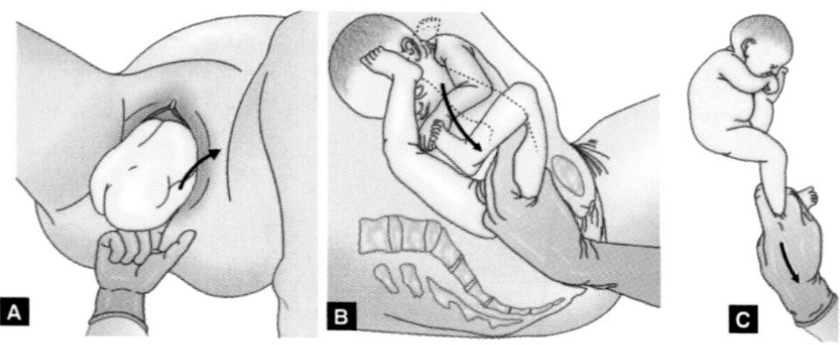

Figures 3.24A to C: Pinard's maneuver: (A) pressure is exerted against the fetal popliteal fossa; (B) Due to application of pressure, the fetal knee gets flexed and abducted; (C) As the fetal leg moves downward, it is pulled out by the clinician

Figure 3.25: Groin traction

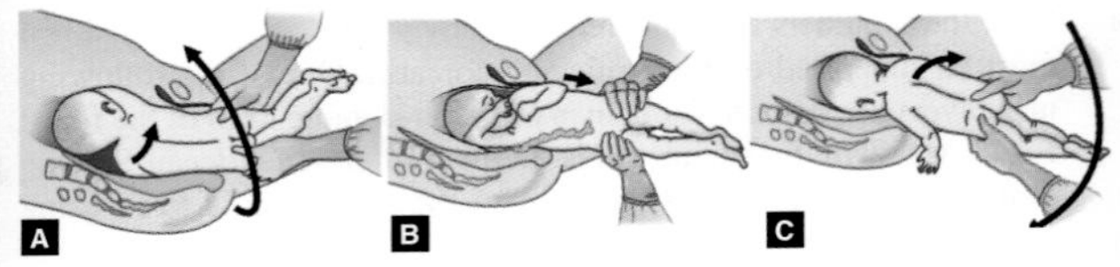

Figures 3.26A to C: Lovset's maneuver: (A) Trunk is rotated through 180° keeping the back anterior. This causes the posterior arm to emerge under pubic arch (B) Posterior arm is hooked out (C) Trunk is rotated in reverse direction to deliver the anterior shoulder

Figure 3.27: Delivery of posterior shoulder

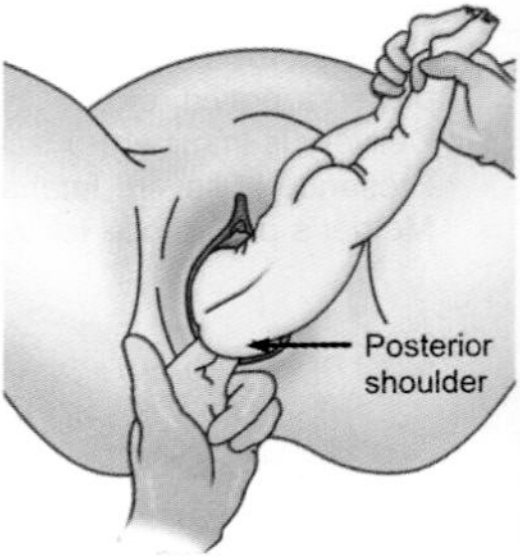

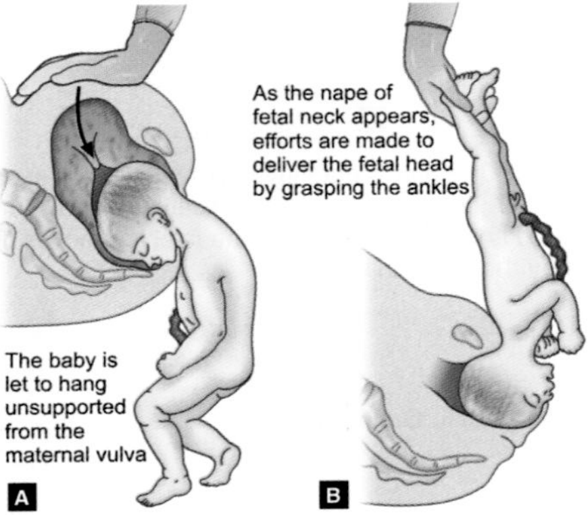

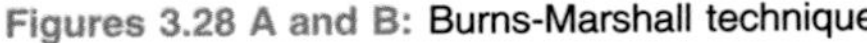

Figures 3.28 A and B: Burns-Marshall technique

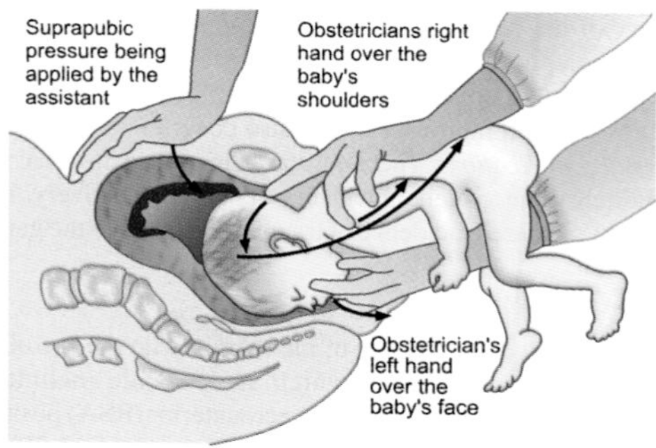

Figure 3.29: Mauriceau Smellie Veit maneuver

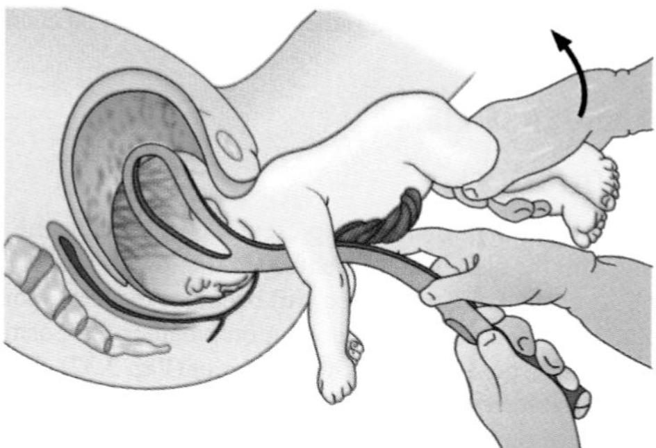

Figure 3.30: Delivery of after-coming head of the breech using forceps

COMPLICATIONS

- *Complications related to ECV*: This has been discussed in the fragment on version
- *Fetal complications*: Breech vaginal delivery can be associated with fetal complications such as low APGAR scores, especially at 1 minute, cord compression, cord prolapse, premature attempts by the baby to breathe while the head is still inside the uterine cavity and delay in the

delivery of the head due to head entrapment. Head entrapment can result in complications such as intracranial hemorrhage and tentorial tears. Neonatal trauma including brachial plexus injuries, hematomas, fractures, visceral injuries, etc. can also occur in about 25% of cases

- *Maternal complications*: There may be an increased maternal morbidity and mortality due to higher incidence of operative delivery. There also may be an increased incidence of traumatic injuries to the genital tract.

CLINICAL PEARLS

- Depending on the relationship of the sacrum with the sacroiliac joint, the positions of the breech which are possible include the left sacroanterior (LSA) position; right sacroanterior (RSA) position; right sacroposterior (RSP) position and left sacroposterior (LSP) position. Of these various positions, LSA is the commonest
- While conducting the breech vaginal delivery, at no point, the clinician must try to pull the baby out, rather the patient must be encouraged to push down.

10. TRANSVERSE LIE

INTRODUCTION

Transverse lie is an abnormal fetal presentation in which the fetus lies transversely with the shoulders presenting in the lower pole of the uterus (**Fig. 3.31**). As a result, the presenting part becomes the fetal shoulder. The denominator is the fetal back. Depending on whether the position of the fetal back is anterior, posterior, superior or inferior (**Fig. 3.32**), the following positions are possible: dorso-anterior (fetal back is anterior); dorso-posterior (fetal back is posterior); dorso-superior (fetal back is directed superiorly) and dorso-inferior (fetal back is directed inferiorly).

ETIOLOGY

Maternal: Maternal risk factors for transverse lie are:

- Cephalopelvic disproportion, contracted maternal pelvis
- Liquor abnormalities (polyhydramnios and oligohydramnios); uterine anomalies (bicornuate, septate, etc.); presence of pelvic tumor
- Space occupying lesions (e.g. fibroids in the lower uterine segment)
- Placental abnormalities (placenta previa, cornuofundal attachment of placenta), multiparity (especially grand multiparas).

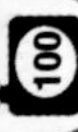

Fetal: Fetal risk factors for transverse lie are:

- Prematurity, twins, hydramnios, intrauterine fetal death, fetal anomalies, etc.

DIAGNOSIS

Abdominal Examination

- Fetal lie is in the horizontal plane with fetal head on one side of the midline and podalic pole on the other

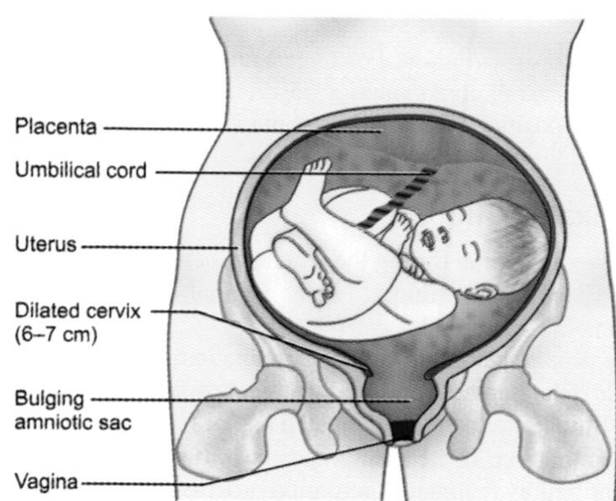

Figure 3.31: Fetus in transverse lie

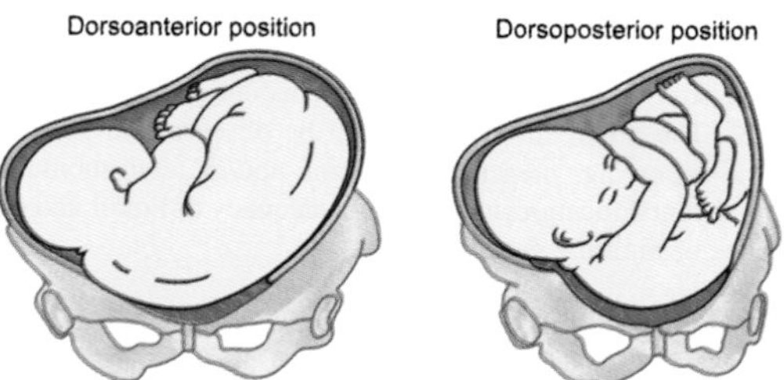

Figure 3.32: Different positions of transverse lie

- The abdomen often appears barrel shaped and is asymmetrical
- Fundal height is less than the period of amenorrhea
- *First Leopold's maneuver/fundal grip*: No fetal pole (either breech or cephalic) is palpable on the fundal grip
- *Second Leopold's maneuver/lateral grip*: Soft, broad, smooth irregular part suggestive of fetal breech is present on one side of the midline, while a smooth hard globular part suggestive of the fetal head is present on the other side of the midline.
- *Third Leopold's maneuver*: Pelvic grip appears to be empty during the time of pregnancy. It may be occupied by the shoulder at the time of labor
- *Fetal heart auscultation*: Fetal heart rate is easily heard much below the umbilicus in dorso-anterior position. On the other hand in dorso-posterior position, the fetal heart may be located at a much higher level and is often above the umbilicus

Vaginal Examination

On vaginal examination during the antenatal period, the pelvis appears to be empty. Even if something is felt on vaginal examination, no definite fetal part may be identified.

At the time of labor, on vaginal examination, fetal shoulder including scapula, clavicle, humerus and grid iron feel of fetal ribs can be palpated. Due to ill-fitting fetal part, an elongated bag of membranes may be felt on vaginal examination. If the membranes have ruptured, the fetal shoulder can be identified by feeling the acromion process, scapula, clavicle, axilla, ribs and intercostal spaces. If the arm prolapse has occurred, the fetal arm might be observed lying outside the vagina.

Investigations

Ultrasound examination: Ultrasound helps in confirming the transverse lie **(Fig. 3.33)**. The other things which can be observed on the ultrasound include the following: presence of uterine and/or fetal anomalies; fetal maturity; placental location and grading; adequacy of liquor and ruling out the presence of multiple gestation.

MANAGEMENT

- *Management during pregnancy*: The management options for transverse lie include ECV during pregnancy or delivery by cesarean section (elective or an emergency). If the version is unsuccessful, the

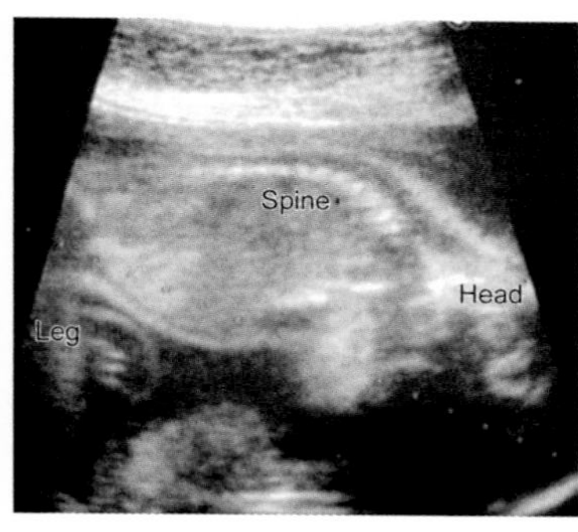

Figure 3.33: Ultrasound examination at 24 weeks showing transverse lie

only option for delivering the fetus in transverse lie is performing a cesarean delivery. Version has been described in details in a subsequent fragment

- *Management during labor*: If the maternal and fetal conditions are stable, the best option in these cases would be to perform a cesarean section.

COMPLICATIONS

- *Complications related to version*: These are described in subsequent fragment
- *Fetal arm prolapse*: Due to the ill-fitting fetal part, the sudden ROM can result in the escape of large amount of liquor and the prolapse of fetal arm, which is often accompanied by a loop of cord
- *Obstructed labor*: If the transverse lie with or without a prolapsed arm is left neglected, a serious complication including obstructed labor can occur. If the uterine obstruction is not immediately relieved, uterine inertia and rupture of the uterus can occur in primigravida and multigravida patients respectively
- *Long-term complications*: Long-term maternal complications include development of genitourinary fistulas, secondary amenorrhea (related to Sheehan's syndrome associated with PPH), hysterectomy, etc.
- *Fetal asphyxia*: Tonic uterine contractions can interfere with uteroplacental circulation resulting in fetal distress. Other fetal complications may include preterm birth, PROM, intrauterine fetal death and increased fetal mortality.

CLINICAL PEARLS

- Ribs and intercostal spaces upon palpation give feeling of grid iron on vaginal examination
- While doing the ECV, the fetus should be moved gently rather than using forceful movements
- There is no mechanism of labor for a fetus in transverse lie, which remains uncorrected until term. A cesarean section is required to deliver the baby with shoulder presentation.

11. OCCIPITOPOSTERIOR POSITION

INTRODUCTION

This is a type of abnormal position of the vertex where the occiput is placed over the left sacroiliac joint (LOP or 4th vertex) or right sacroiliac joint (ROP or 3rd vertex) **(Figs 3.34 A and B)** or directly over the sacrum (direct occipitoposterior position).

ETIOLOGY

- **Presence of an anthropoid or android pelvis**
- **Marked deflexion of fetal head**

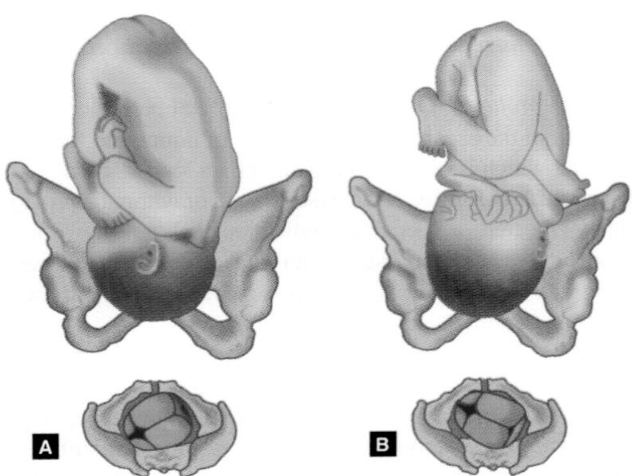

Figures 3.34A and B: (A) Left occipitoanterior position and (B) left occipitoposterior position

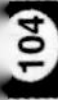

- High pelvic inclination
- Attachment of placenta on the anterior uterine wall
- Brachycephaly of fetal head
- Abnormal uterine contractions.

DIAGNOSIS

Abdominal Examination

- On abdominal inspection there is flattening of the abdomen below the umbilicus
- Fetal limbs are palpated more easily nearly the midline on either side
- Fetal back and anterior shoulders are far away from the midline
- On pelvic grip, the head is not engaged. The cephalic prominence is not felt as prominently as felt in occipitoanterior position **(Figs 3.35 A and B)**. The FHS is difficult to locate and may be best heard in the flanks.

Vaginal Examination

- Presence of an elongated bag of membranes
- Sagittal sutures occupy any of the oblique diameters of the pelvis
- Posterior fontanelle is felt near the sacroiliac joint
- Anterior fontanelle can be felt more easily due to the deflexed head.

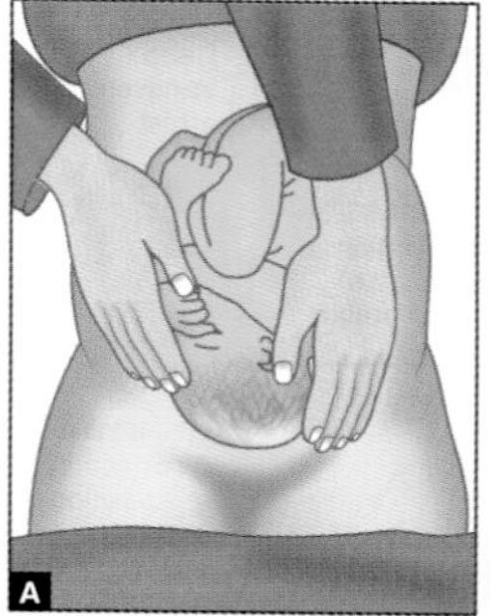

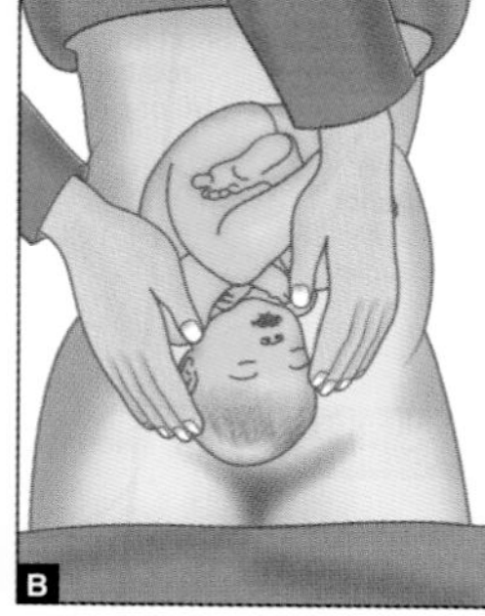

Figures 3.35 A and B: Palpation of the fetal head (third pelvic grip): (A) occipitoanterior position; (B) occipitoposterior position

OBSTETRIC MANAGEMENT

The likely consequences related to occipitoposterior position are shown in **Figure 3.36**. In majority of cases, good uterine contractions result in the flexion of fetal head. Descent occurs and the occiput undergoes rotation by 3/8 of the circle to lie behind the pubic symphysis, resulting in an occipitoanterior position. In a small number of cases, the outcome may be unfavorable, resulting in short anterior rotation, non-rotation and short posterior rotation. In case of short anterior rotation, the occiput rotates through 1/8 of the circle anteriorly so that the sagittal sutures lie in the bispinous diameter. This position is known as the "deep transverse arrest". In case of non-rotation of the occiput, sagittal sutures lie in the oblique diameter. Further progress of labor is unlikely and this is known as oblique posterior arrest. In case of short posterior rotation, posterior rotation of the sinciput occurs by 1/8 of the circle, putting the occiput in the sacral hollow. This position is known as persistent occipitoposterior position. Under favorable conditions with an average-sized baby, spacious pelvis and good uterine contractions, spontaneous face-to-pubis delivery can occur. If conditions are not favorable, delivery may not occur, resulting in an occipitosacral arrest.

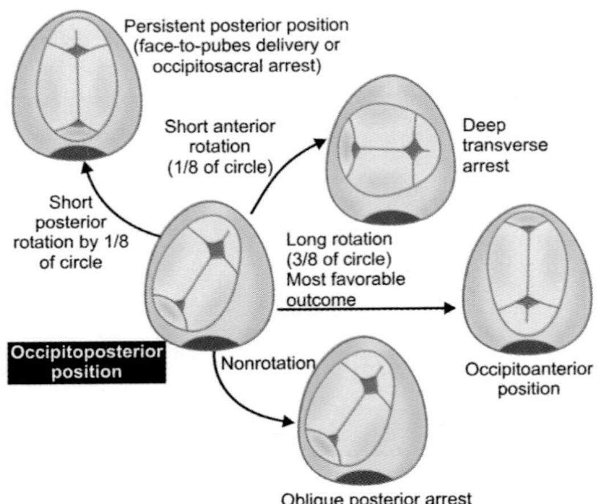

Figure 3.36: Consequences related to occipitoposterior position

Management in the cases of occipitoposterior position comprises of following steps:

- Watchful expectancy hoping for fetal descent and anterior rotation of the occiput
- Intravenous infusion of ringer lactate must be started in anticipation of prolonged labor
- Bed rest must be advised to avoid early ROM
- Pelvis must be assessed for adequacy
- In majority of cases, long anterior rotation of head occurs. Delivery, therefore, in majority of cases occurs spontaneously or with low forceps or ventouse
- Liberal episiotomy should be given to prevent perineal tears
- In cases of occipitotransverse or oblique occipitoposterior positions, ventouse application can be done
- Manual rotation of fetal head or rotation using Keilland's forceps, both of which were previously performed are no longer done nowadays
- Nowadays, cesarean section is the most commonly used mode of delivery in these cases.

COMPLICATIONS

- Prolonged duration of both first and second stages of labor (due to labor dystocia; delayed engagement of the fetal head and abnormal uterine contractions with slow dilatation of cervix
- Early ROM
- Extreme degree of molding of fetal skull can result in tentorial tears
- Increased tendency for postpartum hemorrhage
- High chances of perineal injuries and trauma including complete perineal tears
- High maternal morbidity due to increased rate of operative delivery
- Increased perinatal morbidity and mortality due to asphyxia or trauma.

CLINICAL PEARLS

- Occipitoposterior position can be considered as an abnormal position of the vertex rather than an abnormal presentation
- There are higher chances of perineal injuries with face to pubis delivery because the biparietal diameter stretches the perineum and occipitofrontal diameter emerges out of the introitus
- Cesarean section is not indicated per se in the cases of occipitoposterior position.

12. CORD PROLAPSE

INTRODUCTION

Cord prolapse has been defined as descent of the umbilical cord through the cervix alongside the presenting part (occult presentation) or past it (overt presentation) in the presence of ruptured membranes. In occult prolapse, the cord cannot be felt by the examiner's fingers at the time of vaginal examination. In overt cord prolapse, the cord is found lying inside the vagina or outside the vulva following the ROM **(Fig. 3.37)**. Cord presentation, on the other hand, is the presence of one or more loops of umbilical cord between the fetal presenting part and the cervix, with the membranes being intact **(Fig. 3.38)**.

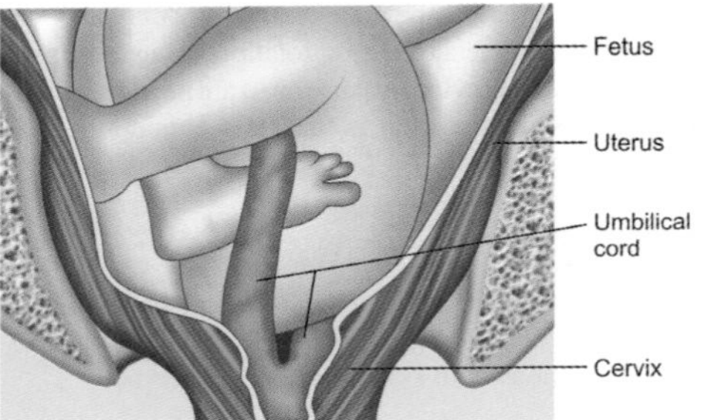

Figure 3.37: Overt cord prolapse

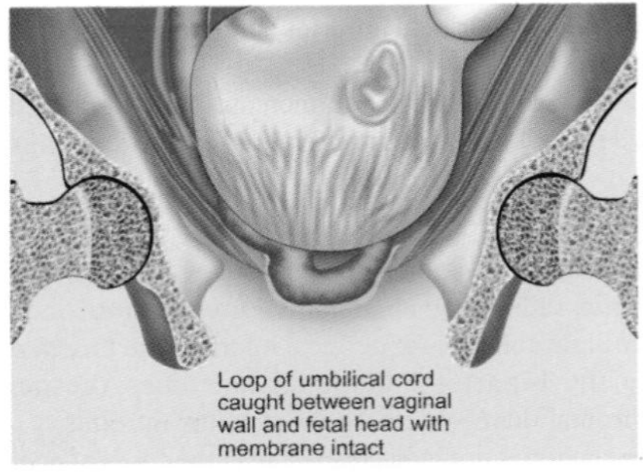

Figure 3.38: Cord presentation

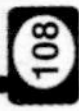

ETIOLOGY

Various probable causes of cord prolapse are listed in the **Table 3.7**.

Table 3.7: Causes of cord prolapse

General causes	*Procedure related causes*
• Multiparity • Low birth weight (< 2.5 kg) • Prematurity (< 37 weeks) • Fetal congenital anomalies • Breech/shoulder presentation • Second twin • Polyhydramnios • Unengaged presenting part • Low placenta and other abnormal placentation • Cord abnormalities (such as true knots or low content of Wharton's jelly)	• Artificial ROM (particularly with unengaged head) • Vaginal manipulation of fetus with ruptured membranes • External cephalic version • Internal podalic version • Stabilizing induction of labor • Application of fetal scalp electrodes or placement of intrauterine catheters

DIAGNOSIS

Clinical Presentation

Clinical findings on vaginal examination have been described in the "introduction".

Investigations

- *Cardiotocography*: There may be variable decelerations of heart rate pattern on continuous electronic fetal monitoring
- *Ultrasound examination*: Ultrasound may help in identification of umbilical cord within the cervix **(Fig. 3.39)**.

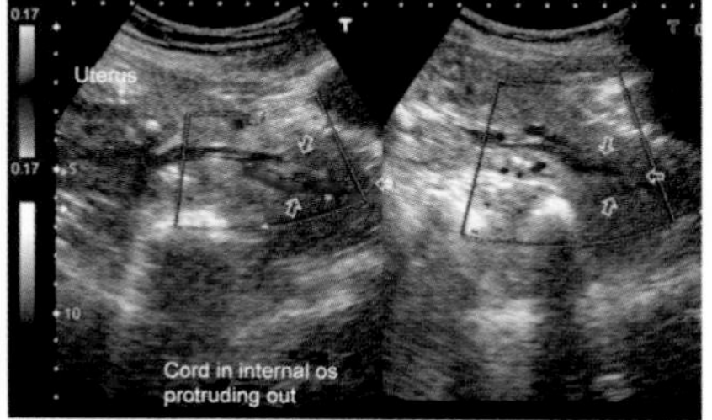

Figure 3.39: Internal os appears dilated with umbilical cord within the cervix; this finding is diagnostic of cord prolapse

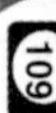

MANAGEMENT

Prevention and First Aid

- Artificial ROM should be avoided whenever possible if the presenting part has yet not engaged or is mobile. In cases where ROM becomes necessary even in such circumstances, this should be performed in an operation theatre with facilities available for an immediate cesarean birth
- In cases of cord prolapse where immediate vaginal delivery is not possible, assistance should be called immediately; venous access should be obtained, consent taken and immediate preparations be made for an urgent cesarean delivery. The following steps can be followed until facilities for cesarean section are made available:
  - To prevent vasospasm, there should be minimal handling of loops of cord lying outside the vagina, which can be covered with surgical packs soaked in warm saline
  - To prevent cord compression, it is recommended that the presenting part be elevated either manually or by filling the urinary bladder with normal saline
  - Cord compression can be further reduced by advising the mother to adopt knee-chest position or head-down tilt (preferably in left-lateral position).

Definitive Management

Definitive management comprises of immediate delivery:

- In cases where vaginal delivery is possible, forceps can be applied in cases of cephalic presentation if the head has engaged. In case of breech presentation, breech extraction can be done. In case of transverse lie, internal version followed by breech extraction must be performed
- A cesarean section is the recommended mode of delivery in cases of cord prolapse when vaginal delivery is not imminent. A cesarean section should ideally be performed within 30 minutes or less (from the point of diagnosis to the delivery of the baby).

COMPLICATIONS

Maternal: These is an increased maternal morbidity due to greater incidence of operative delivery.

Fetal: Cord compression and umbilical artery vasospasm may cause asphyxia, which may result in hypoxic-ischemic encephalopathy and cerebral palsy.

CLINICAL PEARLS

- Incidence of cord prolapse has greatly reduced due to the increased use of elective cesarean deliveries in cases of non-cephalic presentation
- In order to prevent vasospasm of umbilical artery, there should be minimal handling of loops of cord lying outside the vagina.

13. COMPOUND PRESENTATION

INTRODUCTION

In compound presentation, one or two of the fetal extremities enter the pelvis simultaneously with the presenting part. The most common combinations are head-hand **(Fig. 3.40)**; breech-hand and head-arm-foot.

ETIOLOGY

The predisposing factors for the development of compound presentation include the following:

- Prematurity
- Multiparity

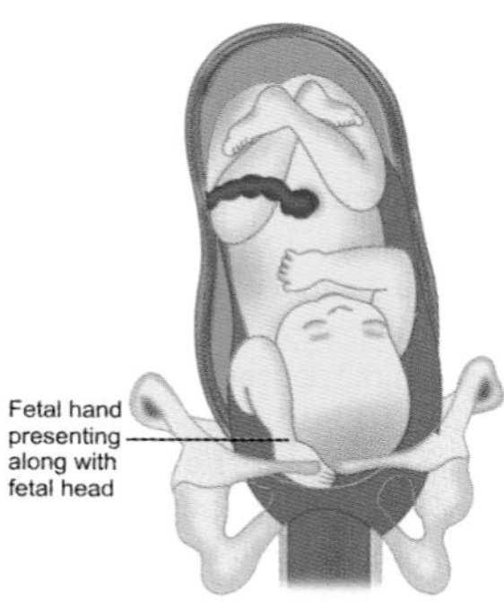

Figure 3.40: Compound presentation where the fetal hand is seen to be entering the pelvis

- Twin/multiple gestation
- Pelvic tumors
- Cephalopelvic disproportion
- Macerated fetus.

DIAGNOSIS

Clinical Presentation

The diagnosis is confirmed on vaginal examination.

OBSTETRIC MANAGEMENT

In most cases, the prolapsed extremity does not cause any interference with the normal progress of labor and vaginal delivery. In most of the cases, the prolapsed limbs spontaneously rise up with the descent of the presenting part.

In presence of cephalopelvic disproportion and/or cord prolapse, cesarean section is required.

COMPLICATIONS

- The most common complication associated with that of compound presentation is cord prolapse (see the previous fragment)
- Temptation to replace the limb early during labor is associated with an increased maternal and fetal mortality and morbidity.

14. FACE PRESENTATION

INTRODUCTION

This is an abnormal fetal position characterized by an extreme extension of the fetal head so that the fetal face rather than the fetal head becomes the presenting part and the fetal occiput comes in direct contact with the back. Denominator in these cases is mentum or chin.

Four positions are possible depending on the position of the chin with left or right sacroiliac joints (**Fig. 3.41**):

- Right mentoposterior position (deflexed LOA)
- Left mentoposterior position (deflexed ROA)
- Left mentoanterior position (deflexed ROP)
- Right mentoanterior position (deflexed LOP).

Commonest type of face presentation is left mentoanterior position.

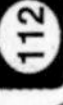

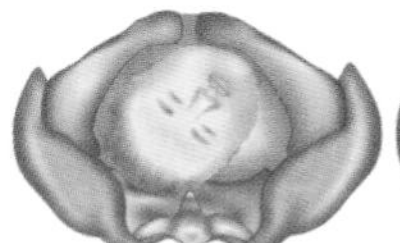

Right mentoanterior

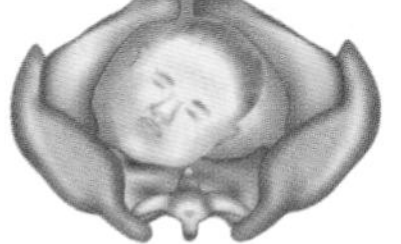

Figure 3.41: Different positions in face presentation

ETIOLOGY

Maternal Causes

- Multiparity with pendulous abdomen
- Contracted pelvis.

Fetal Causes

- Congenital causes (anencephaly, congenital goiter, congenital bronchocele, etc.)
- Several twists of cord around fetal neck
- Dolicocephalic head (with long anterior-posterior diameter)
- Increased tone of extensor group of muscle.

DIAGNOSIS

Clinical Examination

- *Abdominal examination*: In case of mentoanterior positions, the fetal limbs can be palpated anteriorly. Fetal chest is also present anteriorly against the uterine wall. The FHS is thus clearly audible. On abdominal palpation, the groove between the head and neck is not prominent and cephalic prominence lies on the same side as the fetal back. On pelvic grip, the head is not engaged. In case of mentoposterior positions, the back is better palpated towards the front
- *Vaginal examination*: Diagnosis of face presentation is made on vaginal examination. On the vaginal examination, the following structures can be felt: alveolar margins of the mouth, nose, malar eminences, supraorbital ridges and the mentum. There is absence of meconium staining on the examining fingers, unlike in breech presentation.

Investigation

- *Ultrasonography*: Ultrasonography must be performed in order to assess fetal size and to rule out the presence of any bony congenital malformations.

DIFFERENTIAL DIAGNOSIS

Diagnosis of face presentation can often be confused with that of breech presentation. This can be differentiated from breech presentation with the help of following two rules:

1. When the examining finger is inserted into the anus, it offers resistance due to the presence of anal sphincters.
2. Anus is present in line with the anal sphincters, whereas the mouth and malar prominences form a triangle.

OBSTETRIC MANAGEMENT

Delivery occurs spontaneously in most of the cases. In presence of normal cervical dilatation and descent, there is no need for the obstetrician to intervene. Labor will be longer, but if the pelvis is adequate and the head rotates to a mentoanterior position, a vaginal delivery can be expected. The mechanism of delivery and corresponding body movements in case of anterior face presentations are similar to that of the corresponding occipitoanterior position. The only difference being that delivery of head occurs by flexion rather than extension. The engaging diameter is submentobregmatic in case of a fully extended head.

If the head rotates backward to a mentoposterior position, a cesarean section may be required. In case of posterior face presentations, the mechanism of delivery is same as that of occipitoposterior position except that the anterior rotation of the mentum occurs in only 20–30% of the cases. In the remaining 70–80% cases, there may be incomplete anterior rotation, no rotation or short posterior rotation of mentum. There is no possibility of spontaneous vaginal delivery in case of persistent mentoposterior positions. Cesarean section may be required in these cases.

COMPLICATIONS

- Increased chances of cord prolapse
- Delayed labor
- Risk of perineal injuries
- Postpartum hemorrhage

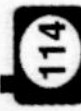

- Caput formation and molding
- Increased rate of operative deliveries
- Fetal cerebral congestion due to poor venous return from head and neck
- Neonatal infection
- Increased maternal morbidity due to operative delivery and vaginal manipulation
- Neglected cases of face presentation may result in obstructed labor and uterine rupture
- Marked caput formation and molding may distort the entire face. This usually subsides within a few days.

CLINICAL PEARLS

- On abdominal examination in case of face presentation, head feels big and is often not engaged
- Although the engaging diameter of the head in flexed vertex and face presentation is the same [submentobregmatic in face (9.5 cm) and suboccipitobregmatic in case of vertex (9.5 cm)], the clinical course of labor is significantly delayed. This could be due to the ill-fitting face in the lower uterine segment, which results in delayed engagement due to the absence of molding
- While conducting a normal vaginal delivery, one should wait for spontaneous delivery. Liberal mediolateral episiotomy must be given to protect the perineum against injuries
- Forceps may be applied in case of delay
- Indications for an elective cesarean section in case of face presentation include co-existing conditions such as contracted pelvis, large sized baby or presence of associated complicating factors.

15. BROW PRESENTATION

INTRODUCTION

This is a type of cephalic presentation where the fetal head is incompletely flexed **(Fig. 3.42)**. The head is short of complete extension, which could have resulted in a face presentation. As a result, presenting part becomes the brow.

ETIOLOGY

The predisposing factors for the brow presentation are similar to that for face presentation.

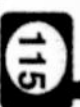

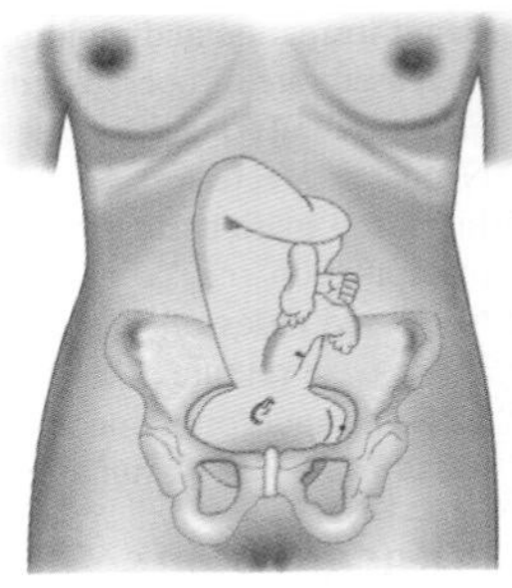

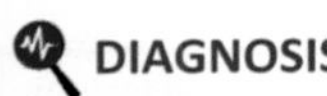

Figure 3.42: Brow presentation

DIAGNOSIS

Abdominal Examination

Findings on abdominal examination are similar to that of face presentation.

Vaginal Examination

Brow presentation can be confirmed on vaginal examination due to the presence of supraorbital ridges and anterior fontanelle.

Investigations

Ultrasonography: This helps in ruling out the presence of any congenital malformations.

OBSTETRIC MANAGEMENT

Since the engaging diameter of the head is mentovertical (14 cm), there would be no mechanism of labor with an average-sized baby and a normal pelvis. Vaginal delivery may be the possible option only in cases where there is spontaneous conversion to face or vertex presentation. Therefore, after ruling out the cephalopelvic disproportion and fetal congenital anomalies, the obstetrician must await spontaneous delivery. In cases where this does not occur, cesarean section is the best method of treatment.

COMPLICATIONS

- Obstructed labor and uterine rupture can occur in cases of neglected brow presentation
- There can be considerable amount of molding and caput formation of the fetal skull.

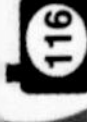

CLINICAL PEARLS

Brow presentation may temporarily persist as it may get converted to either a vertex or face presentation with complete flexion or extension respectively.

16. MULTIFETAL GESTATION

INTRODUCTION

Development of two or more embryos simultaneously in a pregnant uterus is termed as multifetal gestation. Development of two fetuses (whether through monozygotic or dizygotic fertilization) simultaneously is known as twin gestation **(Fig. 3.43)**; development of three fetuses simultaneously as triplets; four fetuses as quadruplets; five fetuses as quintuplets and so on...

ETIOLOGY

The risk factors, which are most likely to result in multifetal gestation, include the following:

- Increased maternal age and parity
- Previous history of twin gestation
- Family history of twin gestation (especially on maternal side)
- Conception following a long period of infertility
- Pregnancy attained through the use of assisted reproductive technology (in vitro fertilization or use of clomiphine citrate)
- Racial origin (twin gestation is more common amongst the women of West African ancestry)

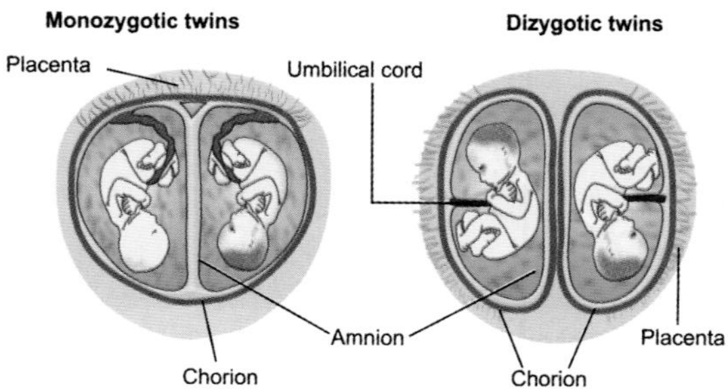

Figure 3.43: Development of twin pregnancy

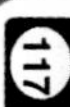

- History of using progestational agents or combined oral contraceptives, which may cause reduction in the tubal mobility
- Previous history of twin gestation.

DIAGNOSIS

Abdominal Examination

- On inspection there may be abdominal over distension or barrel shaped abdomen
- The uterus may be palpable abdominally, earlier than 12 weeks of gestation
- Height of the uterus is greater than period of amenorrhea (fundal height is typically 5 cm greater than the period of amenorrhea in the second trimester)
- Abdominal girth at the level of umbilicus is greater than the normal abdominal girth at term
- Multiple fetal parts may be palpable (e.g. palpation of two fetal heads)
- Hydramnios may be present
- Two FHS can be auscultated, located at two separate spots separated by a silent area in between.

Investigations

- *Ultrasound examination*: There may be presence of two or more fetuses or gestational sacs **(Figs 3.44A and B)**. There may be two or more placentas lying close to one another or presence of a single large placenta with a thick dividing membrane.

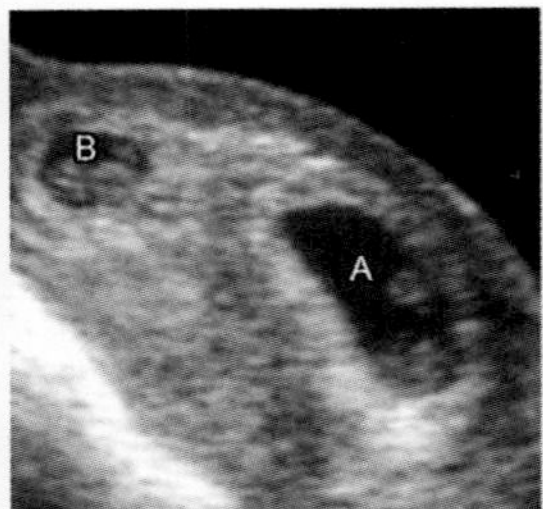

Fig. 3.44A: Presence of two gestational sacs on ultrasound, with sac A = 7.6 weeks and sac B = 5.7 weeks

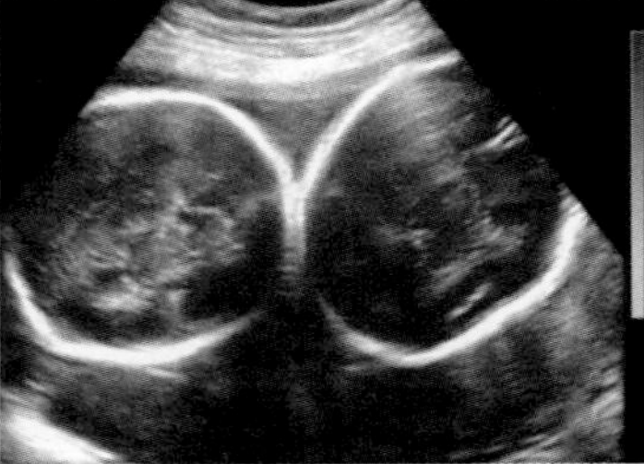

Fig. 3.44B: Ultrasound of the same patient at 30 weeks of gestation showing two fetal heads

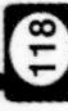

DIFFERENTIAL DIAGNOSIS

- Hydramnios
- Wrong dates
- Hydatidiform mole
- Uterine fibroids
- Adnexal masses
- Fetal macrosomia.

MANAGEMENT

Antenatal Period

- *Steps for prevention of preterm labor*: Some of these include bed rest, administration of tocolytic agents, regular monitoring of uterine activity (if possible using external cardiotocography), prophylactic cervical cerclage, etc.
- *Increased daily requirement for dietary calories, proteins and mineral supplements*: There is an additional calorie requirement to the extent of 300 kcal/day above that required for a normal singleton gestation. Moreover, there is a requirement for increased iron, calcium and folic acid supplements in order to meet the demands of multifetal pregnancy. Iron requirement must be increased to the extent of 60–100 mg/day and folic acid to 1 mg/day
- *Increased frequency of antenatal visits*: The patient should be advised to visit the ANC clinic every 2 weeks, especially if some problem is anticipated
- *Increased fetal surveillance*: Fetal monitoring can be done with the help of serial ultrasound examination, BBP, NST, AFI and Doppler ultrasound examinations.

Intrapartum Period

The following precautions need to be observed in the intrapartum period:

- Blood to be arranged and kept cross matched
- Pediatrician or anesthesiologist needs to be informed
- Patient should be advised to stay in bed as far as possible in order to prevent PROM
- Labor should be monitored with the help of a partogram and the heart rate of both the fetuses must be monitored, preferably using a cardiotocogram
- Prophylactic administration of corticosteroids for attaining pulmonary maturity in cases of anticipated preterm deliveries may be required

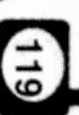

- IV access in the mother must be established
- Careful fetal monitoring is required
- Vaginal examination must be performed soon after the ROM to exclude cord prolapse and to confirm the presentation of first twin.

Time of Delivery

Delivery of the First Baby

- Delivery of the first baby should be conducted according to guidelines for normal pregnancy
- Ergometrine is not to be given at the birth of the first baby
- Cord of the first baby should be clamped and cut to prevent exsanguination of the second twin in case the communicating blood vessels between the twins exist.

Delivery of Second Baby

- After the delivery of the first baby, an abdominal and vaginal examination should be performed to confirm the lie, presentation and FHS of the second baby
- External version can be attempted at the time of abdominal examination, in case the lie is transverse
- Vaginal examination also helps in diagnosing cord prolapse, if present
- According to the ACOG (1998), the interval between the delivery of twins is not critical in determining the outcome of twins delivered
- Depending on the presentation of second twin, various options can be adopted as shown in **Figure 3.45**.

COMPLICATIONS

Maternal

Antenatal Period

- Spontaneous abortion
- Anemia: Due to increased iron requirement by two fetuses, early appearance of anemia is a common complication
- Fatty liver of pregnancy: It is rare complication that occurs more often in multifetal than in singleton pregnancies
- Hyperemesis gravidarum
- Polyhydramnios
- Preeclampsia

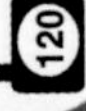

- Antepartum hemorrhage
- Preterm labor
- Varicosities, dependent edema.

Labor

- Fetal malpresentation
- Vasa previa
- Cord prolapse
- Premature separation of placenta, resulting in abruption placenta
- Cord entanglement
- Postpartum hemorrhage
- Dysfunctional uterine contractions
- Increased operative interference.

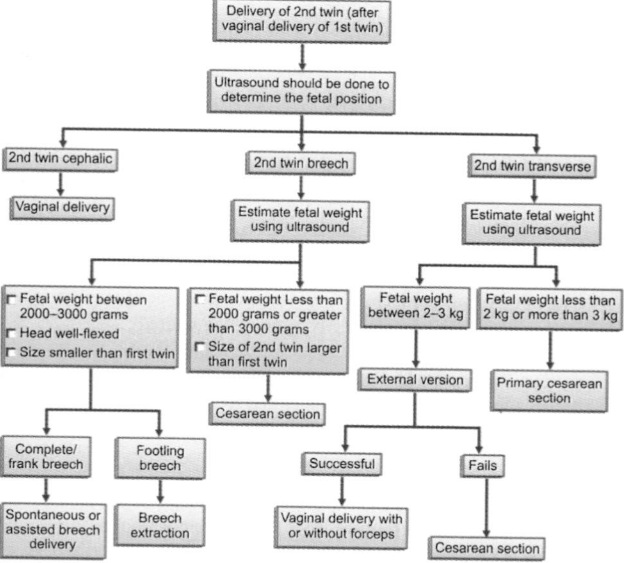

Figure 3.45: Different options for the delivery of second twin

Puerperium

- Subinvolution
- Infection
- Failure of lactation.

Fetal

- Miscarriage
- *Prematurity*: The most frequent neonatal complications of preterm birth are hypothermia, respiratory difficulties, intracranial bleeding, hypoglycemia, necrotizing enterocolitis, infections and retinopathy of prematurity, low birth weight babies, etc.
- *Congenital anomalies*: These can especially occur with the monozygotic twin pregnancies
- Intrauterine death
- Intrauterine growth retardation
- *Fetal complications specific to twin gestation*: These may include complications such as discordant growth, twin to twin transfusion, acardiac twin or twin reversed arterial perfusion (TRAP) syndrome, conjoined twins, etc.

CLINICAL PEARLS

- Routine use of beta-mimetics, cervical cerclage and bed rest has not been supported by good evidence for the prevention of preterm labor in cases of twin gestation
- Cesarean section is not required in routine clinical practice for every case of twin gestation. However, in case of presence of an obstetric or fetal indication, a cesarean delivery may be required
- There are some indications specific to twin gestation for cesarean section, which are as follows: monochorionic twins with twin-to-twin transfusion syndrome; conjoined twins; locking of twins, etc.

17. PRETERM LABOR

INTRODUCTION

Preterm labor is defined as onset of labor (uterine contractions accompanied by cervical dilatation and effacement) before 37 completed weeks of pregnancy (starting from the first day of last menstrual period).

ETIOLOGY

Although the actual cause remains unknown, some risk factors for preterm labor are as follows:

- Previous history of induced or spontaneous abortion or preterm delivery
- Previous history of pregnancy complications such as preeclampsia, antepartum hemorrhage, unexplained vaginal bleeding, PPROM, uterine anomalies such as cervical incompetence, etc.
- History of medical and surgical illnesses such as chronic hypertension, acute pyelonephritis, diabetes, renal diseases, acute appendicitis, etc.
- Previous history of fetal complications such as congenital malformations and intrauterine death
- Previous history of placental complications such as infraction, thrombosis, placenta previa or abruption
- Iatrogenic causes where labor is induced or infant is delivered by a prelabor cesarean section.
- Psychological factors, such as depression, anxiety and chronic stress, have also been implicated as the causative factors
- Twins and higher order multifetal births
- Spontaneous unexplained preterm labor with intact membranes
- Idiopathic PPROM
- PPROM: This can be defined as ROM before onset of labor and prior to 37 weeks of pregnancy. It usually results from intraamniotic infections (especially bacterial vaginosis, ureaplasma urealyticum and mycoplasma hominis).

DIAGNOSIS

Clinical Presentation

The following are clinical presentations suggestive of preterm labor:

- Cervical dilatation of greater than or equal to 1 cm and effacement of 80% or more
- Uterine contractions of greater than or equal to 4 per 20 minutes or greater than or equal to 8 per hour, lasting for more than 40 seconds
- Cervical length on TVS less than or equal to 2.5 cm and funneling of internal os
- Symptoms such as menstrual cramps, pelvic pressure, backache and/or vaginal discharge or bleeding
- Bishop's score may be 4 or greater. Lower uterine segment may be thinned out and the presenting part may be deep in the pelvis.

Based on the findings of clinical examination, preterm labor can be of two types:

- *Early preterm labor*: In cases of early preterm labor, cervical effacement is greater than or equal to 80% and cervical dilatation is greater than or equal to 1 cm, but less than 3 cm
- *Advanced preterm labor*: In cases of advanced preterm labor, cervical dilatation is greater than or equal to 3 cm.

Investigations

Various investigations used for predicting preterm birth are as follows:

- *Uterine activity monitoring*: Hospital-based external cardiotocography has been found to be effective for monitoring uterine contractions for evaluating preterm labor
- *Cervical length measurement*: Presence of short cervix is a poor predictor of preterm birth, whereas funneling of membranes with a history of previous preterm birth is highly predictive of preterm births
- *Measurement of fibronectin levels*: Presence of fibronectin (values > 50 ng/mL) in the cervicovaginal discharge between 24–34 weeks of gestation, prior to ROM is indicative of preterm labor. Negative test implies that delivery is unlikely to occur within the coming 7 days
- *Salivary estriol levels*: The onset of preterm labor is likely to result in an increase in the maternal salivary estriol levels.

OBSTETRIC MANAGEMENT

For a majority of patients, prolonging pregnancy does not offer any benefit because, in a majority of cases, preterm labor serves as a protective mechanism for fetuses threatened by problems such as infection or placental insufficiency. There is no evidence regarding the benefit of bed rest or hospitalization in women with preterm labor.

Preterm labor is often associated with PROM. The management of preterm labor associated with ruptured membranes is reviewed in the fragment on PROM. The following considerations should be given regarding delivery in women with preterm labor:

- For pregnancies less than 34 weeks of gestation in women with no maternal or fetal indication for delivery, expectant management comprising of the following may be used:
    - Close monitoring of uterine contractions
    - Fetal surveillance
    - Corticosteroids may be used for enhancing pulmonary maturity

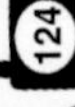

- In these cases, use of magnesium sulfate infusion for 12–24 hours, helps in providing neuroprotection
- Prophylactic therapy for group B streptococcal infection should be administered, especially in the cases where the membranes have also ruptured.

Once the episode of preterm labor has been controlled with tocolytic agents, women in early preterm labor should be managed on OPD basis with the exception to those who have a positive fibronectin test. In these patients, the risk of preterm delivery is substantial and they should be admitted in the hospital for bed-rest

- For pregnancies at 34 weeks or more, women with preterm labor must be monitored for labor progression and fetal well-being. Intrapartum management in these cases comprises of the following steps:
  - Delivery should preferably be undertaken in a tertiary care setting
  - Fetal surveillance to be performed with continuous electronic fetal monitoring
  - At the time of delivery, an episiotomy may be given to facilitate the delivery of fetal head. However, there is no need for routine application of forceps.

MEDICAL MANAGEMENT

The medications prescribed in cases of preterm labor are:

- Use of progesterone therapy to reduce preterm birth
- *Tocolytic therapy*: This may be required to delay delivery for up to 48 hours, thereby buying time to allow the maximum benefit of glucocorticoids in order to reduce the incidence of respiratory distress syndrome
- *Corticosteroid therapy*: The administration of glucocorticoids is recommended in patients with preterm labor, whenever the gestational age is between 24–34 weeks. The recommended dosage of Betamethasone comprises of two 12 mg doses, administered 24 hours apart.

COMPLICATIONS

Maternal

Children of women suffering from chorioamnionitis are more likely to experience complications such as sepsis, respiratory distress syndrome, early-onset seizures, intraventricular hemorrhage and periventricular leukomalacia.

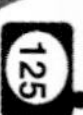

Fetal

Some of the complications which can occur in preterm infants include:

- *Pulmonary complications*: Respiratory distress, bronchopulmonary dysplasia, etc.
- *Gastrointestinal complications*: Hyperbilirubinemia, necrotizing enterocolitis, failure to thrive, etc.
- *Central nervous system complications*: Intraventricular hemorrhage, hydrocephalus, cerebral palsy, neurodevelopmental delay and hearing loss
- *Ophthalmological complications*: Retinopathy of prematurity, retinal detachment, etc.
- *Cardiovascular complications*: Hypotension, patent ductus arteriosus, pulmonary hypertension, etc.
- *Renal complications*: Water and electrolyte imbalance, acid-base disturbances
- *Hematological complications*: Iatrogenic anemia, requirement for frequent blood transfusions, anemia of prematurity, etc.
- *Endocrinological complications*: Hypoglycaemia, transiently low thyroxine levels, cortisol deficiency and increased insulin resistance in adulthood.

CLINICAL PEARLS

- The present threshold of non viability for premature births is weight less than 750 gm and period of gestation less than 26 weeks
- The main goals of obstetric patient management in preterm labor are provision of prophylactic pharmacologic therapy to prolong the period of gestation and avoiding delivery prior to 34 completed weeks of gestation
- In cases of acute or chronic chorioamnionitis, delivery must be achieved rapidly. Signs and symptoms suggestive of acute choriamnionitis include, maternal tachycardia ≥ 100 BPM; fetal tachycardia ≥ 160 BPM; maternal temperature ≥ 37.8° C; uterine tenderness; foul smelling amniotic fluid; maternal leucocytosis ≥ 15,000/ mm^3; C-reactive protein > 0.8 ng/mL.

18. PREMATURE RUPTURE OF MEMBRANES

INTRODUCTION

Premature rupture of membranes can be defined as spontaneous ROM, beyond 28 weeks of pregnancy, but before the onset of labor. ROM occurring beyond 37 weeks of gestation, but before the onset of labor is known as term premature rupture of membranes (PROM). On the other hand, ROM occurring before 37 completed weeks of gestation but before the onset of labor is called preterm premature rupture of membranes (PPROM). If the ROM is present for more than 24 hours before delivery, it is known as prolonged ROM.

ETIOLOGY

- Increased friability and reduced tensile strength of the membranes
- Polyhydramnios
- Cervical incompetence
- Multiple pregnancy
- Intrauterine infection such as chorioamnionitis, urinary tract or lower genital tract infection.

DIAGNOSIS

Clinical Presentation

There may be escape of watery discharge per vaginum either in the form of gush of fluid or slow leakage. The diagnosis of PROM can be confirmed by performing the following tests:

- *Nitrazine paper test*: A per speculum examination must be performed to collect the fluid from posterior fornix (vaginal pool). The pH of the fluid collected from the vaginal fornix must be detected using litmus or nitrazine paper. Since the liquor is normally alkaline in nature (pH 7–7.5), the normally acidic vaginal pH (4.5–5.5) turns alkaline in the presence of PROM, causing the color of the nitrazine paper to change from yellow to blue
- *Ferning*: The liquor smeared slide when examined under the microscope shows appearance of a characteristic ferning pattern
- *Staining of the centrifuged cells with 0.1% nile blue sulfate*: There may be orange-blue discoloration of the cells due to presence of exfoliated fat containing cells from sebaceous glands of the fetus
- *Intra-amniotic injection of lignocaine*: Presence of blue discoloration of the fluid emanating from cervical os, following the injection of 2–3 mL of sterile solution of the dye indigocarmine into the amniotic cavity is indicative of PROM
- *Alpha-fetoproteins*: Presence of alpha-fetoproteins in the vaginal secretions is indicative of PROM.

Investigations

- Full blood count
- White cell count
- Differential count
- Determination of levels of CRP
- Urine routine microscopy and culture
- Speculum examination: This helps in confirming the diagnosis of PPROM, obtaining fluid for determining pulmonary maturity and obtaining endocervical samples for *Chlamydia* and *Neisseria gonorrhea*
- Ultrasound for biophysical profile; estimation of gestational age and weight; measurement of cervical length and amniotic fluid volume
- Non-stress test.

OBSTETRIC MANAGEMENT

Main aim of management in case of PROM is to avoid delivery prior to 34 weeks of gestation. Women who need to be delivered irrespective of the period of gestation include the following:

- Those with acute chorioamnionitis/subclinical infection/inflammation or those at a high risk of infection
- Those with mature lungs or with period of gestation greater than 36 weeks
- Non-reassuring FHS
- Fetuses with lethal congenital anomalies
- Women in advanced labor, with cervical effacement of 80% or more and cervical dilatation of 5 cm or more.

After confirmation of diagnosis of PROM, further management is described in the **Figure 3.46**:

- Cesarean section is not routinely required, but may be required in the presence of an obstetric indication
- The tocolytic agent of choice for women with PPROM is nifedipine. It is given in the initial dosage of 20–30 mg followed by 10–20 mg at every 6 hourly.

COMPLICATIONS

Maternal

- *Infection*: Infection could be related to acute or chronic chorioamnionitis. There are high chances of ascending infection if ROM is present for greater than 24 hours

- *Preterm labor*: PROM is an important cause for preterm labor. In about 80–90% of the cases, labor starts within 24 hours
- *Cord prolapse*: Sudden gush of amniotic fluid may be associated with an increased incidence of cord prolapse and/or premature placental separation (placental abruption) and/or oligohydramnios.

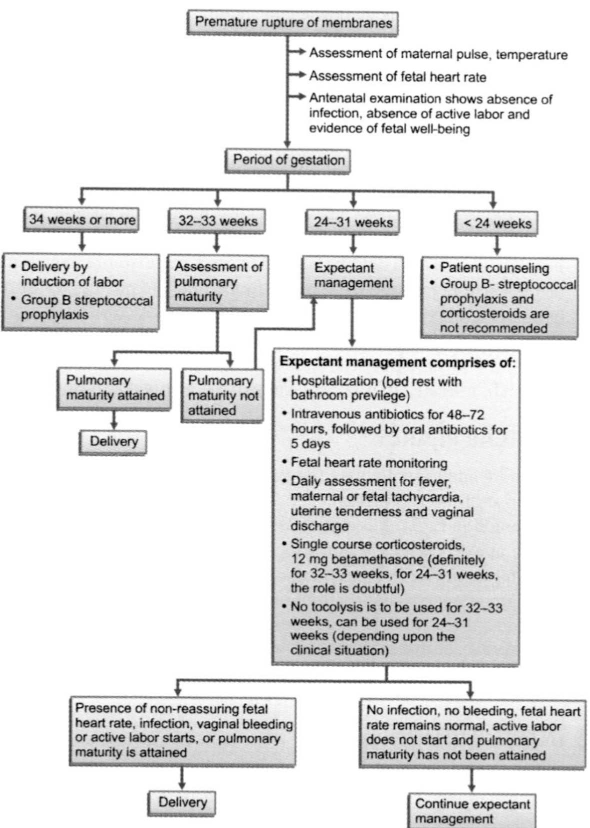

Figure 3.46: Management of premature rupture of membranes

Fetal/Neonatal

- *Respiratory distress syndrome/hyaline membrane disease*: The newborn infant may suffer from severe respiratory distress, thereby requiring ventilator support after birth
- *Non-reassuring fetal heart rate pattern*: Most common abnormality is variable decelerations associated with umbilical cord compression as a result of oligohydramnios. Moderate or severe variable/late decelerations may be present as a result of placental insufficiency and are indicative of intrapartum fetal distress
- *Pulmonary hypoplasia*: This condition may be characterized by the presence of multiple pneumothoraces and interstitial emphysema
- *Cerebral palsy*: This may be the result of intraventricular bleeding, intrapartum fetal acidosis and hypoxia
- *Fetal deformities*: These may especially include facial and skeletal deformities
- *Fetal trauma*: This could be related to fetal macrosomia, which may be responsible for producing injury to the brachial plexus, fracture of humerus or clavicle, cephalic hematomas, skull fracture, etc.
- *Postmaturity syndrome*: This is characterized by the presence of wrinkled skin due to reduced amount of subcutaneous fat. These fetuses are small, tolerate labor poorly and may be acidotic at birth.

CLINICAL PEARLS

- Recommended prophylaxis for group B streptococcal infection may comprise of the following:
  - Penicillin G, 5 million units IV initial dose, then 2.5 million units IV at every 4 hourly intervals until delivery, or
  - Ampicillin, 2 gm IV initial dose then 1 gm IV at every 4 hourly or 2 gm at every 6 hourly until delivery, or
  - Cefazolin, 2 gm IV initial dose, then 1 gm IV at every 8 hourly intervals until delivery.

19. POST-TERM PREGNANCY

INTRODUCTION

Post-term or postmature pregnancy can be defined as any pregnancy continuing beyond 2 weeks of the expected date of delivery (> 294 days).

ETIOLOGY

Although the exact causes of post-dated pregnancy remains unknown, some likely causative factors are as follows:

- *Wrong dates*: This can be considered as the most common cause of postmaturity. In these cases, use of ultrasonography helps in determining the accurate estimation of gestational age
- *Maternal factors*: These include factors such as primiparity, previous history of prolonged pregnancy, sedentary habits and elderly multipara
- *Fetal congenital anomalies*: Fetal congenital anomalies such as anencephaly and adrenal hypoplasia may be implicated in the causation of postmaturity
- *Placental factors*: Placental factors such as sulfatase deficiency may be involved.

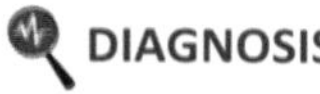

DIAGNOSIS

Clinical Presentation

- *Maternal weight record*: Stationary or falling maternal weight
- *Abdominal girth*: Gradually diminishing abdominal girth due to the gradually reducing liquor volume
- *False labor pains*: Appearance of labor pains which quickly subside
- *Abdominal palpation*: The uterus may feel "full of fetus" due to the diminishing volume of the liquor
- *Internal vaginal examination*: Ripe cervix could be suggestive of fetal maturity. Hard skull bones may be felt through the cervix or vaginal fornix, thereby suggesting fetal maturity.

Investigations

- *Ultrasonography*: Ultrasound parameters, such as crown-rump length (CRL), biparietal diameter (BPD) and femur length (FL), help in the assessment of gestational age. Ultrasound scans performed early in gestation are more helpful in the accurate assessment of gestational age. Amniotic fluid pocket of less than 2 cm and AFI less than or equal to 5 cm on ultrasound examination is an indication for induction of labor or delivery. Absent end-diastolic flow on umbilical artery Doppler is another indicator of fetal jeopardy
- *Tests for fetal well-being*: These include tests, such as NST, biophysical profile and ultrasound assessment of the amniotic fluid volume, which may be performed on a bi-weekly basis.

OBSTETRIC MANAGEMENT

The obstetric management is based on two principles, the first being determination of accurate gestational age and second being increased fetal surveillance. Management of post-term pregnancy has been described in the **Figure 3.47**.

COMPLICATIONS

- *Fetal distress*: Diminished placental function and oligohydramnios due to PROM may result in fetal hypoxia and distress

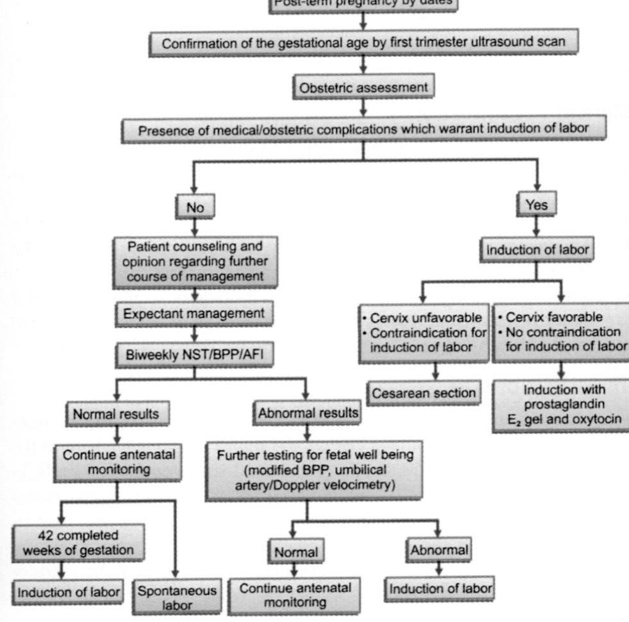

Figure 3.47: Management of post-term pregnancies

- *Macrosomia*: This is associated with an increased incidence of shoulder dystocia and operative delivery
- *Birth trauma*: There is an increased incidence of traumatic birth deliveries due to large size of the baby and non-molding of fetal head due to hardening of skull bones
- *Respiratory distress*: Respiratory distress can occur due to chemical pneumonitis, atelectasis and pulmonary hypertension. This may occur following meconium aspiration and eventually result in hypoxia and respiratory failure
- *Neonatal problems*: After birth, many neonatal complications can arise, such as hypothermia, poor subcutaneous fat, hypoglycemia, hypocalcemia, and increased incidence of injuries such as brachial plexus injuries
- *Increased perinatal mortality and morbidity*: These complications result in an overall increased rate of perinatal morbidity and mortality.

CLINICAL PEARLS

- In uncomplicated cases of post-term pregnancy, where fetal maturity has been attained, expectant attitude may be extended for 7–10 days, following which the labor is induced
- Prolonged labor must be expected due to a large baby and poor molding of the fetal head
- Expectant management is appropriate between 40–41 weeks of gestation
- Delivery becomes mandatory when the period of gestation reaches 42 weeks, because the risk of antepartum stillbirths and maternal complications is significant enough.

20. PRECIPITATE LABOR

INTRODUCTION

Precipitate labor is normally very short, lasting less than 3 hours. It can be defined as the type of labor where the total duration of first and second stage of labor is less than 2 hours.

ETIOLOGY

Precipitate labor occurs due to causes which results in strong uterine contractions and reduced soft tissue resistance, e.g. multiparity.

DIAGNOSIS

Pelvic Examination

Rate of cervical dilatation is 5 cm or more for nulliparous women.

OBSTETRIC MANAGEMENT

Obstetric management in these cases with previous history of precipitate labor comprises of the following steps:

- Uterine contractions can be suppressed by administration of magnesium sulfate or ether
- Delivery of fetal head should be controlled
- Liberal episiotomy should be given to prevent tears
- Augmentation with oxytocin must be avoided.

COMPLICATIONS

Maternal: These include:

- Extensive lacerations of vagina and perineum and cervical tears
- Postpartum hemorrhage from uterine atony
- Uterine inversion or uterine rupture
- Infection
- Amniotic fluid embolism.

Fetal: These include:

- Intracranial hemorrhage
- Erb's/Duchenne brachial palsy
- Injury to the fetal head, especially if delivery occurs in the standing position.

21. VERSION

INTRODUCTION

Version can be defined as a procedure, which helps in changing the lie of the fetus so as to bring the favorable fetal pole to the lower pole of the uterus. Version could be external (involving abdominal manipulation) or internal (involving manipulation by introducing a hand through the vagina). If the cephalic pole is brought down to the lower pole of the uterus through abdominal manipulation, it is known as external cephalic version (ECV). If the podalic pole is brought down through vaginal manipulation, it is known as internal podalic version.

INDICATIONS

- Breech presentation
- Transverse lie.

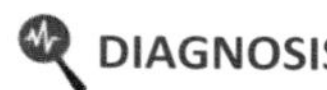

DIAGNOSIS

Clinical Presentation

Clinical presentation with breech and transverse lie has been described in the individual fragments.

SURGICAL MANAGEMENT

Preoperative Preparation

- *Timing for ECV*: It is preferable to wait until term (37 completed weeks of gestation) before external version is attempted because of an increased success rate and avoidance of preterm delivery if complications arise
- Facilities for an immediate cesarean section must be available
- Blood grouping and cross matching should be done
- In case the mother is Rh negative, administration of 50 µg of anti-D immunoglobulin is required after the procedure
- Anesthetists must be informed well in advance
- Maternal intravenous access must be established
- The patient should be NPO for at least 8 hours prior to the procedure
- An ultrasound examination must be performed to confirm the fetal presentation, check the rate of fetal growth, amniotic fluid volume and to rule out any associated anomalies
- A non-stress test or a biophysical profile must be performed to confirm fetal well-being
- A written informed consent must be obtained from the mother
- A tocolytic agent, such as terbutaline in a dosage of 0.25 mg, may be administered subcutaneously
- The patient is placed in a supine or slight trendelenburg position for the procedure.

Obstetric Procedure

- Ultrasonic gel is applied liberally over the abdomen in order to decrease friction and to reduce the chances of an over-vigorous manipulation

- Initially, the degree of engagement of the presenting part should be determined and gentle disengagement of the presenting part be performed, if possible
- While performing ECV, the clinician helps in gently manipulating the fetal head toward the pelvis while the breech is brought up cephalad toward the fundus. Two types of manipulation of fetal head can be performed: a forward roll and a backward roll. The clinician must attempt a forward roll **(Figs 3.48A to D)** first and then a backward roll **(Figs 3.49A to C)**, if the initial attempt is unsuccessful
- The procedure for ECV in case of transverse lie is illustrated in **Figures 3.50A and B**.

Postoperative Care

- Whether the process has been successful or has failed, a non-stress test and ultrasound examination must be performed after each attempt of ECV and after the end of the procedure in order to rule out fetal bradycardia and to confirm successful version
- If unsuccessful, the version can be reattempted at a later time.

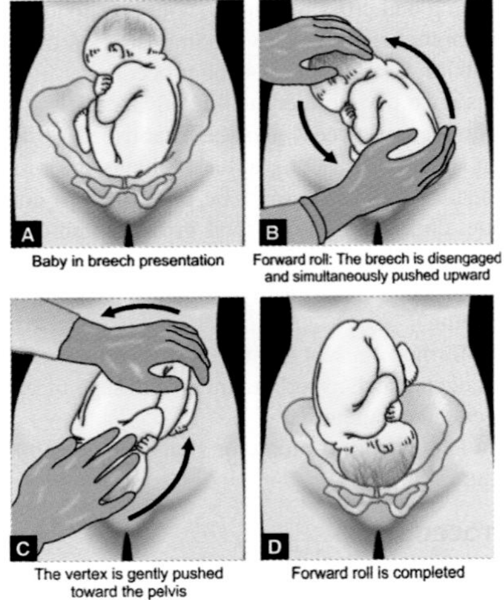

Figures 3.48A to D: ECV through forward roll

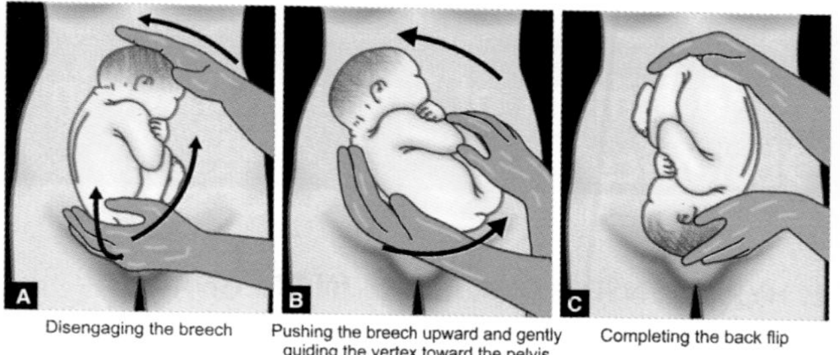

Disengaging the breech | Pushing the breech upward and gently guiding the vertex toward the pelvis | Completing the back flip

Figures 3.49A to C: ECV through back flip

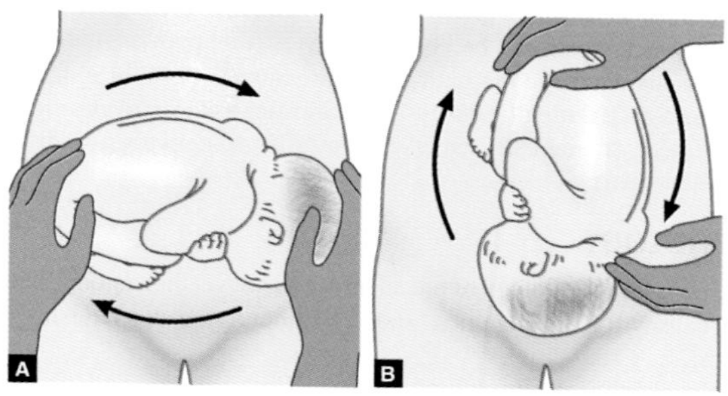

Figures 3.50A and B: Procedure for ECV in case of transverse lie

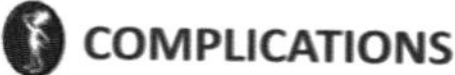

COMPLICATIONS

- Failure of the procedure
- Premature onset of labor, premature rupture of the membranes
- Small amount of fetomaternal hemorrhage, resulting in the development of Rh isoimmunization
- Fetal distress leading to an emergency cesarean delivery
- Risk of cord entanglement and transient reduction of the fetal heart rate.

CLINICAL PEARLS

- In modern obstetrics there is no place for internal podalic version except for the delivery of second twin in transverse presentation
- Forceful attempt at version may result in placental abruption.

CHAPTER 4

Management of Special Cases in Obstetrics

1. HYPERTENSIVE DISORDERS IN PREGNANCY

1.1. PREECLAMPSIA

INTRODUCTION

According to the working group report on high blood pressure in pregnancy (2000), preeclampsia can be considered as a potentially serious disorder, which is characterized by high blood pressure (> 140/90 mm Hg) and proteinuria (> 300 mg/dL or > 1+ on the dipstick). It usually develops after the 20th week of pregnancy and goes away after the delivery (usually within the 12th postpartum week).

ETIOLOGY

The exact pathophysiology of preeclampsia is not yet understood. The most likely causes for preeclampsia and their underlying mechanisms are as follows:

- Inadequate trophoblastic invasion
- Maternal inflammatory response resulting in vascular endothelial dysfunction
- *Hereditary factors*: The exact genetic defect or preeclampsia gene has not yet been identified
- *Immunological factors*: Production of blocking antibodies to various placental antigenic sites is associated with reduced risk
- Endothelial dysfunction and vasospasm due to increased sensitivity to the action of angiotensin II (vasopressor) and due to the imbalance in production of various prostaglandins.

DIAGNOSIS

Clinical Presentation

- *Increased blood pressure*: Presence of an increased BP (> 140/90 mm Hg) for the first time during pregnancy, after 20 weeks of gestation.

- *Proteinuria*: Proteinurea is defined as significant if the excretion of proteins exceeds 300 mg per 24 hours or there is persistent presence of the protein (30 mg/dL or 1 + distick) in random urine sample in the absence of any evidence of urinary tract infection
- *Edema*: Edema of hands and face can commonly occur amongst women with preeclampsia. Since edema is a universal finding in pregnancy, it is not considered as a criterion for diagnosing preeclampsia
- *Other symptoms*: Indicators of severe preeclampsia during pregnancy are headache, visual problems, epigastric or right upper quadrant abdominal pain, oliguria (urine volume $\leq$ 500 mL/24 hours), convulsions, etc.
- *Shortness of breath or dyspnea*: This could be reflective of pulmonary edema or acute respiratory distress syndrome
- *Reduced fetal movements*: This is especially observed in association with IUGR and oligohydramnios
- *Weight gain*: Weight gain of more than 2 pounds per week or 6 pounds in a month can be considered as significant.

Abdominal Examination

There may be evidence of placental insufficiency in the form of oligohydramnios and/or IUGR.

Investigations

- *Hematocrit and CBC*: The decrease in blood volume in preeclampsia can lead to a rise in maternal hemoglobin concentration resulting in an increased hematocrit
- *Platelet count*: Platelet count of less than 150–400 × 10^9/liter could be indicative of the HELLP syndrome
- *Kidney function tests*: In severe preeclampsia, raised serum creatinine and uric acid levels are associated with a worsening outcome both for the mother and baby
- *Liver function test*: An AST level of above 75 IU/L can be considered as significant
- *Ophthalmoscopic examination*: The abnormalities include presence of retinal edema, constrictions of the retinal arterioles and alteration of normal ratio of vein: arteriolar diameter.

DIFFERENTIAL DIAGNOSIS

It is important for the obstetrician to differentiate among preeclampsia, gestational hypertension and chronic hypertension **(Table 4.1)**.

Table 4.1: Characteristic features of various types of hypertensive disorders during pregnancy

	Onset	*Subsidence*	*Blood pressure*	*Proteinuria*
Preeclampsia	Develops after 20th week of pregnancy	Goes away after delivery (usually within 12th postpartum weeks)	> 140/90 mm Hg	Present
Gestational hypertension	Develops after 20th week of pregnancy	Goes away after delivery (usually within 12th postpartum weeks)	> 140/90 mm Hg	Absent
Chronic hypertension	Onset is before pregnancy or before 20th week of pregnancy in absence of gestational trophoblastic disease	The condition does not return to normal within 12 weeks of postpartum period	> 140/90 mm Hg	Absent
Preeclampsia superimposed upon chronic hypertension	Onset is before pregnancy or before the 20th week of pregnancy in absence of gestational trophoblastic disease	The condition does not return to normal within 12 weeks of postpartum period	> 140/90 mm Hg	Onset of proteinuria after 20 weeks of pregnancy

OBSTETRIC MANAGEMENT

- *Antihypertensive medication*: The aim of treatment must be to maintain diastolic BP between 95 mm Hg and 105 mm Hg. The most commonly used first-line drugs include hydralazine (for severe hypertension), alpha-methyldopa, labetalol and nifedipine. Use of diuretics, angiotensin-converting enzyme (ACE) inhibitors and angiotensin II receptor blockers should be preferably avoided during pregnancy
- *Magnesium sulfate*: Magnesium sulfate should be considered for women with preeclampsia, especially in whom there is concern about risk of eclampsia. A total dose of 14 gm is administered in form of loading (4 gm IV) and maintenance dose (5 gm in each buttock by deep IM injection)
- *Conservative therapy*: Initial therapy for mild-moderate preeclampsia is bed rest until fetal maturation becomes adequate. Prescription of the sedatives or tranquilizers is not required. Low-dose aspirin in the dose of 60 mg daily can be prescribed
- *Maternal monitoring*: In severe cases, blood pressure should be checked at every 15 minutes in the beginning, until the woman has stabilized and then after every 30 minutes in the initial phase of assessment. This can be later increased to 4-hourly intervals and then twice daily. Urine should be carefully monitored for proteinuria twice daily. In the presence of significant proteinuria, a 24-hour estimation of urine proteins may be done. Maternal weight must be measured everyday. Tests, like platelet count, kidney function tests and tests of liver function must be done at the time of admission and then twice weekly
- *Fetal surveillance*: Some of the tests for fetal surveillance include daily fetal movement count; weekly measurement of fundal height and abdominal girth in order to detect IUGR; weekly non-stress test; ultrasound examination for evaluating the period of gestation; BPP and/or serial assessment of liquor after every 2 weeks and Doppler ultrasound at every 3–4 weekly intervals. The frequency of the tests can be increased depending upon the severity of the condition
- *Timing of delivery*: The only way to cure preeclampsia is to deliver the baby. The pregnancy should not be allowed to continue beyond EDD. In cases of severe preeclampsia, when the pregnancy is more than 32 weeks of gestation, delivery is the treatment of choice. Prophylactic steroids should be given to induce fetal lung maturity in case the period of gestation is less than 32 weeks. For pregnancies between 26 and 32 weeks of gestation, the obstetrician needs to balance

the risk of prolonging the pregnancy, thereby increasing the maternal risk of developing complications related to severe preeclampsia against the risk of delivering a premature fetus which may not even survive

- *Mode of delivery*: Severe preeclampsia *per se* is not an indication for cesarean section. If the cervix is ripe, labor can be induced by using intravenous oxytocin and ARM. In case of presence of unfavorable cervix or other complications (e.g. breech presentation, fetal distress, etc.), a cesarean section needs to be done
- *Management during labor*: Monitoring of vitals especially maternal pulse and blood pressure at hourly intervals is required. Urine protein levels using a dipstick must be monitored at every 6-hourly intervals
- *Management in the postpartum period*: Antihypertensive drugs should be given if the BP exceeds 150 mm Hg systolic or 100 mm Hg diastolic in the first 4 days of the puerperium.

COMPLICATIONS

Some of the maternal and fetal complications related to preeclampsia are enumerated in **Table 4.2**.

Table 4.2: Complications related to preeclampsia

Maternal	*Fetal*
HELLP syndrome	Oligohydramnios
Abruption placenta	Intrauterine death
Cerebral hemorrhage	Premature delivery (before 37 weeks of gestation)
Sepsis/shock	Intrauterine growth retardation
Eclampsia (described in a separate fragment)	Risk of recurrence of intrauterine asphyxia and acidosis
Preeclampsia in subsequent pregnancies	Infant death
Impaired renal/liver function	
Pulmonary edema maternal death	

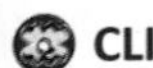

CLINICAL PEARLS

- Management of cases with preeclampsia is important because there is danger of progression to eclampsia, if the blood pressure remains uncontrollably high

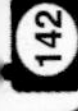

- In case of magnesium sulfate toxicity, 10 mL of 10% calcium gluconate, which serves as an antidote must be slowly administered intravenously
- Umbilical artery Doppler analysis showing absent or reversed end diastolic flow is associated with poor neonatal outcomes and mandates immediate delivery.

1.2. ECLAMPSIA

INTRODUCTION

Eclampsia can be defined as onset of tonic-clonic convulsions in a pregnant patient with preeclampsia, usually occurring in the third trimester of pregnancy, intrapartum period or more than 48 hours postpartum.

ETIOLOGY

Eclampsia is thought to be related to cerebral vasospasm, which can cause ischemia, disruption of the blood brain barrier and cerebral edema.

DIAGNOSIS

Symptoms

- *Premonitory stage*: In this stage there is unconsciousness; twitching of the muscles of face, tongue and limbs; and rolling and fixation of eyeballs
- *Tonic stage*: There is tonic spasm of the body muscles
- *Clonic stage*: There is alternate contraction and relaxation of the skeletal muscles. Twitching starts from the face onto the extremities and soon involves the whole body
- *Coma*: This may be present for a brief period or may persist for a longer time.

Investigations

These are same as that described with preeclampsia.

DIFFERENTIAL DIAGNOSIS

- Epilepsy/hysteria/poisoning
- Meningitis/encephalitis
- Cerebral malaria/thrombosis.

OBSTETRIC MANAGEMENT

- Immediate care involves maintenance of airway, oxygenation, maintenance of circulation and prevention of trauma or injury to the patient. An IV line must be secured and the patient must be given IV Ringer's lactate or 0.9% normal saline solution. The patient should be shifted to the eclampsia room. Injury to the patient can be prevented by placing her on a railed bed and using a tongue blade to prevent her from biting her tongue
- Monitoring of vitals including pulse, blood pressure, respiratory rate and oxygen saturation needs to be done at every 15 minutes. Parameters, such as knee jerks, fluid intake and urine output need to be monitored at every half hourly intervals
- Treatment of choice for convulsions is the administration of magnesium sulfate
- Once the patient has stabilized, an obstetric examination must be performed and fetal status must be evaluated and plan to deliver the patient as soon as possible must be made
- Continued fetal monitoring is required until the baby is delivered
- Intrapartum management: Strict blood pressure monitoring must be continued throughout labor. Eclampsia *per se* is not an indication for cesarean delivery. In case the cervix is not favorable, labor can be induced using vaginal prostaglandins and oxytocin infusion. Second stage of labor should be cut short
- Following delivery, close monitoring should be continued for a minimum of 24 hours.

COMPLICATIONS

Maternal

- Injuries due to fall from bed, tongue bite, etc.
- *Pulmonary complications*: These include pulmonary edema, pneumonia, adult respiratory distress, embolism, etc.
- Hyperpyrexia
- *Cardiac*: Acute left ventricular failure
- Renal failure
- Hepatic necrosis
- *Cerebral complications*: Cerebral anoxia; cerebral edema; cerebral dysrhythmia; cerebral hemorrhage, neurological deficits, etc.

- *Visual complications*: These could be due to retinal detachment or occipital lobe ischemia
- *Hematological complications*: These include thrombocytopenia, DIC, etc.
- *Postpartum complications*: These include shock, sepsis and psychosis.

Fetal

These are same as those described in the fragment of preeclampsia.

CLINICAL PEARLS

- In order to prevent the occurrence of eclampsia, women with severe preeclampsia (BP > 160/110 along with proteinuria) should be given magnesium sulfate as a prophylactic measure
- Occurrence of fits in a quick succession, one after the other is known as status eclampticus.

1.3. CHRONIC RENAL DISEASE DURING PREGNANCY

INTRODUCTION

The most commonly encountered renal diseases during pregnancy are asymptomatic bacteriuria and acute pyelonephritis. Asymptomatic bacteriuria, if left untreated, may develop into symptomatic urinary tract infection including acute pyelonephritis in 25–40% cases.

ETIOLOGY

Most commonly involved pathogenic organism is *Escherichia coli* in both asymptomatic bacteriuria and acute pyelonephritis. Risk factors for the development of both the conditions are shortened, dilated urethra; relative urinary stasis and reduced emptying; glycosuria; dilatation of upper renal tract, etc.

DIAGNOSIS

Clinical Presentation

- Malaise, nausea, vomiting, fatigue
- Fever with or without chills and rigors
- Back pain (localized in the upper lumbar area), with or without uterine contractions

- Fever, dehydration
- Tachycardia, hypotension (in severe cases of pyelonephritis)
- Costovertebral angle tenderness.

Investigations

- *Hemogram*: Heamtocrit including a complete blood count must be done
- *Urine analysis*: There may be presence of red cells, white cell casts, and bacteria on microscopic examination. Diagnosis of asymptomatic bacteriuria is made if upon culturing the urine sample (collected by midstream catch technique), there is a growth of greater than 10^5 colony forming units (CFUs). Urine culture and sensitivity may also be done
- *Tests of renal function*: There may be elevated serum BUN and creatinine levels and an abnormally low creatinine clearance
- *Histological examination*: Histological examination shows infiltration of the renal interstitium and tubules by polymorphonuclear leukocytes in cases of acute pyelonephritis
- *Serum electrolyte levels*: Abnormal serum electrolyte levels may be indicative of renal dysfunction
- *Blood culture*: Blood culture must be obtained when the patient has chills/rigors or temperature elevation.

MANAGEMENT

Asymptomatic bacteriuria: A three-day course of antibiotics is usually useful for treating the episode of asymptomatic bacteriuria. The most commonly used antibiotics are:

- Nitrofurantoin, 100 mg given orally twice daily for 3–7 days
- Trimethoprim-sulfamethoxazole (one single or double strength tablet, orally twice a day for 3 days)
- Amoxycillin (500 mg orally twice a day for 3–7 days)
- Cephalexin (500 mg orally twice a day for 3–7 days).

Acute pyelonephritis: Aggressive treatment is required in order to avoid disease progression and occurrence of complications and comprises of the following steps:

- Admission to the hospital
- Careful monitoring of the patient's vital signs at every 4 hourly
- Maintenance of adequate hydration through administration of IV fluids
- Treatment with intravenous antibiotics (cefazolin in the dosage of 2 gm at every 8 hourly.

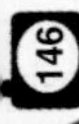

DIFFERENTIAL DIAGNOSIS

- Acute appendicitis/cholecystitis
- Chorioamnionitis/abruption placenta
- Red degeneration of fibroid.

COMPLICATIONS

- Preeclampsia, preterm labor and prematurity
- Miscarriage, intrauterine fetal death (IUD).

CLINICAL PEARLS

- Women with renal disease should be offered low-dose aspirin as prophylaxis against preeclampsia, commencing within the first trimester
- The characteristic renal pathology in preeclampsia is glomerulo-endotheliosis
- Screening for asymptomatic bacteriuria must occur at the time of first prenatal visit
- Acute pyelonephritis is associated with a reduction in glomerular filtration rate, which can be reversed with the treatment of the underlying infection.

2. ANEMIA DURING PREGNANCY

2.1. IRON DEFICIENCY ANEMIA

INTRODUCTION

WHO defines anemia as presence of hemoglobin of less than 11 gm/dL and hematocrit of less than 0.33 gm/dL. Center of Disease Control [CDC, 1990] have defined anemia as hemoglobin levels below 11 gm/dL in the pregnant woman in first and third trimester and less than 10.5 gm/dL in second trimester. Based on the findings of the peripheral smear and the results of various blood indices, anemia can be classified into three types, which have been shown in the **Table 4.3**.

Table 4.3: Classification of anemia based on the blood values

Type	*Lab value*	*Causes*
Macrocytic normochromic anemia	Increased MCV, normal MCHC (MCV > 100 fl; MCHC-34)	Vitamin B_{12} deficiency; folate deficiency

Contd...

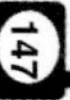

Contd...

Type	*Lab value*	*Causes*
Microcytic hypochromic anemia	Low MCHC; low MCV; (MCV < 80 fl; MCHC < 30)	Thalassemias; iron deficiency anemia; anemia of chronic disease (rare cases)
Normocytic normochromic anemia	Normal MCHC; normal MCV (MCV > 80–99 fl; MCHC-34)	Physiological anemia of pregnancy, anemia due to chronic disease, anemia due to acute hemorrhage; aplastic anemias; hemolytic anemias

ETIOLOGY

Various causes of iron deficiency anemia are listed in **Box 4.1**.

Box 4.1: Causes of iron deficiency anemia

Nutritional causes
Iron deficiency anemia (60%)
Dimorphic anemia both due to deficiency of iron and folic acid

Hemolytic anemia
Hemoglobinopathies

Anemia due to blood loss

Acute: Antepartum hemorrhage, postpartum hemorrhage

Chronic: Hookworm infestation, bleeding piles, malarial infestation.

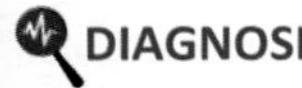

DIAGNOSIS

Symptoms

With mild anemia, the woman may present with vague complaints of ill health, fatigue and diminished capability to perform hard labor, loss of appetite, digestive upset, breathlessness, palpitation, dyspnea on exertion, easy fatigability, fainting, lightheadedness, tinnitus, exhaustion, nocturnal leg cramps, headache, paresthesias and numbness in the extremities; oral and nasopharyngeal symptoms; pica; hair loss, etc.

General Physical Examination

- *Pallor*: There may be pallor in lower palpebral conjunctiva **(Fig. 4.1)**, pale nails, pale palmar surface of hands, pale tongue **(Fig. 4.2)**, lips, nail beds, etc.

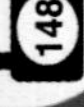

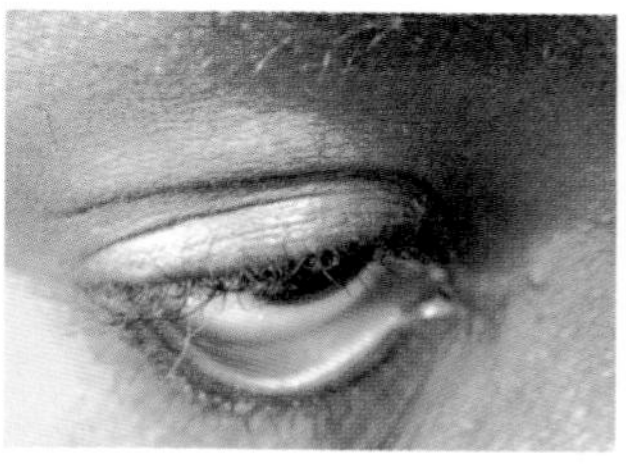

Figure 4.1: Pallor in lower palpebral conjunctiva

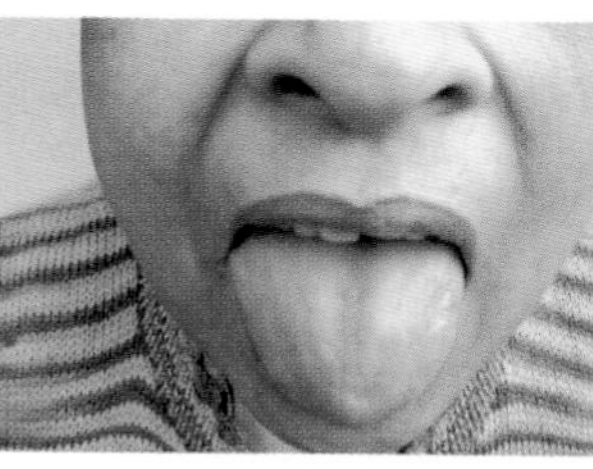

Figure 4.2: Pale tongue

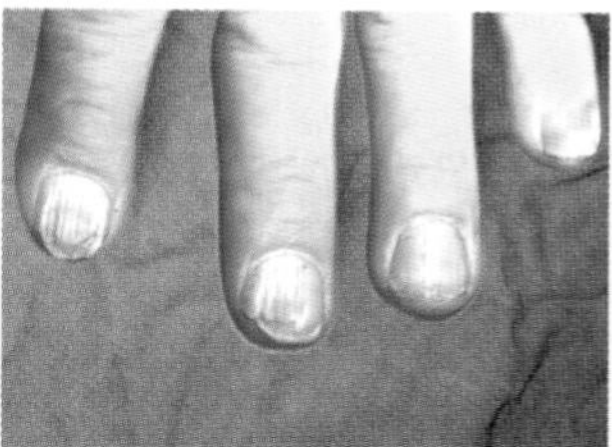

Figure 4.3: Koilonychia

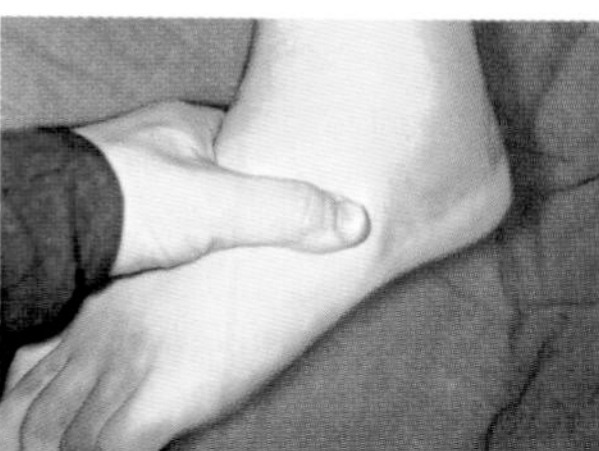

Figure 4.4: Pedal edema

- *Epithelial changes*: The epithelial tissues of nails, tongue, mouth, hypopharynx and stomach are affected resulting in development of nail changes [thinning, flattening and finally development of concave "spoon-shaped nails" or koilonychias, **(Fig. 4.3)**], glossitis, angular stomatitis and atrophic gastritis, etc.
- *Pedal edema*: In severe anemic cases, there may be pedal edema **(Fig. 4.4)**
- *Abdominal examination*: Splenomegaly may occur with severe, persistent, untreated iron deficiency anemia.

Investigations

- *Hemoglobin and hematocrit*: Hemoglobin is less than 11 gm/dL and hematocrit is less than 0.33 gm/dL
- *Blood cellular indices*: Abnormalities in various blood indices with iron deficiency anemia are described in **Table 4.4**

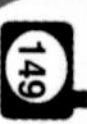

Table 4.4: Abnormalities in blood indices with iron deficiency anemia		
Blood index	*Normal value*	*Value in iron deficiency anemia*
MCH	26.7–33.7 pg/cell (average 30.6 pg/cell)	< 26.7 pg/cell
MCHC	32–36%	< 30 gm%
MCV	83–97 fl (average 90 fl)	< 76 fl
Hemoglobin	12.1–14.1 gm/dL	< 11 gm/dL in 1st and 3rd trimesters and less than 10.5 gm/dL in 2nd trimester
Hematocrit	36.1–44.3%	< 36.1%
Red cell count	3.9–5.0 × 10^6 cells/μL (average 4.42 × 10^6 cells/μL)	< 3.9 × 10^6 cells/μL or normal
Red cell distribution index	31–36%	< 31%

- *Peripheral smear in iron deficiency anemia*: Peripheral smear of blood shows microcytic and hypochromic (**Fig. 4.5**). There may be anisocytosis (abnormal size of cells) in the form of microcytosis and/or poikilocytosis (abnormal shape of cells) in the form of pencil cells and target cells. There may be presence of ring or pessary cells with central hypochromia
- *Osmotic fragility*: RBC osmotic fragility is slightly reduced
- *Serum iron studies*: Changes in the various serum iron parameters are described in **Table 4.5**

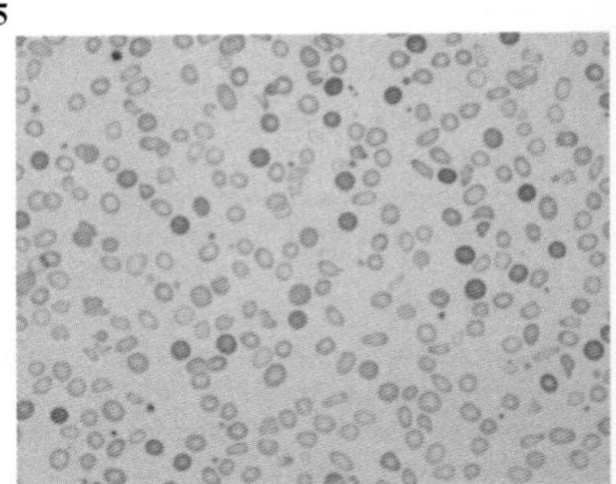

Figure 4.5: Peripheral smear in case of iron deficiency anemia

- *Stool examination*: This helps in excluding out parasitic infestation as a cause of anemia
- *Urine routine/microscopy*: Urine routine/microscopy helps in detecting the presence of pus cells/occult blood or schistosomes
- *Hemoglobin electrophoresis*: Hemoglobin electrophoresis and measurement of hemoglobin A2 and fetal hemoglobin are useful in establishing either beta-thalassemia or hemoglobin C or D as the etiology of the microcytic anemia
- *Bone marrow examination*: A bone marrow aspirate stained for iron (Perls stain) can be diagnostic of iron deficiency.

Table 4.5: Changes in serum iron studies with iron deficiency anemia

Blood parameter	*Normal value*	*Value in iron deficiency anemia*
Serum transferrin levels	200–360 mg/dL	> 360 mg/dL
Serum iron concentration	60–175 µgm/dL	< 60 µgm/dL
Transferrin saturation	25–60%	< 25%
Ferritin levels	50–145 ng/mL	< 20 ng/mL
Serum protoporphyrin	30–70 µgm/dL	> 70 µgm/dL

DIFFERENTIAL DIAGNOSIS

Differentiation between various types of anemia is described in **Table 4.3**.

OBSTETRIC MANAGEMENT

Antenatal Period

Dietary changes: Eating a healthy and a well-balanced diet during pregnancy helps in maintaining the iron stores.

Iron supplements: If the period of gestation is less than 30 completed weeks of gestation, oral iron supplements (containing 200–300 mg of iron salt with 500 µg of folic acid) must be prescribed in divided doses. The main problems associated with the use of oral iron supplements are occurrence of side effects including anorexia, diarrhea, epigastric discomfort, nausea, etc. Sometimes parenteral iron therapy (by intramuscular or intravenous routes) is started in cases where there is intolerance to oral form of iron; when iron deficiency is not correctable with oral treatment; there is non-compliance on part of the patient; the patient is unable to absorb iron orally

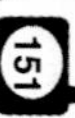

or the patient is near term. The two most commonly used parenteral iron preparations include, iron sorbitol citric acid complex (jectofer) and iron dextran (imferon).

Blood transfusion: This may be required when there is not enough time to achieve a reasonable hemoglobin level before delivery, for example, patient presents with severe anemia beyond 36 weeks; there is acute blood loss or associated infections and anemia is refractory to iron therapy.

Intrapartum Period

- *First stage of labor*: The following need to be done:
  - Patient's blood grouping and cross-matching
  - Adequate pain relief must be provided
  - Oxygen inhalation through face mask must be provided
  - Digitalization may be required especially if the patient shows a potential to develop congestive heart failure
  - Antibiotic prophylaxis must be given as the anemic women are prone to develop infections
- *Second stage of labor*: In order to shorten the duration of second stage of labor, forceps or vacuum can be applied prophylactically
- *At the time of delivery*: The following precautions must be taken during the time of delivery in order to reduce the amount of blood loss:
  - Routine administration of oxytocics (methergine, oxytocin, etc.) following the delivery of baby, as well as the placenta
  - Late clamping of cord at the time of delivery.

COMPLICATIONS

Maternal

- *Throughout the pregnancy*: These include high-maternal mortality rate, cerebral anoxia, cardiac failure, increased susceptibility to develop infection, abortions, preterm labor, etc.
- *During antenatal period*: Poor weight gain, preterm labor, PIH, placenta previa, accidental hemorrhage, eclampsia, PROM, etc.
- *During intranatal period*: Dysfunctional labor, intranatal hemorrhage, shock, anesthesia risk, cardiac failure, etc.
- *During postnatal period*: Postnatal sepsis, subinvolution, embolism.

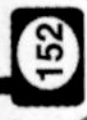

Fetal

- Preterm birth, low-birth-weight and IUGR babies
- Fetal distress and neonatal distress requiring prolonged resuscitation
- Impaired neurological and mental development
- Tendency of the infants to develop conditions, such as iron deficiency anemia, failure to thrive, poor intellectual development, delayed milestones and other morbidities later in life.

CLINICAL PEARLS

- Out of the various blood indices used, mean corpuscular volume and mean corpuscular hemoglobin concentration are the two most sensitive indices of iron deficiency
- The earliest hematological response to treatment is reticulocytosis
- The WHO recommends universal iron supplementation comprising of 60 mg elemental iron and 400 μg of folic acid once or twice daily for 6 months in pregnancy, in countries with prevalence of anemia less than 40% and an additional 3 months postpartum in countries where prevalence is greater than 40%.

2.2. MEGALOBLASTIC ANEMIA

INTRODUCTION

Megaloblastic anemia is characterized by the presence of megaloblasts, which are large cells having an increased nuclear to cytoplasmic ratio with delayed nuclear maturation and more advanced cytoplasmic maturation. There is a defect in DNA synthesis amongst the rapidly dividing cells. RNA and protein synthesis are also impaired to a certain extent. This results in the production of abnormal precursors called megaloblasts in the bone marrow.

ETIOLOGY

- Isolated deficiency of vitamin B_{12} or folate (more common during pregnancy)
- Combined deficiency of both vitamin B_{12} and folate.

DIAGNOSIS

Symptoms

These are same as those described in the fragment of iron deficiency anemia. Some symptoms specific to megaloblastic anemia include memory loss, depression, personality changes, psychosis, peripheral neuropathy, etc.

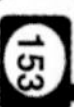

General Physical Examination

- Pallor
- Ulceration in mouth (glossitis) and tongue
- Hemorrhagic patches under the skin and conjunctiva
- Enlarged liver and spleen.

Investigations

- *Complete blood count, hemoglobin and hematocrit*: Hemoglobin is less than 11 gm/dL and hematocrit is less than 0.33 gm/dL. There may be associated leucopenia and thrombocytopenia
- *Peripheral smear*: This may reveal the presence of macrocytes and megaloblasts; hypersegmentation of neutrophils (showing five lobes or more (**Fig. 4.6**); fully hemoglobinized red blood cells and Howell Jolly bodies
- *Blood indices*: MCV and MCH are both increased to values greater than 100 mm^3 and 33 pg respectively
- *Serum iron studies*: Serum iron is normal or high, and iron binding capacity is low
- *Serum folate and B_{12} levels*: Serum folate levels may be less than 3 ng/mL, and B_{12} levels less than 90 pg/mL
- *Bone marrow studies*: Examination of bone marrow may show megaloblastic erythropoiesis.

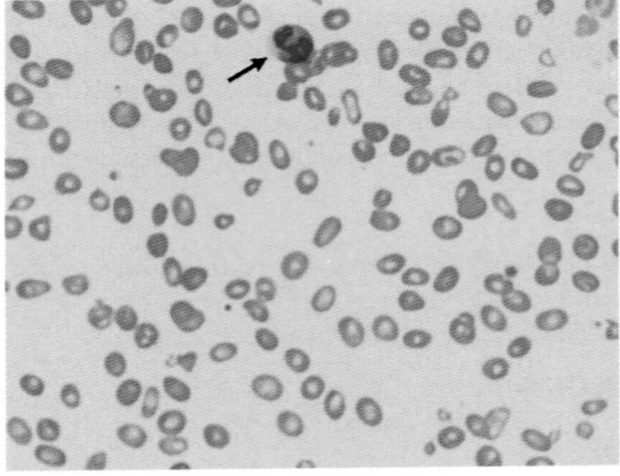

Figure 4.6: Peripheral smear in case of megaloblastic anemia

The arrow points toward persegmented neutrophil

DIFFERENTIAL DIAGNOSIS

Differentiation between various types of anemia has been described in **Table 4.3**.

MANAGEMENT

- Prescription of diet rich in folic acid
- Folate supplements: This should be in the form of daily administration of folic acid in the dosage of 4 mg orally, continued until 4 weeks following delivery
- In case of B_{12} deficiency, intramuscular injections of vitamin B_{12} in the dosage of 100 μg daily can be given.

COMPLICATIONS

These are similar to those described in the fragment of iron deficiency anemia. Some complications specific to megaloblastic anemia include abortion, IUGR, prematurity, abruptio placentae, fetal malformations (cleft lip, neural tube defects, etc.).

CLINICAL PEARLS

- Folate deficiency can cause serious neural tube defects and other developmental anomalies
- Folate supplementation, 1 month before conception and then throughout the first trimester, help in the prevention of neural tube defects.

3. GESTATIONAL DIABETES

INTRODUCTION

Gestational diabetes is defined by the WHO as "carbohydrate intolerance resulting in hyperglycemia of variable severity with onset or first recognition during pregnancy". Gestational diabetes now includes both gestational impaired glucose tolerance and gestational diabetes mellitus (GDM).

ETIOLOGY

The risk factors, which predispose a woman to develop gestational diabetes, are listed in **Box 4.2**.

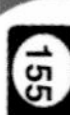

Box 4.2: Risk factors for the development of diabetes

- Body mass index above 30 kg/m^2
- Previous macrosomic baby weighing 4.5 kg or above
- Previous history of gestational diabetes
- Family history of diabetes
- Ethnic origin with a high prevalence of diabetes (e.g. South Asian, Middle Eastern, etc.)

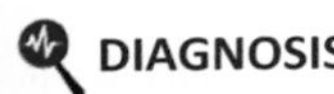

DIAGNOSIS

Clinical Presentation

Signs suggestive of preeclampsia may be present as the women with GDM are especially prone to develop preeclampsia (refer to the previous fragments)

Abdominal Examination

Women with GDM are especially prone to develop polyhydramnios (refer to the fragment on polyhydramnios for suggestive signs on abdominal examination).

Investigations

- *Glucose challenge test (GCT)*: Glucose challenge test is a screening test for gestational diabetes, in which plasma blood glucose levels are measured 1 hour after giving a glucose load of 50 gm to the woman, irrespective of the time of the day or last meals. A value of 140 mg/dL or higher indicates high risk for development of gestational diabetes. An abnormal result on glucose challenge test must be followed by a 100 gm oral glucose tolerance test
- *Oral glucose tolerance test (OGTT)*: This test involves measurement of blood glucose levels at fixed time intervals following the intake of prefixed quantities of glucose (usually 100 gm). Further diagnosis can be established either using the Carpenter and Coustan criteria **(Table 4.6)** or criteria defined by the National Diabetes Data Group **(Table 4.7)**

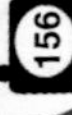

Table 4.6: 100 gm glucose load by O'Sullivan and Mahan: criteria modified by Carpenter and Coustan

Status	*Plasma/serum glucose (mmol/liter)*	*Plasma/serum glucose levels (mg/dL)*
Fasting	≥ 5.8	95
1 hr.	≥ 10.0	180
2 hr.	≥ 9.1	155
3 hr.	≥ 8.0	140

Source: Carpenter MW and Coustan DR. Criteria for screening tests for gestational diabetes. Am J Obstet Gynecol. 1982;144:768-73.

Table 4.7: National Diabetes Data Group criteria for 100 gm OGTT

Status	*Plasma/serum glucose levels (mmol/liter)*	*Plasma/serum glucose levels (mg/dL)*
Fasting	> 5.3	105
1 hr.	> 10.0	190
2 hr.	> 8.6	165
3 hr.	> 7.8	145

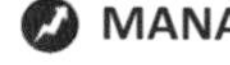

MANAGEMENT

Management during the Antenatal Period

- *Diabetes education and information*: Education and information regarding diabetes, hypoglycemia, self-monitoring of blood glucose levels, etc. needs to be provided to the patient
- *Maintenance of blood glucose levels*: This can be done with the help of monthly measurement of the glycosylated hemoglobin levels and self-monitoring of blood glucose levels using a glucose meter
- *Requirement for hypoglycemic therapy*: In case of previously diabetic women, oral diabetes medication needs to be changed to insulin. In case of women with gestational diabetes, initial control of blood glucose levels must be through exercise and nutritional advice. If these options do not work, insulin may be advised. The objective of the antidiabetic treatment is to maintain the fasting capillary glucose values under 95 mg/dL and 1 or 2 hour postprandial values under 140 mg/dL and 120 mg/dL respectively. The aim should be to maintain her HbA1c levels below 7.0% and glucose levels within 4–7 mmol/liter

- *Maintenance of adequate body weight*: Women with diabetes who are planning to become pregnant and who have a body mass index above 27 kg/m^2 should be offered advice on how to lose weight
- *Regular intake of folic acid*: Women with diabetes who are planning to become pregnant should be advised to take folic acid in the dose of 5 mg/day, starting right from the periconceptional period and extending throughout the period of gestation
- *Insulin therapy*: Insulin therapy may include regular insulin, or rapid-acting insulin analogues (aspart and lispro). During pregnancy, women are usually prescribed 4-daily insulin injections (3 injections of regular insulin to be taken before each meal and one injection of isophane insulin to be taken at night time)
- *Fetal monitoring*: These include tests, such as daily fetal movement count, NST, fetal biophysical profile and monthly ultrasound scans for estimation of fetal weight starting at 32–36 weeks of gestation
- *Screening for congenital malformations*: First trimester ultrasound scan at 11–13 weeks must be done to look for nuchal translucency as there is an increased risk of neural tube defects. Maternal serum screening for α-fetal proteins at 16–18 weeks must be done to rule out the risk for neural tube defects. Second trimester ultrasound scan for detailed scanning for fetal congenital anomalies must be performed at 18–20 weeks
- *Timing and mode of birth*:
    - Low-risk patients: These women may be allowed to develop spontaneous labor and to deliver by 38–40 weeks of gestation
    - High-risk patients: High-risk gestational diabetic patients should have their labor induced when they reach 38 weeks.

Management during the Intrapartum Period

During the time of labor and birth, capillary blood glucose should be monitored on an hourly basis in women with diabetes and maintained at levels between 4 and 7 mmol/liter by using intravenous dextrose and insulin infusion.

Postnatal care: Immediately after birth, the insulin requirements may fall; therefore, insulin doses must be reduced immediately to pre-pregnancy levels, in order to avoid hypoglycemia.

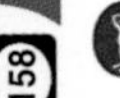

COMPLICATIONS

Diabetes in pregnancy is associated with numerous risks to the mother and the developing fetus, which are enumerated in **Table 4.8**.

Table 4.8: Maternal and fetal complications related to gestational diabetes

Maternal complications	*Fetal complications*
• Miscarriage • Preeclampsia • Preterm labor • Prolonged labor • Polyhydramnios (could be associated with fetal polyuria) • Shoulder dystocia • 35–50% risk of developing type 2 diabetes later in the life • Increased risk of traumatic damage during labor • Increased risk of shoulder dystocia • Diabetic retinopathy and nephropathy can worsen rapidly during pregnancy	• Fetal distress and birth asphyxia • Brachial plexus injuries • Mactrosomia (birth weight more than 4 kg) • Increased risk for perinatal death, birth trauma and rates of cesarean section • Cephalohematoma, resulting in more pronounced neonatal jaundice • Stillbirth, congenital malformations, macrosomia, birth injury, perinatal mortality • Hypoxia and sudden intrauterine death after 36 weeks gestation • Congenital malformations (caudal regression sequence; congenital heart diseases; GI abnormalities; renal defects; neural tube defects; cystic fibrosis, etc.) • Fetal/neonatal hypoglycemia, polycythemia, hyperbilirubinemia and renal vein thrombosis • Stillbirths • An increased long-term risk of obesity and diabetes in the child

CLINICAL PEARLS

- Diabetes should not in itself be considered a contraindication for attempting VBAC. The ACOG recommends an elective cesarean section in women with sonographically estimated fetal weight of 4.5 kg
- Early feeding of the neonate is recommended for reducing the risk of neonatal hypoglycemia.

4. CARDIAC DISEASE IN PREGNANCY

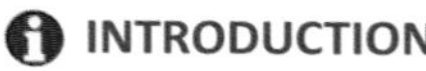

INTRODUCTION

Pregnancy is associated with significant hemodynamic changes (**Fig. 4.7** and **Table 4.9**) that can pose a substantial demand on cardiac function in patients with valvular heart disease and may require the initiation or titration

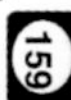

of cardiovascular medications to manage volume overload, hypertension or arrhythmias. Furthermore, pregnancy is a state of relative hypercoagulability, which clearly increases the risk of thromboembolic events.

Table 4.9: Hemodynamic changes during normal pregnancy

Hemodynamic parameter	*Change during normal pregnancy*	*Change during labor and delivery*	*Change during postpartum*
Blood volume	Increases by 40–50%	Increases	Decreases (auto-diuresis)
Heart rate	Increases by 10–15 beats/min.	Increases	Decreases
Cardiac output	Increases by 30–50% above the base line	Additional increase by 50%	Decreases
Blood pressure	Decreases by 10 mm Hg	Increases	Decreases
Stroke volume	Increases during the first and second trimesters; decreases during the third trimester	Additional increase of 300–500 mL with each uterine contraction	Decreases
Systemic vascular resistance	Decreases	Increases	Decreases

The most common valvular heart disease encountered during pregnancy is mitral stenosis. Chronic mitral regurgitation, most commonly encountered as a result of rheumatic heart disease is usually well-tolerated during pregnancy.

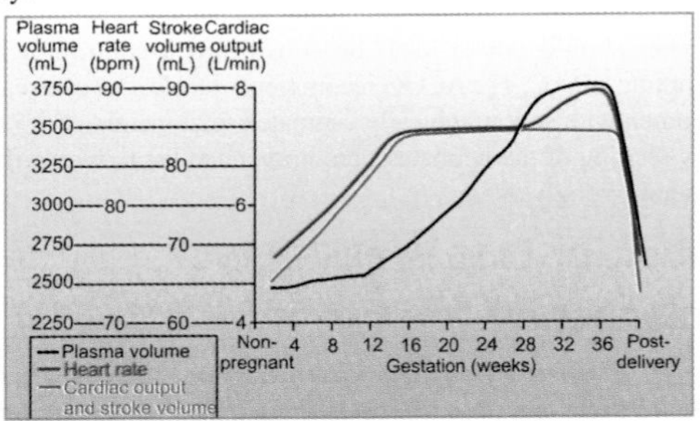

Figure 4.7: Normal hemodynamic changes during pregnancy

DIAGNOSIS

Clinical Presentation

- Fatigue; dizziness
- Dyspnea, orthopnea
- Nonspecific chest pain
- Peripheral edema
- *Palpitations*: May be due to ectopic beats, atrial fibrillations, supraventricular tachycardia, thyrotoxicosis, anxiety, etc.
- Abdominal discomfort and distention
- Light-headedness or fainting.

General Physical Examination

- *Pulse*: Abnormalities in pulse pattern may be suggestive of underlying cardiac disease. Presence of radiofemoral delay could be suggestive of coarctation of aorta
- *Respiratory rate*: The patient's dyspnea may be revealed
- *Finger clubbing*: Clubbing of fingers may be associated with the diseases of heart or lungs
- *Cyanosis*: Presence of cyanosis suggests that arterial oxygen saturation is less than 85%. Peripheral cyanosis is detected in the fingertips including underneath the nail beds, whereas central cyanosis may be present in the lips and tongue
- *Features indicative of infective endocarditis*: These may include features, such as splinter hemorrhages, Janeway lesions, Osler's nodes, etc.
- *Peripheral edema*: Presence of edema in the feet or sacral region could occur as a result of congestive cardiac failure.

Abdominal Examination

- *Hepatomegaly*: Presence of hepatomegaly or ascites on abdominal examination could be due to congestive heart failure.

Examination of Cardiovascular System

- *Palpation*: The cardiac apex (normally palpated in the left fifth intercostal space, one centimeter medial to the midclavicular line) may be shifted downward and outward in cases of left ventricular enlargement
- *Auscultation*: Upon auscultation of the precordial area, normal heart sounds (S1 and S2) can be heard. Upon auscultation, it is important to note whether or not an additional sound (e.g. murmur, opening snap, click, third or fourth heard sounds, etc.) are present.

Investigations

- A 12-lead electrocardiogram and a chest radiograph
- A transthoracic echocardiogram
- An arterial oxygen saturation measurement by percutaneous oximetry.

MANAGEMENT

Antenatal Care

Management of mitral stenosis: Drugs, like digoxin and beta-blockers, can be used to reduce heart rate, and diuretics can be used to reduce the blood volume and left atrial pressure. With development of atrial fibrillations and hemodynamic deterioration, electrocardioversion can be performed safely. Anticoagulation must be initiated with the onset of atrial fibrillations in order to reduce the risk of stroke.

Heart surgery may be necessary when medical treatment fails to control heart failure or symptoms remain intolerable to the patients despite medical therapy. While open heart surgery may be associated with risks to the fetus, closed mitral valvuloplasty (CMV), a relatively safe procedure, may be performed in case of severe pulmonary congestion unresponsive to drugs, profuse hemoptysis and any episode of pulmonary edema before pregnancy. Most patients with mitral stenosis can undergo vaginal delivery.

- *Fetal surveillance*: Careful fetal monitoring, mainly in the form of clinical and ultrasound examinations may be required when signs of hemodynamic compromise are present
- *Increased frequency of antenatal visits*: In general, prenatal visits should be scheduled every month in women with mild disease and every 2 weeks in women with moderate or severe disease, until 28–30 weeks and weekly thereafter until delivery
- *Use of antiarrhythmic medicines during pregnancy*: Pharmacologic treatment is usually reserved for patients with severe symptoms
- Management by a multidisciplinary team
- Bed rest.

Intrapartum Care

- The main objective of management should be to minimize any additional load on the cardiovascular system from delivery and puerperium by aiming for spontaneous onset of labor and providing effective pain relief with low-dose regional analgesia
- Vaginal delivery over cesarean section is the preferred mode of delivery for most women with heart disease—whether congenital or acquired.

Cesarean section is considered only in the presence of specific obstetric or cardiac considerations

- Positioning the patient on the left lateral side helps in reducing associated hemodynamic fluctuations
- *Intrapartum antibiotic prophylaxis*: Presently, American Heart Association guidelines do not recommend the routine use of endocarditis prophylaxis for cesarean section delivery or for uncomplicated vaginal delivery without infection
- *Management of the third stage of labor*: During the third stage of labor in women with heart disease, bolus doses of oxytocin can cause severe hypotension and should therefore be avoided. Low-dose oxytocin infusions are safer and may be equally effective. Ergometrine is best avoided in most cases as it can cause acute hypertension. Misoprostol may be safer but it can cause problems such as hyperthermia.

COMPLICATIONS

Maternal: These include the following:

- Pulmonary edema and arrhythmias
- Increased maternal morbidity
- An increased risk for cardiac complications, such as heart failure, arrhythmias and stroke.

Fetal: These include the following:

- IUGR (mild in cases of patients with rheumatic heart valve disease and severe in cases of lesions associated with cyanosis in the mothers)
- Neonatal asphyxia
- Respiratory distress and fetal or neonatal death.

CLINICAL PEARLS

- Confidential enquiry into the causes of maternal death in the UK (1997–1999) has shown maternal cardiac disease to be the cause for greatest number of maternal deaths
- ACE inhibitors are safe to use in breastfeeding mothers
- There is a small increased risk of IUGR with the use of beta blockers during pregnancy.

5. SPONTANEOUS ABORTION OR MISCARRIAGE

INTRODUCTION

A miscarriage (also known as spontaneous abortion) is any pregnancy, which undergoes spontaneous termination before reaching the period of viability (20 weeks). Different types of miscarriages are as follows:

- *Threatened abortion*: The process of abortion has started, but has not progressed toward completion
- *Inevitable abortion*: The process of abortion has progressed to a stage from where continuation of pregnancy is impossible
- *Incomplete abortion*: In this type of abortion, products of conception have not been fully expelled out of the uterine cavity and can be felt through the cervical os
- *Complete abortion*: There is expulsion of products of conception en masse, following which there is subsistence of pain or bleeding. On per vaginal examination, the cervical os is closed and uterus is smaller than the period of amenorrhea
- *Missed abortion*: The fetus is dead and gets retained inside the uterine cavity.

ETIOLOGY

Although the actual cause of the miscarriage is frequently unclear, the most common reasons include the following:

- *Genetic factors*: These include chromosomal anomalies such as trisomy, polyploidy, monosomy, structural chromosomal aberrations, etc.
- *Endocrine and metabolic disorders*: Endocrine disorders, such as luteal phase defects, thyroid anomalies, diabetes mellitus, etc.
- *Infections*: Acute viral infections, such as German measles, cytomegalovirus, variola, vaccinia, HIV, mycoplasma, etc. and bacterial infections such as ureaplasma, chlamydia, brucella, spirochaetes, etc. can also cause miscarriage
- *Anatomical abnormalities*: These include diseases and abnormalities of the internal genital organs, such as cervical incompetence, congenital malformations of the uterus (bicornuate or septate uterus), submucous fibroids, intrauterine adhesions (Asherman's syndrome)
- *Immunological disorders*: Autoimmune and alloimmune disorders including antiphospholipid syndrome are usually responsible for causing second trimester miscarriage
- *Other factors*: These may include emotional factors or factors causing stress, certain drugs, caffeine, alcohol, tobacco, cocaine, etc.

DIAGNOSIS

Symptoms

- *Signs of shock*: In case of excessive bleeding, signs of shock may be present

- Bleeding per vaginum
- *Pain or cramping per abdomen*: The pain can be referred the lower back, buttocks and genital area
- *Disappearance of the symptoms of pregnancy*: Symptoms, e.g. nausea, breast tenderness, etc., which were previously present may disappear
- *Abdominal examination*: The uterus may appear tender on palpation.

Vaginal Examination

- Bleeding may be present. Products of conception may be observed to be coming out in case of incomplete and inevitable abortion
- The uterus may appear smaller than the period of gestation in cases of incomplete, missed and complete abortion
- The cervical os may be open.

Investigations

- *Hematocrit and complete blood count*: Hemoglobin levels are indicative of the degree of anemia, whereas leucocytosis is indicative of the presence of infection
- *Ultrasound examination*: Ultrasound examination may reveal a healthy gestational sac, features of missed abortion, anembryonic pregnancy, blighted ovum, etc.
- *Urine or blood for β-hCG level determination*: Especially in cases where there is a suspicion of ectopic pregnancy
- *Urine routine or microscopy and culture or sensitivity*: This may be especially required in cases where an infection is suspected.

DIFFERENTIAL DIAGNOSIS

Different types of abortions as described in the "introduction" need to be differentiated from one another.

MANAGEMENT

- Monitoring of the amount of bleeding and daily inspection of the vulval pad to see if there is expulsion of any products of conception, needs to be done
- Correction of shock by infusion of IV fluids or blood transfusion
- Bed rest must be prescribed for a few days till the bleeding stops
- Sedation and relief of pain must be provided
- Administration of methergine, 0.2 mg to reduce the amount of bleeding
- Prescription of antibiotics in case of presence of infection

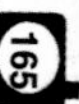

- Use of hCG supplements has been thought to improve pregnancy-related outcomes
- *Administration of anti-Rh immunoglobulins*: This helps in prevention of Rh isoimmunization
- In case, size of the uterus is less than 12 weeks, the uterine cavity can be emptied either using blunt curettage or suction evacuation followed by curettage under anesthesia. After 12 weeks of gestation, the uterus can be induced using oxytocin drip or prostaglandins.

COMPLICATIONS

- Continued bleeding
- Sepsis
- Continuation of pregnancy is associated with an increased risk of complications, such as preterm labor, placenta previa, IUGR, fetal anomalies, etc.

CLINICAL PEARLS

- The commonest type of abortion is an incomplete abortion
- In about two-thirds of the patients, pregnancy continues beyond 28 weeks. In nearly one-third of the patients, pregnancy terminates in inevitable or missed abortion
- Use of progesterone supplements (natural/synthetic) has not been found to be associated with an improved outcome
- Abnormalities in the fetus are responsible for almost all miscarriages during the first trimester of pregnancy; whereas miscarriage during the second trimester is usually related to an abnormality in the mother rather than in the fetus.

6. MEDICAL TERMINATION OF PREGNANCY

INTRODUCTION

Medical termination of pregnancy (MTP) most commonly uses the surgical method, primarily suction evacuation or vacuum aspiration for legal termination of pregnancy during the first trimester of pregnancy. Nowadays, a number of drugs, such as mifepristone/misoprostol or misoprostol alone or in combination with methotrexate, considered safe for termination of pregnancy are also being used. According to the MTP law (1971), termination of pregnancy in India by registered medical practitioners can be done as follows:

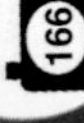

- When the length of the pregnancy is less than 12 weeks, it can be terminated by a registered medical practitioner
- If the length of the pregnancy is between 12 and 20 weeks, termination can be done if at least two registered medical practitioners have given their approval for it in good faith.

The termination of the pregnancy can be done on the basis of medical indications, eugenic and social causes (e.g. pregnancy due to rape, failure of contraception, etc.).

SURGICAL MANAGEMENT

Preoperative Preparation

- Adequate counseling of the woman and her partner is essential, in order to enable her to make a free and fully informed decision
- The clinician can estimate the gestational age by calculating the period of amenorrhea, bimanual examination or a routine ultrasound examination
- A complete medical history must be taken in order to rule out the presence of medical diseases, such as asthma, diabetes and history of drug allergies
- Simple investigations, such as hemoglobin estimation, urine analysis and blood grouping (ABO, Rh), need to be done prior to the procedure
- Cervical priming using 400 μg of the vaginal or anal misoprostol can be done prior to the procedure
- The procedure is usually carried out under local anesthesia, using a paracervical block with 20 mL of 0.5% lignocaine
- Bladder must be emptied prior to the procedure
- After taking all aseptic precautions, the area of perineum, mons and lower part of the abdomen must be cleaned and draped, using povidone-iodine or chlorhexidine solution. The surgeon must use the "no-touch" technique at the time of surgery.

Steps of Surgery

The procedure of vacuum aspiration comprises of the steps described in **Figures 4.8A to D**:

Postoperative Care

- Methergine 0.25 mg IM may be administered after the procedure
- The aspirated tissue must be sent for histopathological examination to confirm for the presence of chorionic villi in the aspirated tissues

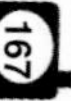

- The patient must be observed in the recovery room for 2–3 hours before discharge
- In case of pain, analgesic drugs may be prescribed
- Women who are Rhesus-negative can be given Rh immune globulins immediately following the procedure
- A woman who has undergone MTP must be counseled regarding the use of contraception in future, in order to prevent the recurrence of unwanted pregnancies

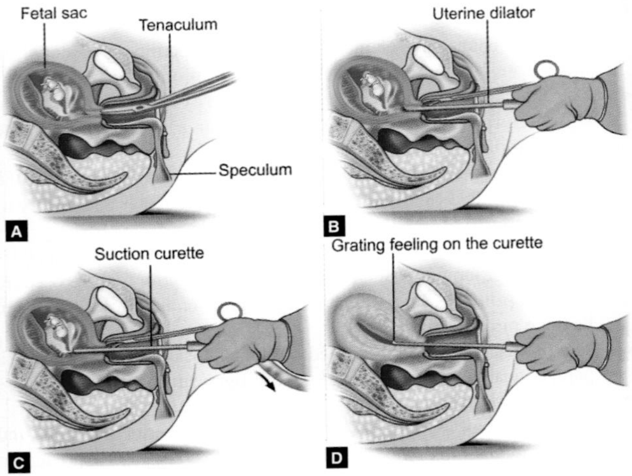

Fetal sac
Tenaculum
Speculum
A
Uterine dilator
B
Suction curette
C
Grating feeling on the curette
D

Figures 4.8A to D: Steps of the procedure of vacuum aspiration: (A) retracting the posterior wall of the uterus with Sim's speculum and grasping the anterior lip with tenaculum; (B) dilating the external cervical os with Hegar's dilator; (C) insertion of Karman's cannula for producing suction; once the cannula has been inserted, the clinician must connect the cannula to a suction machine, which generates pressure equivalent to 60–70 mm Hg. The cannula is rotated at an angle of 360° and moved back by 1–2 cm, back and forth, till the entire uterine cavity has been evacuated (D) the evacuation of the uterine contents is almost complete resulting in a grating feeling

- The patients are scheduled for a follow-up visit, 1–2 weeks after abortion, to check for the presence of any potential MTP related complications.

COMPLICATIONS

- *Minor complaints*: Mild-to-moderate amount of cramping, pain, nausea and vomiting, and bleeding can commonly occur for 2–3 days following the procedure
- *Uterine perforation*: The most dreaded complication of the procedure is uterine perforation
- *Infection*: This can be easily avoided by the administration of broad-spectrum antibiotics
- *Incomplete evacuation*: The most common presentation in these cases is prolonged bleeding. Ultrasound examination helps in confirming the diagnosis
- *Bleeding during and following the abortion*: Uterine atony is the most likely cause of heavy and prolonged bleeding in these cases. Intravenous ergometrine (0.2 mg) or oxytocin (10–20 units) may be used to contract the uterus. Alternatively misoprostol, in the dosage of 400 μg, may be prescribed either through oral or rectal route
- *Failure of the procedure*: The procedure, if not performed properly, may result in the continuation of the pregnancy
- *Hypotension*: This could be related to excessive blood loss or due to a vasovagal response to pain
- *Asherman's syndrome*: This is delayed complication, which can occur as a result of vigorous curettage
- *Cervical lacerations/cervical incompetence*: Rarely, vigorous dilatation may result in cervical lacerations and/or cervical incompetence.

CLINICAL PEARLS

- For MTP using medicines, the following regimen is used: mifepristone in the dosage of 200 mg on day 1 and misoprostol in the dose of 400–800 μg orally or vaginally on day 3
- While medical abortion should be only used in cases the pregnancy is less than or equal to 7 weeks, vacuum aspiration can be performed all through the 12 weeks in the first trimester.

7. GESTATIONAL TROPHOBLASTIC DISEASES

7.1. COMPLETE HYDATIDIFORM MOLE

INTRODUCTION

Hydatidiform mole (H. mole) belongs to a spectrum of disease known as gestational trophoblastic disease (GTD), resulting from overproduction of the chorionic tissue, which is normally supposed to develop into the placenta. It can be considered as an abnormal pregnancy in which placental villi become edematous (hydropic) and start proliferating, resulting in the development of a cystic, grape-like structure filled with watery fluid. There are two types of benign form of GTD: complete (CHM) and partial H. mole (PHM). **Figure 4.9** shows gross clinical specimen of hydatidiform mole, whereas comparison between a complete mole and partial mole has been illustrated in the **Table 4.10**.

Table 4.10: Comparison between complete and partial mole

Parameter under consideration	*Complete mole*	*Partial mole*
Cytogenetic studies	Karyotype 46XX	Triploid karyotype 69XXY
Etiology	Duplication of the haploid sperm following fertilization of an "empty" ovum or dispermic fertilization of an "empty" ovum	These contain two sets of paternal haploid genes and one set of maternal haploid genes. They usually occur following dispermic fertilization of an ovum
Histopathological analysis	There is no evidence of fetal tissue	There may be an evidence of fetal tissue or red blood vessels
Invasive potential and propensity for malignant transformation	Persistent trophoblastic disease following uterine evacuation may develop in about 15% cases with a complete mole	Persistent trophoblastic disease may develop in < 5% of cases of partial mole

ETIOLOGY

Normal process of fertilization is shown in **Figure 4.10**. Etiology of a complete mole is described in **Table 4.10** and **Figure 4.11**.

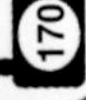

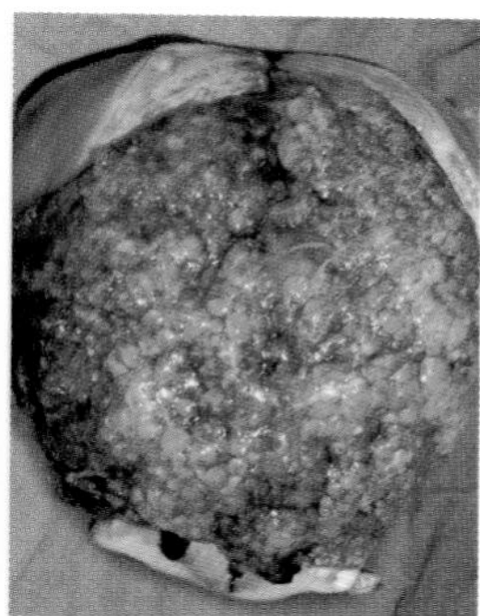

Figure 4.9: Clinical specimen of complete hydatidiform mole

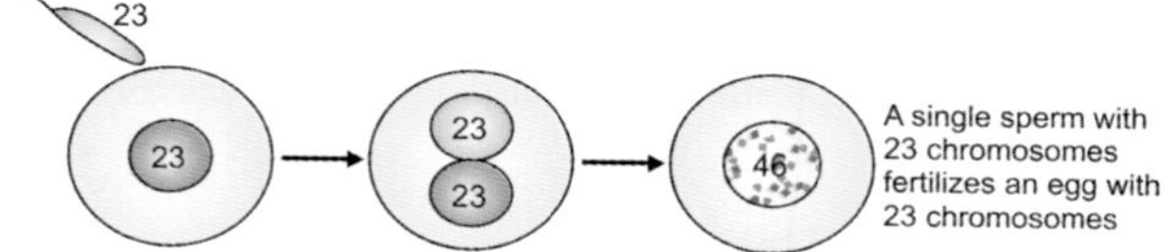

Figure 4.10: Normal process of fertilization

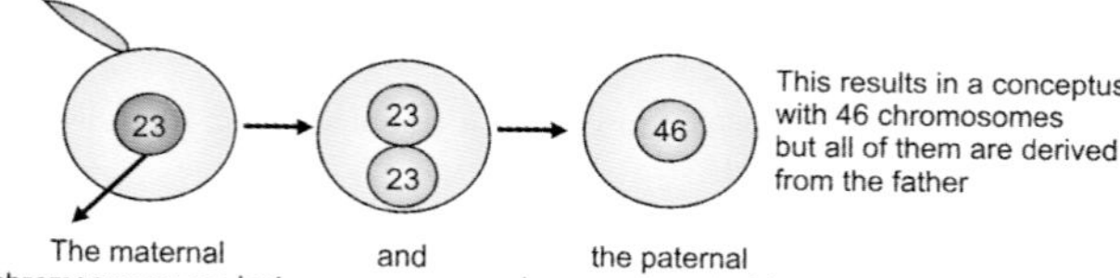

Figure 4.11: Etiology of a complete mole

DIAGNOSIS

Clinical Presentation

- Initially, the symptoms may be suggestive of early pregnancy; however, the uterus is often larger than the period of gestation. The fetal movements and heart tones are usually absent. The uterus may appear doughy in consistency due to lack of fetal parts and amniotic fluid. External ballottement is absent

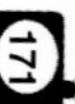

- There may be history suggestive of vaginal bleeding or passage of grape-like tissue early in pregnancy
- There may be excessive nausea and vomiting. Hyperemesis may commonly occur
- There may be symptoms suggestive of hyperthyroidism
- H. mole may be associated with early appearance of preeclampsia.

General Physical Examination

- Signs suggestive of preeclampsia, hyperthyroidism and/or early pregnancy
- Extreme pallor: The patient's pallor may be disproportionate to the amount of blood loss due to concealed hemorrhage.

Vaginal Examination

There may be some vaginal bleeding or passage of grape-like vesicles. Internal ballottement cannot be elicited due to lack of fetus. Unilateral or bilateral enlargement of the ovaries in the form of theca lutein cysts may be palpable.

Investigations

- Complete blood count, blood grouping and cross-matching
- *Serum β-hCG levels*: β-hCG levels in both serum and urine are raised. In cases of complete mole, β-hCG levels may be more than 100,000 mIU/mL
- *Ultrasound of the pelvis*: In case of a complete mole, the following features are observed:
    - Features of missed miscarriage or anembryonic pregnancy (blighted ovum) may be observed on ultrasound examination
    - Characteristic vesicular pattern, also known as "snowstorm appearance" may be present due to generalized swelling of the chorionic villi and presence of multiple, small cystic spaces
    - There may be presence of an enlarged uterine endometrial cavity containing homogeneously hyperechoic endometrial mass with innumerable anechoic cysts **(Fig. 4.12)**
    - Ultrasound may also show the presence of theca lutein cysts in the ovaries
- *Histopathological examination*: Pathologic evaluation may demonstrate swollen chorionic villi having a grape-like appearance, along with presence of hyperplastic trophoblastic tissue.

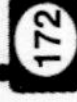

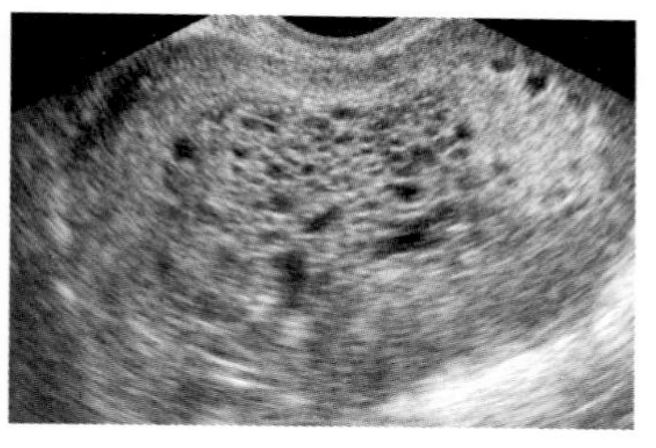

Figure 4.12: Transvaginal sonogram of a second trimester complete hydatidiform mole (transverse section). There is presence of numerous anechoic cysts with intervening hyperechoic material

DIFFERENTIAL DIAGNOSIS

- *Anembryonic gestation*
- *Threatened abortion*: Both the conditions are associated with vaginal bleeding and similar sonographic findings
- *Presence of fibroid or an ovarian tumor with pregnancy*: They may cause the uterine size to be larger in relation to the period of gestation
- *Multiple gestations*: Both the conditions may be associated with early onset of preeclampsia before 20 weeks.

OBSTETRIC MANAGEMENT

The two main treatment options in case of H. mole are suction evacuation and hysterectomy.

Suction Evacuation

Due to the lack of fetal parts, a suction catheter, up to a maximum size of 12 mm, is usually sufficient to evacuate all complete molar pregnancies. In order to ensure that complete sustained remission has been achieved, serial assays of serum and urine β-hCG levels should be carried out on 2 weekly basis until three negative levels are obtained. Post evacuation, contraceptive measures should be instituted and the patient advised to avoid pregnancy until hCG values have remained normal for 6 months.

Hysterectomy with Mole In Situ

Hysterectomy may serve as an option in elderly multiparous women (age > 40 years) who do not wish to become pregnant in the future; women with H. mole desiring sterilization, those with severe infection or uncontrolled bleeding, and patients with nonmetastatic persistent disease who have completed childbearing or are not concerned about preserving their fertility.

Chemotherapy following evacuation may be required in cases of persistent disease as evidenced by rising or plateauing of β-hCG levels.

COMPLICATIONS

- Risk of development of persistent gestational trophoblastic neoplasia (GTN) (described in later text).

7.2. PARTIAL MOLE

INTRODUCTION

Partial H. mole is another form of benign disease belonging to the spectrum of GTD. Difference between the complete and partial mole has already been described in the **Table 4.10**.

ETIOLOGY

Etiology of partial mole is explained in **Table 4.10** and is illustrated in **Figure 4.13**.

DIAGNOSIS

Clinical Presentation

The clinical features are same as that with CHM, described in the previous fragment.

Investigations

- *Ultrasound examination*: These include the following:
    - Presence of a large placenta, cystic spaces within the placenta, an empty gestational sac or sac containing amorphous echoes or growth retarded fetus
    - Increase in ratio of transverse to anterior-posterior dimension of the gestational sac to a value greater than 1.5

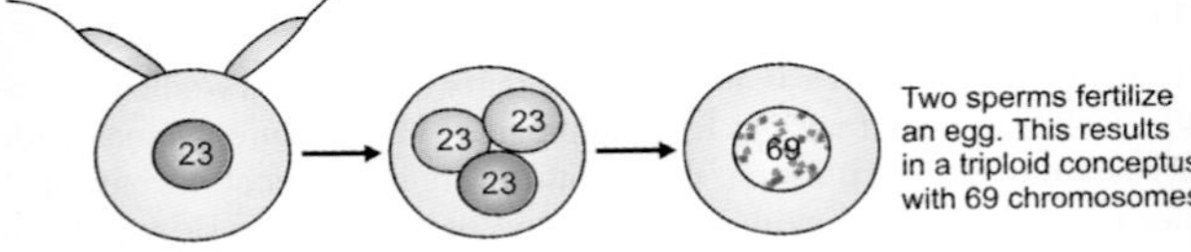

Figure 4.13: Etiology of partial mole

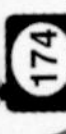

- *Histopathological examination*: Although complete mole does not contain any fetal tissue, non-viable fetal tissue may sometimes be present in PHM.

DIFFERENTIAL DIAGNOSIS

The conditions from which a PHM needs to be differentiated are same as that for CHM (as described in the previous fragment).

MANAGEMENT

This is same as that described with CHM.

COMPLICATIONS

This is same as that described with CHM.

7.3. GESTATIONAL TROPHOBLASTIC NEOPLASIA

INTRODUCTION

Gestational trophoblastic neoplasia (GTN) represents a spectrum of malignant diseases associated with the spectrum of GTDs. These include:

- Invasive mole
- Choriocarcinoma
- Placental site trophoblastic tumor (PSTT)
- Epithelioid trophoblastic tumor.

If the β-hCG level does not normalize within 10 weeks, the disease is classified as persistent. If metastasis is detected on various investigations (chest X-ray, CT, MRI, etc.), the disease is classified as metastatic. If no metastasis is detected, the disease is classified as nonmetastatic.

DIAGNOSIS

Clinical Presentation

The metastatic disease can spread through the blood stream to lungs (80%); vagina (30%); pelvis (20%); brain (10%) and liver (10%). Metastasis to the lungs may result in symptoms like dyspnea, cough, hemoptysis, chest pain, etc.

Investigations

- *Investigations to detect the metastatic disease*: Besides the investigations described in the fragment of CHM, in the cases of GTN,

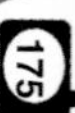

investigations, such as chest X-ray and CT scan of brain, chest, abdomen and pelvis, need to be done in order to detect the metastatic disease. On chest X-ray the lungs may show presence of distinct nodules or cannon ball appearance
- *β-hCG titers*: Women who have the malignant form of GTD may show β-hCG titers, which either plateau or rise and remain elevated beyond 8 weeks.

MANAGEMENT

Nonmetastatic Disease

In most of the cases, nonmetastatic disease can be treated with a single chemotherapeutic drug, either methotrexate (more commonly used) or dactinomycin (used in cases of resistance to methotrexate). If single drug chemotherapy is ineffective, hysterectomy or multidrug chemotherapy can be tried.

Metastatic Disease

The system adopted by the WHO and Federation International of Gynecologists and Obstetricians (FIGO) for classifying gestational trophoblastic tumors (GTT) and treatment protocols is shown in **Table 4.11**. Low-risk group has a score of 0–6; the moderate-risk group has a score between 5 and 7; and the high-risk group will have a score of 7 or higher.

Table 4.11: The classification system by the WHO and FIGO for classifying gestational trophoblastic tumors and treatment protocols

Risk factor	*0*	*1*	*2*	*4*
Age (years)	< 40	≥ 40	—	—
Antecedent pregnancy	Mole	Abortion	Term	—
Interval (end of antecedent pregnancy to chemotherapy in months)	< 4	4–6	7–13	> 13
Human chorionic gonadotropin (IU/L)	$< 10^3$	10^3–10^4	10^4–10^5	$> 10^5$
Number of metastasis	0	1–4	5–8	> 8
Site of metastasis	Lung	Spleen, Kidney	Gastrointestinal tract	Brain, Liver
Largest tumor mass	—	3–5 cm	> 5 cm	—
Previous chemotherapy	—	—	Single drug	≥ 2 drugs

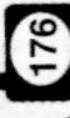

Low-risk metastatic disease is treated with single or multiple drug chemotherapy (intramuscular methotrexate or a combination of intravenous dactinomycin and etoposide). Moderate-risk metastatic disease is usually treated with multiagent chemotherapy. Women with high-risk GTT usually require combination chemotherapy along with selective use of surgery and radiotherapy. The standard multiagent chemotherapy regimen in high-risk group is EMA/CO in which the drugs, like etoposide, dactinomycin and methotrexate, are alternated at weekly intervals with vincristine and cyclophosphamide.

COMPLICATIONS

The development of GTT may result in conditions like invasive mole, choriocarcinoma and PSTT, all of which may metastasize and are potentially fatal if left untreated.

CLINICAL PEARLS

- The lungs are the most common site for metastasis in case of malignant GTD.

8. ANTEPARTUM HEMORRHAGE

8.1. PLACENTA PREVIA

INTRODUCTION

Antepartum hemorrhage (APH) can be defined as hemorrhage from the genital tract occurring after the 28th week of pregnancy, but before the delivery of baby. It does not include bleeding, which occurs after the delivery of the baby (postpartum hemorrhage). It can occur due to placental and extra-placental causes. Besides this, some cases of APH could be due to unexplained causes (indeterminate APH).The placental causes of bleeding are termed as true APH and can be due to placenta previa or placental abruption. Placenta previa can be defined as abnormal implantation of the placenta in the lower uterine segment. Depending on the location of placenta in the relation of cervical os, there can be four types of placenta previa, which are described in the **Figure 4.14**.

ETIOLOGY

The various causes of APH have been described in the "introduction".

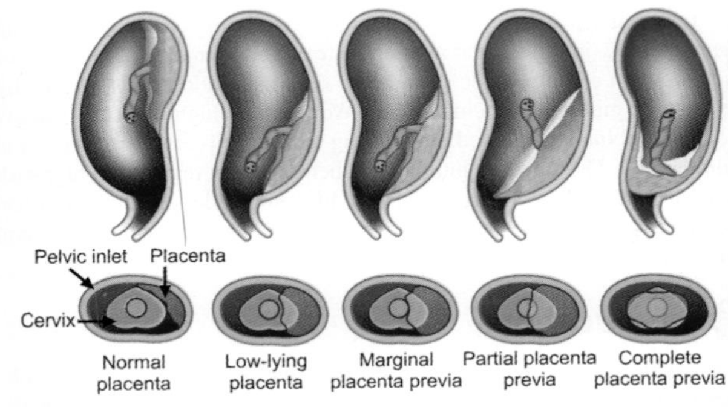

Figure 4.14: Relationship of various types of placenta previa with the cervix

DIAGNOSIS

Clinical Presentation

Bleeding: Placenta previa is typically associated with sudden, painless, apparently causeless, recurrent and profuse bleeding, which is bright red in color and occurs after 28 weeks of gestation. The amount of bleeding may range from light to heavy.

The patient's physical condition is proportional to the amount of blood loss. Repeated bleeding can result in anemia, whereas heavy bleeding may cause shock, in hypotension and/or tachycardia.

Abdominal Examination

- Uterus is soft, relaxed and non-tender
- Uterine contractions may be palpated
- Size of the uterus is proportional to the period of gestation
- The fetal presenting part may be high and cannot be pressed into the pelvic inlet due to the presence of placenta
- There may be abnormal fetal presentation (e.g. breech presentation, transverse lie, etc.)
- Fetal heart rate is usually within normal limits.

Vaginal Examination

Vaginal/rectal examination must never be performed in suspected cases of placenta previa. Instead, an initial inspection must only be performed. On inspection and per speculum examination, the amount and color of the bleeding must be noted. Any local cause of bleeding per vaginum (e.g. cervical erosions, polyps, etc.) must also be ruled out.

Investigations

- *ABO/Rh compatibility*: At least four units of blood need to be cross-matched and arranged. At any time, if severe hemorrhage occurs, the patient may require a blood transfusion
- *Imaging studies*: The main way of confirming the diagnosis of placenta previa is, by imaging studies, both transabdominal **(Fig. 4.15)** and transvaginal ultrasound (more accurate). Color flow Doppler imaging may also prove to be helpful
- *Magnetic resonance imaging (MRI)*: This may be required when the images obtained by ultrasound (both TAS and TVS) are unsatisfactory.

DIFFERENTIAL DIAGNOSIS

Various causes for antepartum vaginal bleeding, of which the exact cause needs to be delineated have been described in the "introduction".

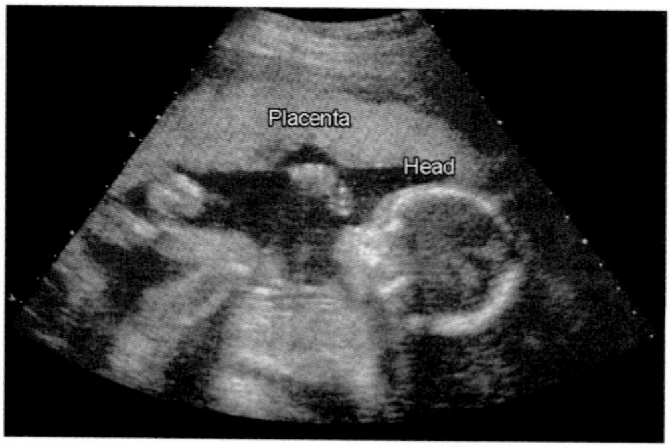

Figure 4.15: Placental localization on transabdominal imaging

OBSTETRIC MANAGEMENT

Intrapartum Period

- *Management of patients with severe bleeding*: In case of severe bleeding, the most important step in management is to stabilize the patient; arrange and cross-match at least four units of blood and start blood transfusion, if required. All efforts must be made to shift her to the operating theater as soon as possible for an emergency cesarean delivery
- *Management of patients with mild-moderate bleeding*: If the period of gestation is between 32 and 36 weeks in patients with mild-moderate bleeding, assessment of fetal lung maturity needs to be done using the L:S ratio. The L:S ratio of greater than or equal to 2 indicates fetal lung maturity, implying that the fetus can be delivered in these cases. If L:S ratio is less than 2, the fetal lungs have yet not attained maturity. In these cases, expectant management comprising of complete bed rest, intramuscular corticosteroid injection, intensive fetal monitoring and use of tocolytic agents to prevent uterine activity, can be undertaken if the patient remains stable for next 24–48 hours. All Rh negative women with placenta previa who bleed must be offered anti-D immunoglobulin injections in order to prevent the risk of Rh isoimmunization
- *Mode of delivery*: Cesarean delivery is necessary for most cases of placenta previa, especially the major degree placenta previa including Type II (posterior); Type III and Type IV. Indications for immediate delivery by an emergency cesarean section irrespective of the period of gestation or type of placenta previa are listed in **Box 4.3**.

Box 4.3: Indications for an emergency cesarean section

- Bleeding is heavy and/or uncontrolled
- Major degree placenta previa (Type II posterior, Type III and Type IV)
- Fetal distress
- Obstetric factors like CPD, fetal malpresentation, etc.

COMPLICATIONS

Maternal

- *Bleeding*: The bleeding can be heavy enough to cause maternal shock or even death
- *Placenta accreta, increta, percreta*: These occur due to the pathological adherence of placenta

- *Anemia and infection*: Excessive blood loss can result in anemia and increased susceptibility to infections.

Fetal

- *Premature birth*: Severe bleeding may force the obstetrician to proceed with an emergency preterm cesarean delivery
- *Fetal death or fetal distress*: Severe maternal bleeding in cases with placenta previa is sometimes also responsible for producing fetal distress.

CLINICAL PEARLS

- Vaginal examination should be strictly avoided in cases of placenta previa because it can provoke an episode of torrential bleeding. In case vaginal examination needs to be done, a double set-up examination must be performed at a place with facilities of an emergency cesarean section
- Women having placenta previa with a previous history of uterine scar are at an increased risk of developing a morbidly adherent placenta.

8.2. ABRUPTION PLACENTA

INTRODUCTION

Placental abruption, also known as accidental hemorrhage, can be defined as abnormal, pathological separation of the normally situated placenta from its uterine attachment. As a result, bleeding occurs from the opened sinuses present in the uterine myometrium. Clinical classification of placental abruption is described in **Table 4.12**.

Table 4.12: Clinical classification of placental abruption

Parameter	*Grade 0*	*Grade 1*	*Grade 2*	*Grade 4*
External bleeding	Absent	Slight	Mild to moderate	Moderate to severe
Uterine tenderness	Absent	Uterus irritable, uterine tenderness may or may not be present	Uterine tenderness is usually present	Tonic uterine contractions and marked uterine tenderness

Contd...

Contd...

Parameter	*Grade 0*	*Grade 1*	*Grade 2*	*Grade 4*
Abdominal pain	Absent	Abdominal pain may or may not be present	Abdominal pain is usually present	Severe degree of abdominal pain may be present
FHS	Present, good	Present, good	Fetal distress	Fetal death
Maternal shock	Absent	Absent	Generally absent	Present
Perinatal outcome	Good	Good	May be poor	Extremely poor
Complications	Absent	Rare	May be present	Complications like DIC and oliguria
Volume of retroplacental clot	Absent	< 200 mL	150–500 mL	> 500 mL

 ETIOLOGY

The specific cause of placental abruption is often unknown. Separation of the normally situated placenta results in hemorrhage into decidua basalis. A retroplacental clot develops between the placenta and the decidua basalis, which interferes with the supply of oxygen to the fetus, resulting in the development of fetal distress. Based on the type of clinical presentation, there can be three types of placental abruption:

- *Concealed type*: In this case the blood loss is not visible because it collects between the fetal membranes and decidua in form of the retroplacental clot
- *Revealed type*: In this type, the blood does not collect between the fetal membranes and the decidua but moves out of the cervical canal and is visible externally
- *Mixed type*: This is the most common type of placental abruption and is associated with both revealed and concealed hemorrhage.

 DIAGNOSIS

Clinical Presentation

- *Vaginal bleeding*: The most common symptom of placental abruption is dark-red vaginal bleeding with pain, usually occurring after 28 weeks of gestation

- *Abdominal pain*: Abdominal and back pain often begins suddenly. Uterine tenderness may be present
- *Other symptoms*: Some women may experience slightly different symptoms including, faintness and collapse, nausea, thirst, reduced fetal movements, etc.
- *Shock*: The patient may be in shock (tachycardia and low blood pressure)
- *Preeclampsia*: There may be signs and symptoms suggestive of preeclampsia.

Abdominal Examination

- Uterine hypertonicity and frequent uterine contractions are commonly present. It may be difficult to feel the fetal parts due to presence of uterine hypertonicity
- Severe degree of placental abruption may be associated with fetal bradycardia and other fetal heart rate abnormalities. In extreme cases, fetal demise may even be detected at the time of examination.

Vaginal Examination

Although presence of placental abruption is not a contraindication for vaginal examination, it should not ideally be performed in patients with history of APH due to the risk of placenta previa.

Investigations

Ultrasound examination: This helps in showing the location of the placenta and thereby making or ruling out the diagnosis of placenta previa; visualization of retroplacental clot **(Fig. 4.16)**; checking the fetal viability and presentation.

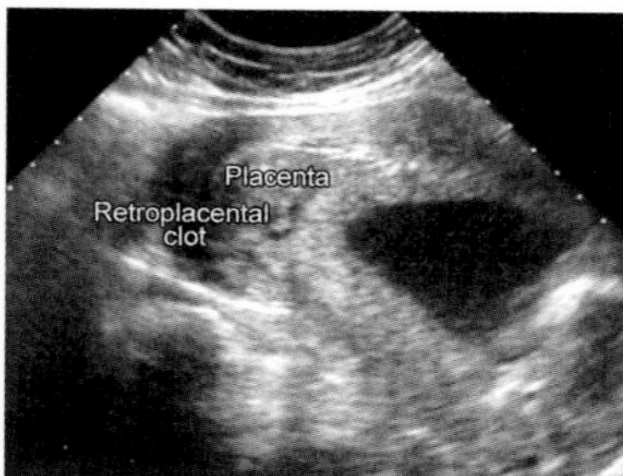

Figure 4.16: Ultrasound examination in case of placental abruption showing presence of a retroplacental clot

DIFFERENTIAL DIAGNOSIS

The differential diagnosis includes various causes for antepartum vaginal bleeding, which have been described in the "indroduction" section of previous fragment. The main differential diagnosis is placenta previa.

OBSTETRIC MANAGEMENT

The management plan depends on grade of placental abruption and fetal maturity. In cases with mild abruption, where fetal maturity has not yet been attained, expectant management can be undertaken until the fetus attains maturity. A moderate case of placental abruption requires hospitalization and constant fetal monitoring. The expectant management can be continued if the mother remains stable. If at any time, maternal or fetal distress appears in these cases or the women present with severe placental abruption, the following steps need to be urgently undertaken:

- Urgent admission to the hospital
- Insertion of a central venous pressure line, IV line and a urinary catheter
- Blood to be sent for ABO and Rh typing, cross-matching and CBC. Blood transfusion must be started if signs of shock are present
- Inspection of vaginal pads and monitoring of vitals (pulse, blood pressure, etc.) at every 15–30 minutes intervals depending upon the severity of bleeding needs to be done
- Blood coagulation profile needs to be done at every 2 hourly intervals
- The placental position must be localized using an ultrasound scan
- The fetal heart sounds must be monitored continuously
- Intramuscular corticosteroids need to be administered to the mother in case of fetal prematurity
- Definitive treatment in these cases is the delivery of the baby. In case of severe abruption, delivery should be performed by the fastest possible route. Cesarean delivery needs to be performed for most cases with severe placental abruption. Other indications for an emergency cesarean delivery are listed in **Box 4.4**.

Box 4.4: Indications for emergency cesarean section in case of placental abruption

- Appearance of fetal distress
- Bleeding continues to occur or there is an abnormal progress of labor despite of artificial rupture of membranes and oxytocin infusion
- Fetal malpresentation
- Appearance of complications (DIC, oliguria, etc.)
- Associated obstetric factors.

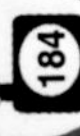

COMPLICATIONS

Maternal

- Maternal shock due to severe bleeding
- *Maternal death*: This may be due to severe bleeding, shock and DIC
- *Renal failure*: Severe shock resulting from Grade 3 placental abruption and/or DIC can be responsible for the development of renal failure
- *Couvelaire uterus or uteroplacental apoplexy*: This condition is characterized by massive intravasation of blood into the uterine musculature up to the level of serosa
- Risk of recurrence of abruption in future pregnancies
- Postpartum uterine atony and postpartum hemorrhage
- *DIC*: DIC is a syndrome associated with both thrombosis and hemorrhage. It can result in development of hypoxia, ischemia and necrosis, which ultimately results in end stage organ damage, especially renal and hepatic failure.

Fetal

- Fetal distress, premature delivery
- Stillbirth and fetal death.

CLINICAL PEARLS

- Once placental detachment has occurred, presently there is no treatment to replace the placenta back to its original position
- Concealed type of placental abruption carries higher risk of maternal and fetal hazards in comparison to the revealed type because patient's clinical condition may often be disproportionate to the amount of blood loss, especially in cases of concealed hemorrhage.

9. ABNORMALITIES OF AMNIOTIC FLUID

9.1. OLIGOHYDRAMNIOS

INTRODUCTION

Oligohyramnios can be defined as having less than 200 mL of amniotic fluid at term or an amniotic fluid index (AFI) of less than 5 cm or presence of the largest pocket of fluid, which does not measure more than 1 cm at its largest diameter.

ETIOLOGY

Known causes of oligohydramnios include the following:

- Premature rupture of the membranes
- *Birth defects*: Birth defects, especially those involving the kidneys and urinary tract, e.g. renal agenesis, or obstruction of the urinary tract (posterior urethral valves)
- *Post-term pregnancy (≥ 40 weeks)*
- *Placental dysfunction*: Presence of amnion nodosum (squamous metaplasia of amnion) on the placenta
- *Maternal health conditions*: GDM, preeclampsia, chronic hypertension, etc.
- *Certain medications*: Medications including ACE inhibitors, prostaglandin inhibitors (aspirin, etc.) can cause oligohydramnios
- Fetal chromosomal abnormalities
- IUGR associated with placental insufficiency

DIAGNOSIS

Clinical Presentation

- The patient may give a history of experiencing reduced fetal movements
- Fundal height is less than that estimated on the basis of LMP
- Uterus appears full of fetus
- Evidence of IUGR may be present.

Investigations

Ultrasound examination: Findings are same as that described in "introduction" **(Fig. 4.17)**.

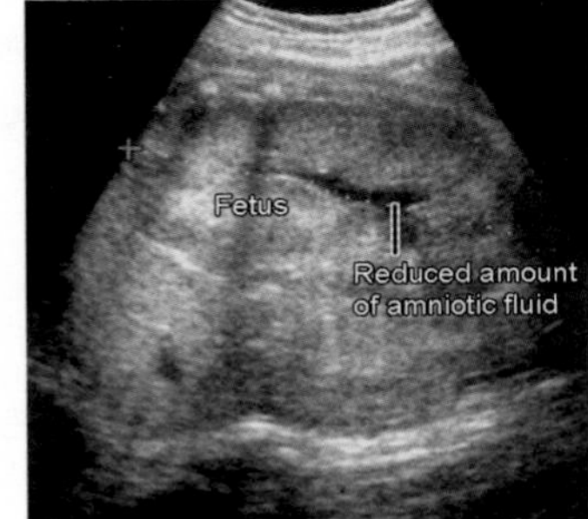

Figure 4.17: Ultrasound scan of 26 weeks old fetus showing oligohydramnios

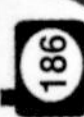

OBSTETRIC MANAGEMENT

- Women with otherwise normal pregnancies who develop oligohydramnios near term probably need no treatment because in most of these cases, oligohydramnios would resolve itself without treatment
- Hospitalization may also be sometimes required in severe cases
- *Reduced physical activity*: Many providers advise women to observe bed rest
- *Maternal hydration*: Simple maternal hydration has been suggested as a way of increasing amniotic fluid volume
- *Amnioinfusion*: This method, involves infusion of sterile water through the cervix into the uterine cavity. This treatment may help to reduce complications during labor and delivery and reduce the requirement for cesarean section
- *Fetal surveillance*: Close fetal surveillance of these patients in the form of weekly (or more frequent) ultrasound examinations to measure the level of amniotic fluid, tests of fetal well-being, such as the non-stress test, biophysical profile, etc. may also be required. If one of these tests shows abnormality, early delivery by fastest route may be required even if the fetus is preterm.

COMPLICATIONS

Complications during early pregnancy: These include the following:

- Restriction of the amount of free space inside the uterine cavity
- Amniotic adhesions causing deformities or constriction of the umbilical cord
- Pressure deformities such as clubfeet.

Complications during the late pregnancy: These include the following:

- Fetal distress, IUGR
- Cord compression, resulting in fetal hypoxia and asphyxia
- Prolonged rupture of membranes
- Fetal malformations (renal agenesis, polycystic kidneys, urethral obstruction, etc.)
- Postmaturity syndrome
- Birth defects (compression of fetal organs, resulting in lung and limb defects)
- Miscarriage, premature birth, stillbirth
- Increased risk of meconium aspiration syndrome
- Increased requirement for operative delivery.

CLINICAL PEARLS

- Normal amount of amniotic fluid varies from 700 mL to 1 L in amount, whereas the normal AFI ranges between 5 cm and 25 cm
- Induction of labor may not always be the best option in all cases of oligohydramnios due to increased chances of fetal distress
- Early onset oligohydroamnios, in comparison to that with a late onset, often results in poor outcomes.

9.2. POLYHYDRAMNIOS

INTRODUCTION

Polyhydramnios is defined as presence of amniotic fluid volume of 2,000 mL or greater at term **(Fig. 4.18)**. The varying degrees of polyhydramnios **(Table 4.13)** are based on the measurement of the largest vertical pocket of liquor.

Table 4.13: Degrees of polyhydroamnios

Grading	*Criteria*
Mild	Largest vertical pocket of liquor measures 8–11 cm
Moderate	Largest vertical pocket of liquor measured 12–15 cm
Severe	Largest vertical pocket of liquor measures ≥ 16 cm

ETIOLOGY

In about two-thirds of cases, the cause of polyhydramnios is unknown. Polyhydramnios is more likely to occur due to the following causes:

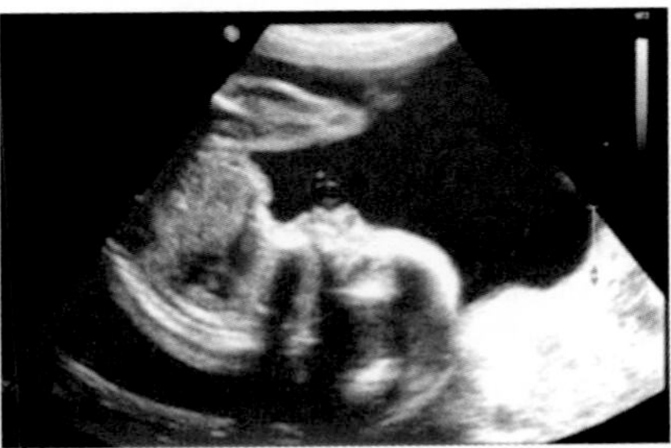

Figure 4.18: Fetus with polyhydramnios

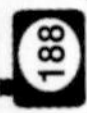

Fetal causes: These include the following:

- *Congenital abnormalities*: The most common birth defects that cause polyhydramnios are those that hinder fetal swallowing, such as birth defects involving the gastrointestinal tract and central nervous system (e.g. esophageal atresia, anencephaly, etc.)
- *Twin-twin transfusion syndrome*
- *Parvovirus B19 infection.*

Maternal causes: These include multiple gestations, maternal diabetes, and Rh blood incompatibilities between mother and fetus.

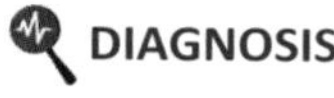

DIAGNOSIS

Clinical Presentation

Women with minor polyhydramnios experience few symptoms. Those who are more severely affected may experience the following symptoms:

- Difficulty in breathing
- Presence of large varicosities in the legs and/or vulva
- Presence of new hemorrhoids or the worsening of those present previously.

Abdominal Examination

- Abdomen is markedly enlarged, along with fullness of flanks
- The skin of the abdominal wall appears to be tense, shiny and may show appearance of large striae
- Clinically, the patients have a fundal height greater than the period of amenorrhea
- Fetal heart sounds may appear muffled as if coming from a distance
- A fluid thrill may be commonly present
- It may be difficult to palpate the uterus or the fetal presenting parts due to presence of excessive fluid.

Investigations

Ultrasound examination: The various grades of polyhydramnios based on the ultrasound findings have been previously described in **Table 4.13**.

MANAGEMENT

Mild degree of hydramnios usually resolves on its own without any treatment. No active management may be required in patients with

asymptomatic hydramnios. For patients showing symptomatic hydramnios, the following treatment options are available:

- *Treatment of the underlying cause*
- *Decompression by amniocentesis*: Amniocentesis is a procedure involving the removal of a sample of amniotic fluid in order to provide relief against symptoms, such as respiratory embarrassment, excessive uterine activity or premature opening of cervical os, etc.

COMPLICATIONS

Maternal

- Respiratory compromise
- Antepartum and postpartum hemorrhage
- Abnormal fetal presentations
- Uterine dysfunction, gestational diabetes
- Increased incidence of operative intervention
- Increased risk of premature delivery and PROM
- Increased risk of placental abruption and stillbirth.

10. Rh NEGATIVE PREGNANCY

INTRODUCTION

Rh blood group system (rhesus blood group classification system) is the most important blood group system after the ABO blood group system. Although the Rh system contains five main antigens (C, c, D, E and e), antigen D is considered to be the most immunogenic. According to the rhesus classification, the blood groups can be classified as Rh positive (those having D antigen) and Rh negative (those not having D antigen).

ETIOLOGY

The pathogenesis of Rh isoimmunization is shown in **Figure 4.19**.

DIAGNOSIS

Clinical Presentation

Clinical manifestations in the neonate can include the following:

- Hydrops fetalis, icterus gravis neonatorum and congenital anemia of the newborn
- Hemolysis often results in hyperbilirubinemia, which may cause kernicterus

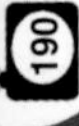

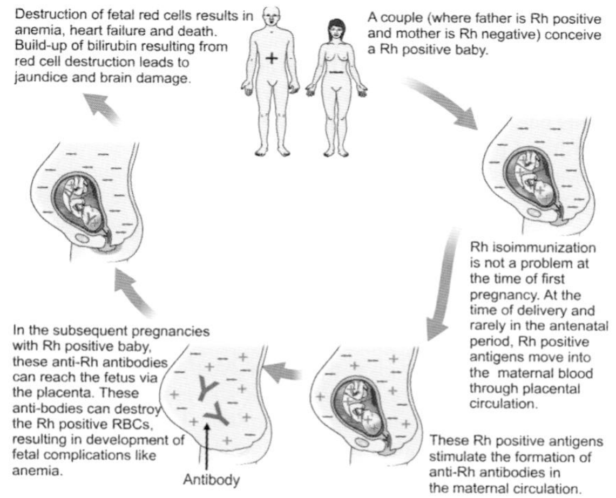

Figure 4.19: Pathogenesis of Rh isoimmunization

Investigations

- Blood grouping (both ABO and Rh)
- *Coomb's test*: In this test the maternal serum is incubated with Rh positive erythrocytes and Coomb's serum (antiglobulin antibodies). The red cells will agglutinate, if Rh antibodies are present in the maternal plasma
- *Kleihauer-Betke test*: This is a blood test for measuring the amount of fetal hemoglobin transferred from a fetus to mother's bloodstream as a result of fetomaternal hemorrhage.

OBSTETRIC MANAGEMENT

Antenatal Management

The Rh negative women whose husbands are Rh positive can be divided into two groups: Rh negative non-immunized women and the Rh negative immunized women:

- *Rh negative non-immunized women*: The indirect Coomb's test in order to detect the presence of any new antibodies, which may develop during the pregnancy, needs to be carried out at 20, 24 and 28 weeks of gestation. In case, the antibody screen is negative, the patient should

be administered 300 μg of immunoglobulins at 28 weeks of gestation. After delivery of the baby, the Rh status of the newborn is to be checked. If the baby is Rh positive, 300 μg of anti-D immunoglobulins must be administered within 72 hours of delivery. In case the antibody screen turns out to be positive, the woman must be further managed as Rh sensitized pregnancy

- *Rh negative immunized women*: In Rh negative immunized women, the main objective of the management is to diagnose and treat fetal anemia as soon as possible. This can be done through one of the following ways: measurement of the peak systolic velocity (PSV) of the fetal middle cerebral artery; Doppler ultrasound; amniocentesis and amniotic fluid analysis; ultrasound examination of the fetus and percutaneous umbilical cord blood sampling (cordocentesis).

Amniotic fluid analysis involves determination of bilirubin concentration in the amniotic fluid and spectrophotometric analysis. The OD 450 values are plotted on Liley's chart **(Fig. 4.20)**. Zone 3 on the Liley's curve corresponds to severely affected infants, zone 2 to moderately affected infants and zone 1 to unaffected or mildly affected infants. If bilirubin levels in amniotic fluid remain normal, the pregnancy can be allowed to continue to term and the clinician can await spontaneous labor. If bilirubin levels are elevated, indicating impending intrauterine death, the fetus can be given intrauterine blood transfusions at 10-day to 2-week intervals, generally until 35–36 weeks of gestation, following which the delivery is usually performed by 37–38 weeks. If at any time, the OD 450 value lies in the zone 3 or shows a rising trend, the fetus is in imminent danger of the intrauterine death. In these cases cordocentesis must be done and fetal hemoglobin values must be determined. If fetal hematocrit values are less than 30%, intrauterine transfusion is indicated. Treatment of fetal anemia can be in the form of in-utero transfusion (intraperitoneal or intravascular), if fetal anemia is severe or exchange transfusion after birth.

Intrapartum Management

- *Precautions to be taken at the time of delivery*: Following steps must be taken to minimize the chances of fetomaternal bleeding during the time of delivery:
  - Prophylactic ergometrine with the delivery of the anterior shoulder must be withheld
  - If the manual removal of the placenta is required, it should be performed gently

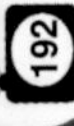

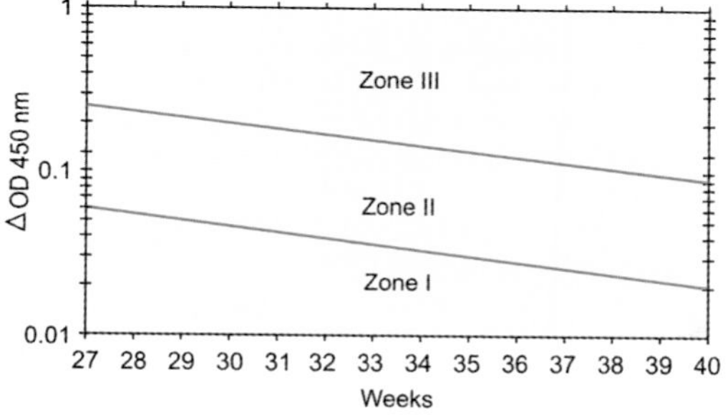

Figure 4.20: Liley's chart

- ○ Rh positive blood transfusion must be preferably avoided in Rh negative woman right from birth until menopause
- ○ Invasive procedures, like amniocentesis, chorionic villus sampling, etc., should be followed by administration of 300 µg of anti-Rh immunoglobulins, except for the cases of first trimester abortion where the dose required in 50 µg
- ○ Careful fetal monitoring needs to be performed during the time of labor
- ○ Delivery should be as nontraumatic as possible
- ○ The clinician should remain vigilant regarding the possibility for the occurrence of PPH
- ○ Umbilical cord should be clamped as soon as possible to minimize the chances of fetomaternal hemorrhage
- ○ At the time of cesarean section, all precautions should be taken to prevent any spillage of blood into the peritoneal cavity.

COMPLICATIONS

Fetal

- *Erythroblastosis fetalis*: Clinical manifestations of erythroblastosis fetalis include hydrops fetalis, icterus gravis neonatorum and congenital anemia of the newborn. Excessive destruction of fetal RBCs results in hyperbilirubinemia, jaundice and/or kernicterus, which can lead to deafness, speech problems, cerebral palsy or mental retardation

- *Hydrops fetalis*: This is a condition, characterized by an accumulation of fluids within the baby's body, resulting in development of ascites, pleural effusion, pericardial effusion, skin edema, etc.

Maternal

- Recurrent miscarriages and intrauterine deaths
- Complications, such as abortion and preterm labor, are related to procedures, such as fetal cord blood sampling.

CLINICAL PEARLS

- Rh positive ABO compatible blood can be transfused to Rh negative males in case of emergency as a life saving procedure. However, such transfusions must be avoided in Rh negative females from birth until menopause due to the risk of acceleration of the process of Rh isoimmunization process in case the Rh negative woman marries an Rh positive man and conceives an Rh positive child
- Cordocentesis, is a diagnostic test which aims at detection of fetal anomalies (e.g. chromosomal anomalies like Down's syndrome; blood disorders like hemolytic anemia, etc.) through direct examination of fetal blood.

11. VOMITING IN PREGNANCY

INTRODUCTION

Nausea and vomiting in pregnancy, commonly known as "morning sickness", affects approximately 75–85% of pregnant women. Morning sickness is generally a mild, self-limited condition, commonly encountered between 4th and 7th week of pregnancy, diminishing greatly in intensity by 14–16 weeks of pregnancy. On the other hand, a severe form of morning sickness, hyperemesis gravidarum (HG) is a syndrome defined as severe nausea and vomiting in early pregnancy associated with weight loss of more than 5% during early pregnancy.

ETIOLOGY

The exact pathology behind morning sickness remains unknown; however, many theories have been proposed:

- Relaxation of gastrointestinal muscles occurring as a result of hormones such as estrogen and relaxin
- Possible role of the bacteria, such as, *Helicobacter pylori*

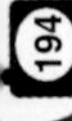

- HG may be caused by high serum hCG and estradiol concentrations (e.g. pregnancy-related conditions like multiple pregnancies, H. mole, etc.).

DIAGNOSIS

Clinical Presentation

HG is characterized by severe persistent vomiting, dehydration, ketosis, electrolyte disturbances and weight loss (> 5% of body weight). Morning sickness, on the other hand, is associated with nausea and vomiting of mild-moderate degree.

Investigations

- Serum electrolytes, urine for ketones
- Thyroid function tests.

DIFFERENTIAL DIAGNOSIS

Various causes of severe vomiting during pregnancy are listed in **Table 4.14**.

Table 4.14: Differential diagnosis of severe vomiting during pregnancy

Common pregnancy related causes of hyperemesis gravidarum	*Common non-pregnancy related causes of severe vomiting*
• Gestational trophoblastic disease • Triploidy, Trisomy 21 • Hydrops fetalis • Multiple gestation • History of hyperemesis gravidarum in previous pregnancy	• Gastrointestinal disorders (e.g. gastroenteritis, hepatitis, etc.) • Genitourinary disorders (e.g. pyelonephritis, kidney stones, etc.) • Metabolic disorders (e.g. diabetic ketoacidosis, hyperthyroidism, etc.) • Neurological disorders (e.g. CNS tumors, etc.)

Source: Quinlan JD, Hill DA. Nausea and vomiting of pregnancy. Am Fam Physician. 2003;68(1):121-8.

OBSTETRIC MANAGEMENT

Management of cases of morning sickness is described in **Figure 4.21**, **Box 4.5** and **Table 4.15**.

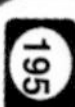

Box 4.5: Lifestyle and dietary changes

- Chewing a piece of dry food (toasted bread, etc.) before getting out of bed
- Avoiding fatty and spicy foods
- Consuming five portions of fresh foods and vegetables and drinking eight glasses of water daily
- Eating small meals multiple times a day
- Eating a protein rich snack at bed-time
- Sucking on some candy, a piece of lemon, etc. in between meals
- Emotional and psychological support.

Table 4.15: Commonly prescribed therapeutic options for morning sickness

Medicine	*Dosage*	*Route*
Pyridoxine (vitamin B6)	25 mg, 3 times/day (or 75 mg/day)	Oral
Metoclopramide (antimotility drug)	5–10 mg, 3–4 times/day	Oral
Promethazine (phenergan)	25 mg at every 4 hourly or 150 mg/day	Orally or rectally
Prednisolone (corticosteroids)	40–60 mg/day reducing by half at every 3 days followed by tapering over 2 weeks	Oral
Ondansetron (zofran)	4–8 mg, 2–3 times/day	Oral
Ginger	1 gm/day (powdered ginger) in divided doses	Can be used in the following forms: biscuits, ginger crystals, powder, tablets, capsules,fresh ginger, teas, preserves, ginger ale, etc.

 COMPLICATIONS

Morning sickness usually has no negative maternal or fetal consequences. Complications associated with HG are as follows:

Maternal: These include the following:
- Increased incidence of maternal mortality

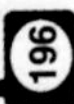

- Splenic avulsion, esophageal rupture, Mallory-Weiss tears, pneumothorax, Wernicke-Korsakoff syndrome
- Increase in the incidence of preeclampsia.

Fetal: These include fetal growth retardation and fetal anomalies.

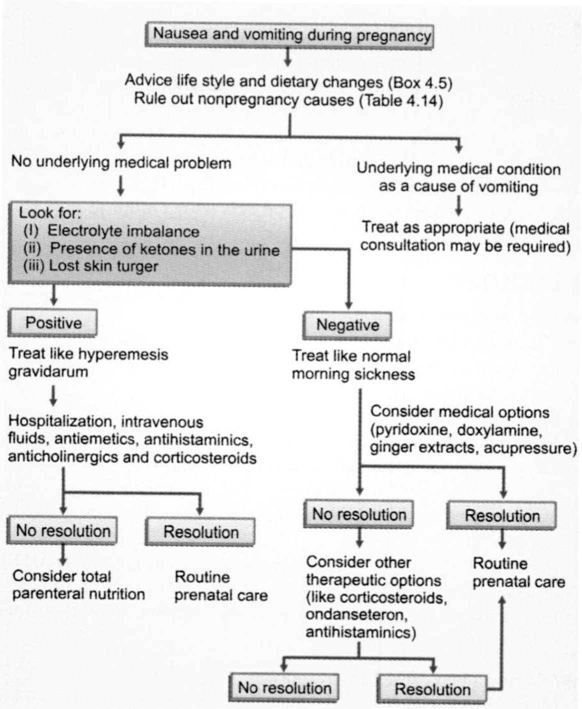

Figure 4.21: Algorithm for the suggested evaluation and management of women with nausea and vomiting of pregnancy

CLINICAL PEARLS

- Emotional support from family, especially the spouse, helps the women in effectively dealing with the condition.

12. INTRAUTERINE GROWTH RETARDATION

INTRODUCTION

IUGR refers to low-birth-weight infants whose birth weight is below the 10th percentile of the average for the particular gestational age. Even if the infant's birth weight is less than 10th percentile, he/she may not be pathologically growth restricted. These infants are termed as small for gestational age and have simply failed to achieve a specific weight or biometric size in accordance with the gestational age. However, if the growth restriction is due to some pathological process (either intrinsic or extrinsic), it is known as IUGR.

ETIOLOGY

Maternal: Maternal causes are as follows:

- Constitutionally small mothers or low maternal weight
- Excessive alcohol intake
- Strenuous physical exercise
- Poor socioeconomic conditions
- Maternal anemia, especially sickle cell anemia
- Tobacco smoking, drug abuse during pregnancy
- Chronic placental insufficiency due to preeclampsia, chronic hypertension, renal disease, connective tissue disorders, gestational diabetes, etc.
- Maternal hypoxia (e.g. pulmonary diseases, cyanotic congenital heart disease, etc.)
- Endocrine disorders (e.g. diabetic nephropathy, hyperthyroidism, Addison's disease).

Fetal: Various fetal causes are as follows:

- Multiple pregnancy
- Congenital malformations (e.g. congenital heart disease, renal agenesis, etc.)
- Chromosomal abnormalities (e.g. trisomy 13, 16, 18, 21, etc.)
- Chronic intrauterine infection, e.g. congenital syphilis, TORCH, viral, bacterial, protozoal and spirochetal infections.

Placental: Placental abnormalities including chorioangioma, circumvallate placenta, marginal or velamentous cord insertion, placenta previa, placenta abruption, etc. may also be responsible.

DIAGNOSIS

Abdominal Examination

- A lag of 4 cm or more on symphysis-fundal height measurement is suggestive of fetal growth restriction
- Reduced size of the fetus (in lieu of the gestational age) can be estimated on abdominal examination
- Palpation of fetal head gives an estimation of fetal size and maturity.

Investigations

Ultrasound biometry: This includes measurement of crown-rump length (**Fig. 4.22**); biparietal diameter (**Fig. 4.23**); abdominal circumference (**Fig. 4.24**); femur length (**Fig. 4.25**); transverse cerebellar diameter (**Fig. 4.26**); and ultrasound estimated fetal weight. Ratio of various diameters, such as head circumference or abdominal circumference (HC/AC ratio); transverse cerebellar diameter/abdominal circumference (TCD/AC ratio) and femoral length/abdominal circumference (FL/AC ratio), can also be used. Fetal ponderal index (FPI) is another ultrasound measured fetal index (FPI) for predicting IUGR, which is calculated with the help of the following formula:

$$FPI = \frac{\text{Estimated fetal weight}}{\text{Femur length}^3}$$

Biophysical tests: These tests help in assessing fetal wellbeing:

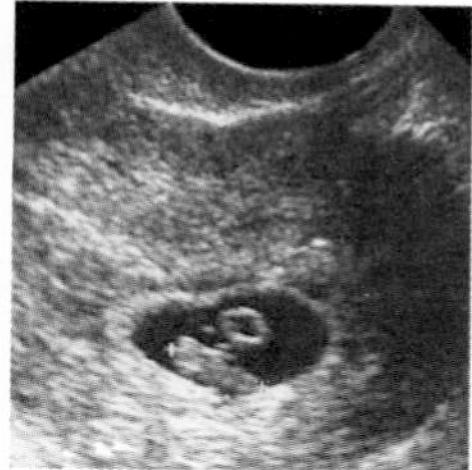

Figure 4.22: Ultrasound measurement of CRL

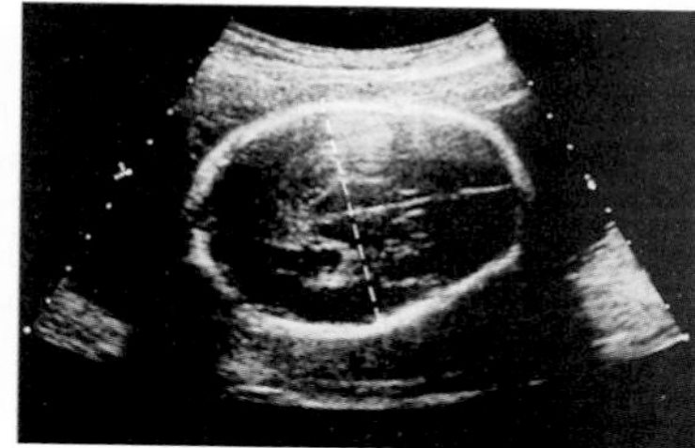

Figure 4.23: Ultrasound measurement of BPD

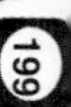

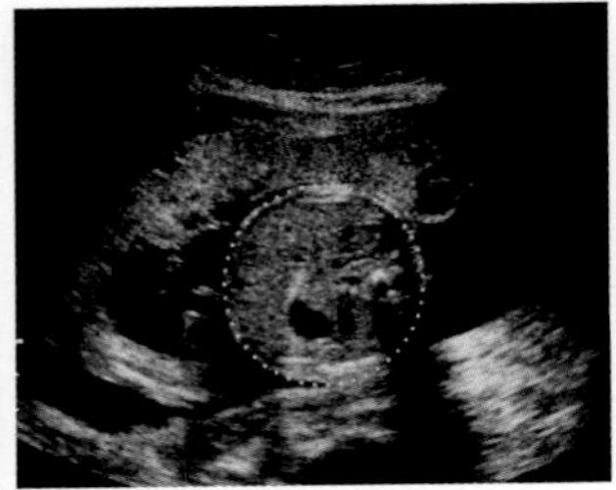
Figure 4.24: Ultrasound measurement of abdominal circumference

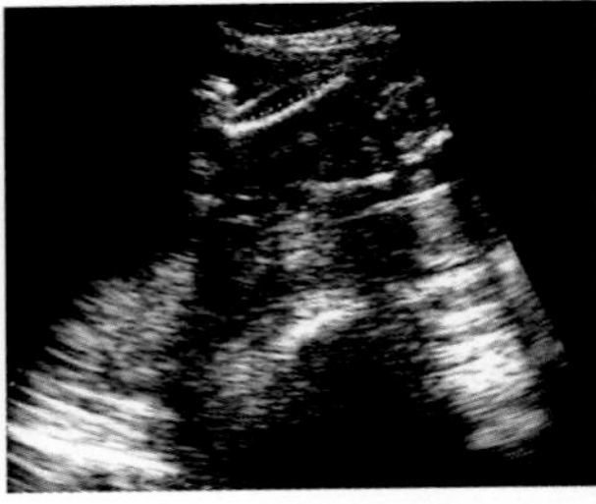
Figure 4.25: Ultrasound measurement of femur length

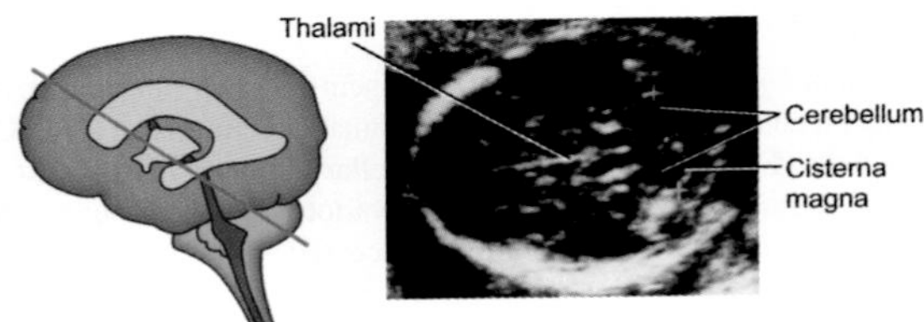

Figure 4.26: Measurement of transverse cerebellar diameter

- Non-stress test
- Biophysical profile, amniotic fluid volume
- Ultrasound Doppler flow velocimetry
- Fetal cardiotocography.

OBSTETRIC MANAGEMENT

Antenatal Period

- Identifying the underlying cause for IUGR
- Women must be advised to take rest in the left lateral position for a period of at least 10 hours everyday
- *Daily fetal movement count*: In case the woman perceives less than 6 fetal movements within 2 hours, she should be advised to immediately consult her doctor.

Intrapartum Period

Since the growth restricted fetus is especially prone to develop asphyxia, continuous fetal monitoring using external or internal cardiotocographic examination needs to be done in the intrapartum period. If, at any time, the fetal heart rate appears to be non-reassuring, an emergency cesarean may be required. However elective cesarean section is not justified for delivery of all IUGR fetuses. Administration of intramuscular corticosteroids is required in case the delivery takes place between 24 and 36 weeks of gestation. Presently the RCOG (2002) recommends that the clinician needs to individualize each patient and decide the time for delivery by weighing the risk of fetal demise due to delayed intervention against the risk of long-term disabilities resulting from preterm delivery due to early intervention.

COMPLICATIONS

Fetal

Antepartum: This includes:

- Fetal hypoxia and acidosis
- Stillbirth
- Oligohydramnios.

Intrapartum: This includes:

- Neonatal asphyxia and acidosis
- Respiratory distress syndrome
- Meconium aspiration syndrome
- Persistent fetal circulation
- Intraventricular bleeding, neonatal encephalopathy.

Neonatal period: This includes:

- Hypoglycemia (glucose levels of < 30 mg/dL): It can be associated with symptoms like jitteriness, twitching, apnea, etc.
- Hypoinsulinemia, hypertriglyceridemia
- Hypocalcemia and hyperphosphatemia
- Meconium aspiration and/or birth asphyxia
- Hypothermia
- Hyperbilirubinemia, polycythemia, hyperviscosity syndrome
- Sepsis, necrotizing enterocolitis
- Complications, such as cerebral palsy in long term.

CLINICAL PEARLS

- The fetal abdominal circumference (AC) and expected fetal weight can be considered as the most accurate parameters for predicting IUGR
- Crown-rump length of 15–60 mm (corresponding to gestational period varying from 8 to 12.5 weeks) is found to have greatest accuracy in determining the period of gestation in the first trimester

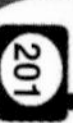

- The major Doppler detectable modifications in the fetal circulation associated with IUGR and fetal hypoxemia include increased resistance in the umbilical artery, fetal peripheral vessels and maternal uterine vessels, in association with decreased resistance in the fetal cerebral vessels.

13. THYROID DISORDERS DURING PREGNANCY

INTRODUCTION

The major changes related in thyroid function during normal pregnancy are increase in serum thyroxine-binding globulin (TBG) concentrations; stimulation of the thyrotropin receptor by chorionic gonadotropin; TBG excess resulting in an increase in the concentration of both serum total thyroxine (T4) and triiodothyronine (T3), whereas free serum T4 and T3 concentrations remain within normal range. Moreover, the levels of thyroid stimulating hormone (TSH) do not change during pregnancy. Maternal thyroxine is transferred to the fetus throughout pregnancy. This hormone is important for normal fetal brain development especially before the development of fetal thyroid glands.

ETIOLOGY

- *Hyperthyroidism*: The commonest cause is Grave's disease
- *Hypothyroidism*: Common causes are autoimmune thyroiditis (e.g. Hashimoto's thyroiditis); radiotherapy or surgery; drugs (e.g. lithium, amiodarone, etc.); iodine deficiency; pituitary or hypothalamic disease; etc.

DIAGNOSIS

Clinical Presentation

- *Hypothyroidism*: The various symptoms include dry skin with yellowing especially around eyes, hair loss, weakness, tiredness, fatigue, hoarseness, constipation, sleep disturbance, depression, cold intolerance, muscle cramps, weight gain , edema, dry skin, prolonged relaxation phase of deep tendon reflexes and/or a pathologically enlarged thyroid gland or goiter (in cases of endemic iodine deficiency or Hashimoto's thyroiditis).

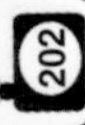

- *Hyperthyroidism*: The various symptoms include palpitations, nervousness, irritability, breathlessness, tachycardia, tremors in hands, heat intolerance, insomnia, increased bowel movements, light or absent menstrual periods, weight loss, muscle weakness, warm moist skin, hair loss, nervousness, etc.

Investigations

- *Hyperthyroidism*: The diagnosis of hyperthyroidism in pregnant women should be based primarily on serum TSH value less than 0.01 mU/ liter and a high serum free T4 value
- *Hypothyroidism*: Hypothyroidism is characterized by low T4 levels and raised TSH levels.

MANAGEMENT

- *Hyperthyroidism*: Thionamides [propylthiouracil (PTU), methimazole and carbimazole] are recommended for the treatment of moderate to severe hyperthyroidism complicating pregnancy. Beta blockers may be given to ameliorate the symptoms of moderate to severe hyperthyroidism in pregnant women
- Ablation with radioiodine is absolutely contraindicated during pregnancy due to the possibility of the ablation of thyroid tissue as well, which is usually present by 10–12 weeks of gestation
- Replacement therapy with levothyroxine is administered in the dosage of 1–2 μg/kg/day (approximately 100 μg/day) in cases of hypothyroidism.

COMPLICATIONS

- *Hyperthyroidism*: This includes complications, such as spontaneous abortion or miscarriage, premature labor, low-birth-weight, stillbirth, preeclampsia, heart failure, thyroid storm (rarely), fetal or neonatal hyperthyroidism or hypothyroidism, with or without a goiter, non-immune hydrops and fetal demise
- *Hypothyroidism*: This includes complications, such as preeclampsia, gestational hypertension, placental abruption, nonreassuring fetal heart rate tracing, preterm delivery, low birth weight, increased rate of cesarean section, neuropsychological and cognitive impairment, postpartum hemorrhage, and overall increased rate of perinatal morbidity and mortality.

CLINICAL PEARLS

- Serum TSH is the most reliable indicator of genuine hypothyroidism
- Overt hypothyroidism complicating pregnancy is unusual because hypothyroidism may be associated with anovulation, as well as a high rate of first trimester spontaneous abortion.

14. CONNECTIVE TISSUE DISEASES DURING PREGNANCY

INTRODUCTION

Connective tissue disorders are characterized by production of antibodies to components of cell nucleus, resulting in autoantibody mediated connective tissue abnormalities. There is a deposition of immune complexes at specific organ or tissue sites, thereby affecting them. Systemic lupus erythematosus (SLE), a heterogeneous autoimmune disorder is one of the commonest connective tissue disorders characterized by the presence of antinuclear antibodies (ANA) directed against components of cell nucleus.

ETIOLOGY

- Unknown
- Genetic factors (high concordance rate among twins)
- Environmental factors such as sunlight (UV rays), stress, etc.
- Viral or other type of infection
- Drugs (e.g. hydralazine, procainamide and isoniazid).

DIAGNOSIS

Clinical Presentation

Diagnosis of SLE is clinical and may be made using the revised criteria of the American Rheumatism Association (1997) **(Box 4.6)**. The diagnosis is made, if four or more classification criteria are present.

Box 4.6: The revised criteria of the American Rheumatism Association

1. *Malar (butterfly) rash*: Fixed erythema, flat or raised, over malar eminences, with a tendency to spare nasolabial folds
2. *Discoid lupus*: Erythematous raised patches with scaling and follicular plugging
3. *Photosensitivity*: Skin rash resulting from hypersensitivity reaction to sunlight

Contd...

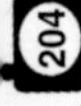

Contd...

4. *Oral or nasopharyngeal ulcers*: These are usually painless
5. *Non-erosive arthritis*: Involving two or more peripheral joints, often accompanied with tenderness, and swelling
6. *Serositis*: This could be manifested in the form of pleuritis or pericarditis
7. *Renal involvement*: Persistent proteinuria (> 0.5 gm/day or 3+ on dipstick) or cellular casts (red cell, hemoglobin, granular, tubular or mixed)
8. *Neurological disorders*: Seizures or psychosis without any underlying organic cause
9. *Hematologic disorder*: This may be characterized by hemolytic anemia with reticulocytosis, or leukopenia (leukocyte count < 4,000 on two occasions) or lymphopenia (absolute lymphocyte count < 1,500/mm^3 on at least two occasions) or thrombocytopenia (platelet count < 100,000/mm^3 without any history of using thrombocytopenic drugs)
10. *Immunologic disorder*: This may be characterized by the presence of anti-DNA antibodies (anti-dsDNA) in abnormal titer, anti-Sm antibodies, false-positive VDRL test or positive finding of antiphospholipid antibodies, such as IgG or IgM anticardiolipin antibodies, or positive test for lupus anticoagulant using standard method
11. *Antinuclear antibodies*: Abnormal titers of ANAs in the absence of drugs.

Source: Hochberg MC. Updating the American College of Rheumatology revised criteria for the classification of systemic lupus erythematosus. Arthritis Rheum. 1997;40(9):1725.

Investigations

- *Detection of autoimmune antibodies*: Identification of ANAs is the best screening test. However, this test is not specific for lupus. Other antibodies which can be present include antidouble stranded (ds)-DNA, anti-Sm (Smith antigen), anti-SSA (anti-Ro), anti-SSB (anti-La), anti-histone, antiphospholipid antibodies, etc. Of these, antibodies, such as anti-Sm and ds-DNA, are quite specific
- *Blood investigations*: The following findings may be observed:
  - Positive Coomb's test (hemolysis may be observed)
  - Anemia
  - Thrombocytopenia
  - Leucopenia
  - *D-dimer levels*: Elevated serum D-dimer levels may commonly follow a flare or infection
  - *Liver function tests*: Hepatic involvement is suggested by increased serum levels of bilirubin or serum transaminase activity
  - Rheumatoid factor
- *Urine for proteins*: New-onset or worsening of pre-existing proteinuria could be suggestive of the disease.

OBSTETRIC MANAGEMENT

- *Preconceptional counseling*: Women must be counseled regarding the effect of the disease on the pregnancy outcome
- *Prenatal visits*: Frequent follow-up with prenatal visits (weekly visits after 28 weeks) are required
- *Fetal surveillance*: In pregnant women, close monitoring of fetal growth needs to be done (e.g. weekly NST after 28 weeks)
- *Patient monitoring*: The patient needs to be regularly monitored for thrombocytopenia and proteinuria
- *Mode of delivery*: There is no need for a routine cesarean delivery in these cases. Cesarean section may be required in cases of obstetric complications or fetuses with congenital heart block
- There is no cure for the disease and complete remission is rare. The drugs, which can be used include NSAIDs (for relief from mild aches and pains); corticosteroids (for severe flare-ups); immunosuppressive agents (azathioprine); cyclophosphamide; methotrexate (for arthritis); antimalarials (e.g. hydroxychloroquine to control skin disease), etc.
- *Breastfeeding*: Breastfeeding is recommended even for women with SLE.

COMPLICATIONS

Maternal: These include the following:
- Preeclampsia
- Fetal loss, low-birth-weight infant
- Deep vein thrombosis or pulmonary embolism
- Renal impairment, chronic hypertension
- Recurrence: Risk of neonatal lupus in subsequent pregnancies is 17%

Fetal: These include the following:
- Preterm delivery
- Fetal growth restriction
- Stillbirths
- Neonatal lupus: This is characterized by lupus dermatitis (red, raised rash on the scalp and around the eyes), a number of hematological and systematic derangements, congenital heart block, etc.
- SLE complications in babies: Complete heart block and learning disabilities.

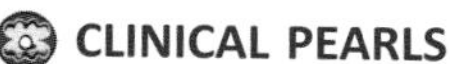

CLINICAL PEARLS

- Outcome is best for mother and baby when SLE has been controlled for at least 6 months prior to pregnancy
- Approximately one-third of the women with SLE may have flare-ups during pregnancy.

15. PREVIOUS CESAREAN DELIVERY

INTRODUCTION

With the increasing incidence of operative abdominal deliveries (cesarean births), the number of patients with the previous history of one or more previous cesarean births, being encountered in clinical practice is progressively on rise. As a result the obstetrician must be well-versed in dealing with the complications related to previous cesarean birth.

DIAGNOSIS

Clinical Presentation

A complete history of previous cesarean births must be taken including the type of the scar given (classical or the lower segment); any technical difficulties encountered during the procedure; the reason for which the cesarean birth was performed; and whether there was any history of complications during the surgery.

General Physical Examination

The obstetrician must be particularly vigilant regarding the detection of signs of impending scar rupture, which include the following:

- Dull suprapubic pain or severe abdominal pain, especially, if persisting in-between the uterine contractions
- Slight vaginal bleeding or hematuria
- Bladder tenesmus or frequent desire to pass urine
- Unexplained maternal tachycardia
- Maternal hypotension
- Chest pain, shoulder tip pain or sudden onset of shortness of breath.

Abdominal Examination

- Besides the routine obstetric abdominal examination, careful examination of the abdominal scar and elicitation of scar tenderness is important
- Abnormal fetal heart rate pattern may be observed on external carditocography.

Investigations

- Routine ANC investigations including blood grouping (ABO and Rh typing)
- Complete blood count
- Ultrasound examination.

MANAGEMENT

In the past, management of the patient with a history of cesarean scar was considered as "once a cesarean, always a cesarean". This dictum has now been changed to "once a cesarean, always hospitalization". Presently, the two most commonly used options for delivery in these patients comprise of vaginal birth after cesarean (VBAC) delivery and elective repeat cesarean section (ERCS).

Vaginal Birth after Cesarean

The criteria for VBAC are described in **Box 4.7**. With VBAC, the following steps must be observed during the intrapartum period:

- Blood should be sent for grouping, cross-matching and complete blood count (including hemoglobin and hematocrit levels). One unit of blood should be arranged
- IV access to be established and ringer lactate can be started
- Clinical monitoring of the mother for the signs of scar dehiscence needs to be done
- Careful monitoring of fetal heart rate, preferably using continuous external CTG
- The use of prostaglandins for induction of labor in women with the previous history of cesarean section must be best avoided
- Epidural analgesia can be safely given at the time of labor
- Intrapartum monitoring regarding the progress of labor must be done using a partogram
- Second stage of labor can be cut short by using prophylactic forceps or ventouse

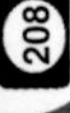

- Routine uterine exploration following VBAC is not recommended. If the patient shows signs of uterine rupture, uterine exploration may be done. Laparotomy may be required, if a uterine rent is found on the uterine exploration.

Box 4.7: Criteria for vaginal birth after cesarean birth

- Previous history of one uncomplicated lower segment transverse cesarean section
- Pelvis is adequate
- Patient is willing for VBAC
- Facilities for continuous fetal monitoring during labor are available
- No other contraindication for cesarean section
- Previous cesarean was performed for a nonrecurrent cause (e.g. fetal distress or non progress of labor)
- Facilities for emergency cesarean section are present.

Elective Repeat Cesarean Section

For the physician, ERCS may offer a few advantages including convenience, saving of time and reduced fear of legal litigation in case of complications with VBAC.

In case of previous history of classical scar, the woman must preferably be hospitalized at 36 weeks and posted for an elective cesarean section at 38 weeks. In patients with previous history of lower segment uterine scar, the planned surgery should be preferably done after 39 weeks.

COMPLICATIONS

- If VBAC turns out to be unsuccessful, an emergency cesarean section may be required
- There is a risk of the scar dehiscence and rupture, which may be associated with increased maternal and perinatal mortality
- Pelvic floor dysfunction
- ERCS may be associated with difficult surgery due to the presence of adhesions.

CLINICAL PEARLS

- The patient must be considered as high risk and frequent antenatal check-ups are required
- The identification or suspicion of uterine rupture is a medical emergency and must be followed by an immediate and urgent response

from the obstetrician. An emergency laparotomy is usually required to save the patient's life
- According to recommendations by RCOG (2007), women with the history of previous two uncomplicated low transverse cesarean sections can also be considered for the planned VBAC.

16. BAD OBSTETRIC HISTORY

INTRODUCTION

This can be defined as a condition in which the present obstetric outcome is likely to be adversely affected by the cause of previous obstetric mishap.

ETIOLOGY

In most cases the causes remain undetermined. Some important causes of BOH are as follows:
- Genetic causes (Robertsonian translocations)
- Abnormal maternal immune response
- Hormonal causes (luteal phase defect, polycystic ovary syndrome, hypothyroidism, diabetes mellitus, hyperprolactinemia, etc.)
- Maternal infection (infections by TORCH complex, syphilis, bacterial vaginosis, etc.)
- Environmental factors (radiation exposure, occupational hazards, addictions, etc.)
- Autoimmune causes (antiphospholipid syndrome)
- Inherited thrombophilias (factor V Leiden mutation, deficiency of protein C and S, hyperhomocysteinemia)
- Structural anomalies of cervix (septate uterus, cervical incompetence)
- Anatomical causes (uterine malformations, Asherman's syndrome, uterine fibroids).

DIAGNOSIS

Clinical Presentation

Bad obstetric history could be related to recurrent miscarriage or a history of previous unfavorable fetal outcome in terms of two or more consecutive spontaneous abortions, early neonatal deaths, stillbirths, IUDs, congenital anomalies, etc.

Investigations

- Parental karyotype
- Thyroid function test

- Serum prolactin levels
- Blood glucose levels
- Blood grouping
- VDRL test for syphilis
- TORCH test
- High vaginal swab for detection of infections
- Ultrasound examination: For evaluation of uterine cavity and cervix
- Antiphospholipid antibodies such as lupus anticoagulant and anticardiolipin antibodies (IgG or IgM)
- Thrombophilia Screening for factor V Leiden, prothrombin time
- Tests for cervical incompetence: Using ultrasound examination and passage of No. 6–8 Hegars dilator through the internal os without any pain or resistance especially in the premenstrual period.

MANAGEMENT

- Diagnosis and treatment of abnormality (e.g. diabetes, thyroid dysfunction, cervical incompetence, etc.), if possible
- Provision of psychological support and alleviation of patient's anxiety
- To remain vigilant till the delivery
- Patients with positive antiphospholipid antibodies and thrombophilias must be treated with aspirin in the dosage of 50 mg daily
- In case of a thrombotic event, subcutaneous heparin in the dosage of 5,000 IU BD should be administered. Low molecular weight heparin may also prove to be useful.

COMPLICATIONS

- Recurrent fetal loss, IUD
- IUGR
- Severe preeclampsia/eclampsia/HELLP syndrome
- Placental abruption
- Recurrent thrombotic events, thrombocytopenia.

CLINICAL PEARLS

- If the cause remains undetermined, constant vigilance followed by hospitalization during the early and later months of pregnancy usually works
- If a mishap occurs in two subsequent pregnancies, it is likely to occur in the third pregnancy as well. Therefore, the obstetrician must remain vigilant regarding the same.

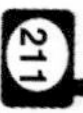

17. LIVER DISEASE DURING PREGNANCY

INTRODUCTION

Acute viral hepatitis is the most common cause of jaundice during pregnancy, the second being intrahepatic cholestasis. Other causes of jaundice specific to pregnancy include severe preeclampsia, eclampsia, HELLP syndrome, acute fatty liver, severe HG, endotoxic shock (DIC).

ETIOLOGY

The causative organisms for various types of hepatitis include hepatitis virus A, B, C, D and E.

DIAGNOSIS

Clinical Presentation

- Generalized pruritis
- Weakness, nausea, vomiting
- Jaundice: This is evident as the yellowing of sclera, nail beds and the palmer creases of hands.

Investigations

- *Increased serum bilirubin levels*: Serum bilirubin levels greater than 2 mg %
- *Liver function tests*: Increased levels of liver enzymes, such as AST, ALT and alkaline phosphatase
- *Liver biopsy*: Liver biopsy may show evidence of intrahepatic cholestasis. However, there is no evidence of hepatic necrosis.

OBSTETRIC MANAGEMENT

- General measures for prevention of hepatitis include precautions, such as provision of safe drinking water and improved sanitation; adequate care of personal hygiene; use of disposable syringes for blood collection and screening of the blood donors for HBsAg
- Infants of HBsAg-positive mothers should receive hepatitis B immune globulins (dosage 0.06 mg/kg, intramuscular)
- These infants must receive immunoprophylaxis at birth with hepatitis B vaccine (1 ml, 3 doses) at 1 week, 1 month and 6 months after birth
- The rate of vertical transmission of the neonatal hepatitis B infection is the greatest when the maternal infection occurs during the third trimester or the immediate postpartum period

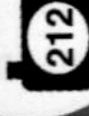

- Diphenhydramine is used for intense pruritis
- Cholestyramine or ursodeoxycholic acid is also used for itching.

There is no specific treatment for viral hepatitis; it is usually supportive and comprises of steps such as hospitalization and bed rest; patient isolation and prescription of diet rich in proteins and carbohydrates.

COMPLICATIONS

- Preterm labor, low-birth-weight babies
- Meconium stained liquor
- Intrauterine death
- Postpartum hemorrhage.

CLINICAL PEARLS

- Preeclampsia may be associated with hepatic complications, such as HELLP syndrome, acute fatty liver of pregnancy, hepatic infarction and rupture
- The course of most viral hepatitis infections, e.g. hepatitis A, B, C and D except for hepatitis E and disseminated herpes simplex virus remains unaltered by pregnancy.

18. OBSTETRIC HYSTERECTOMY

INTRODUCTION

Obstetric hysterectomy refers to the removal of the uterus at the time of a planned or unplanned cesarean section. It involves either the removal of pregnant uterus with pregnancy in situ, or the recently pregnant uterus due to some complications of delivery. Sometimes hysterectomy may be required following delivery, either vaginal or cesarean in order to save mother's life. When hysterectomy is performed at the time of cesarean delivery, the procedure is termed as the cesarean hysterectomy. If performed within the short time after vaginal delivery, it is termed as postpartum hysterectomy.

ETIOLOGY

Some important causes for emergency obstetric hysterectomy are enumerated in **Box 4.8**.

Box 4.8: Indications for obstetric hysterectomy

Obstetric emergencies
- Postpartum hemorrhage
- Intractable uterine atony
- Inverted uterus
- Coagulopathy
- Laceration of a pelvic vessel
- Sepsis (chorioamnionitis)
- Myometrial abscesses.

Cesarean delivery
- Ruptured uterus:
  - Traumatic
  - Spontaneous
- Extending pelvic hematoma
- Lateral extension of the uterine incision with the involvement of uterine vessels.

Non-emergency situations

Coexisting gynecological disorders:
- Leiomyomas
- Stage I cervical carcinoma
- Cervical intraepithelial neoplasia
- Ovarian malignancy.

Previous gynecological disorders:
- Endometritis
- PID
- Heavy and irregular menstrual bleeding
- Pelvic adhesions.

SURGICAL MANAGEMENT

Preoperative Preparation

- Hematocrit assessment
- *Blood transfusion*: Pregnant women having CS for antepartum hemorrhage, abruption, uterine rupture and placenta previa are at increased risk of blood loss greater than 1,000 mL and may require blood transfusion
- *Informed consent*: The indications for the procedure and its possible outcomes must be discussed with the patient and her partner, and an informed consent be obtained
- *Prophylactic antibiotics*: Antibiotics (single dose of first-generation cephalosporin or ampicillin) must be prescribed prior to the procedure

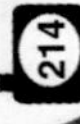

- *Prophylaxis for thromboembolism*: This could be in the form of graduated stockings, hydration, early mobilization and low molecular weight heparin
- *Preanesthetic preparation*: In order to reduce the risk of aspiration pneumonitis, the patient must be kept nil per mouth at least 12 hours prior to the surgery
- *Catheterization*: This helps in preventing injury to the urinary bladder at the time of surgery
- *Maternal position*: The woman should be positioned with left lateral tilt to avoid aortocaval compression
- *Anesthesia*: The procedure can be performed under either general or regional anesthesia (epidural or spinal block)
- *Preparation of the skin*: The pubic hair in the area around the proposed incision site must be clipped
- *Cleaning and draping*: The skin at the operation site must be cleaned with antiseptic solution and then draped in order to reduce risk of postoperative wound infections.

Steps of Surgery

- If a cesarean section has not been performed prior to the hysterectomy, a vertical midline incision must be given below the umbilicus until the pubic hairline, through the skin and to the level of the fascia
- After giving a vertical fascial incision (about 2–3 cm in length), the edges of the fascia must be held with the forceps and the incision lengthened up and down using scissors
- The rectus muscles must be separated using fingers or the scissors. Once the peritoneum has been identified, the fingers must be used for making an opening in the peritonium near the umbilicus. The incision must carefully be extended in the upward and downward direction, using a scissors
- A bladder retractor must be placed over the pubic bone and self-retracting abdominal retractors must be placed to retract the abdominal skin
- If a cesarean section has already been performed, there is no need for the above mentioned steps. In these women, following the delivery of the baby and the placenta, the uterine incision may be stitched in cases where appreciable amount of bleeding is occurring. Instead of stitching the uterine incision, sponge holding forceps or green armytage forceps can be applied at the margin of uterine incision for achieving hemostasis
- The uterus is lifted out of the abdomen and gently pulled in order to maintain erection

- The next steps of surgery are illustrated in **Figures 4.27A to G**
- Following the closure of vaginal vault, there is no need to close the bladder or abdominal peritoneum. Fascia must be closed using continuous No. 0 chromic catgut or polyglycolic sutures
- If there are no signs of infection, the skin can be closed using vertical mattress sutures of 3-0 nylon or silk and a sterile dressing may be applied.

Postoperative Care

- *Prophylactic antibiotics*: Immediately after the cord is clamped, a single dose of prophylactic antibiotics must be given intravenously
- *Monitoring the vitals*: After surgery is completed, the woman's vital parameters, amount of bleeding per vaginum, bleeding from the incision site and whether the uterus remains well-contracted or not, must be monitored in a recovery area for about 4–8 hours
- *Analgesics*: Adequate postoperative pain control is of prime importance
- *Diet*: If the surgical procedure was uncomplicated, the woman can be started on a liquid diet from the next day onward
- *Early ambulation*: The woman must be encouraged to ambulate as soon as possible, usually within 24 hours in order to prevent the development of complications such as thromboembolism
- *Dressing over the incision site*: The dressing over the incision site must be kept for the first few days after the surgery in order to protect the woman against infection.

COMPLICATIONS

- *Mortality and morbidity*: The procedure is associated with a high rate of mortality and morbidity
- *Hemorrhage*: There is an increased risk of the blood loss due to the presence of hypertrophied pelvic vessels in the pregnant women
- *Injury to the urinary tract*: Bladder injury may occur while dissecting the bladder from the scarred lower uterine segment
- *Infections*: These commonly include vaginal cuff cellulitis, abdominal incisional infections and urinary infections.

CLINICAL PEARLS

- Hysterectomy is the second most common major surgery among reproductive-aged women, after cesarean delivery
- This procedure is usually performed under emergency situations such as catastrophic uterine rupture or refractory uterine atony with life threatening hemorrhage.

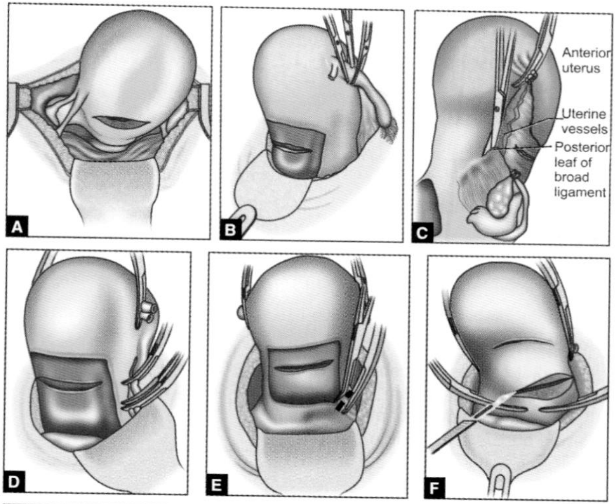

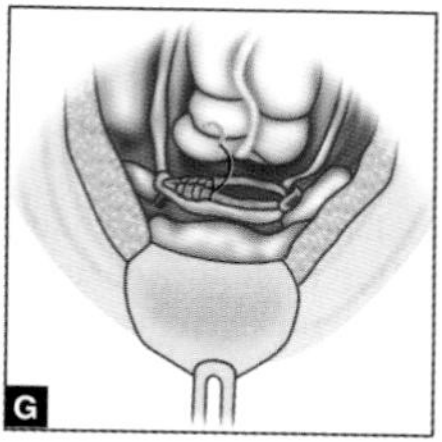

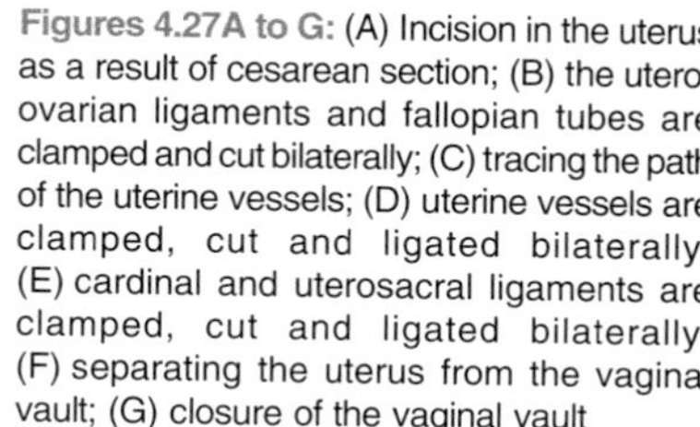

Figures 4.27A to G: (A) Incision in the uterus as a result of cesarean section; (B) the utero-ovarian ligaments and fallopian tubes are clamped and cut bilaterally; (C) tracing the path of the uterine vessels; (D) uterine vessels are clamped, cut and ligated bilaterally; (E) cardinal and uterosacral ligaments are clamped, cut and ligated bilaterally; (F) separating the uterus from the vaginal vault; (G) closure of the vaginal vault

19. INTRAUTERINE DEATH

INTRODUCTION

Intrauterine fetal death can be defined as the diagnosis of the stillborn infant (with the period of gestation being ≥ 28 weeks and fetal weight ≥ 500 gm). Fetal deaths may be divided into two: (1) antepartum IUD (fetal deaths occurring in the antenatal period) and (2) intrapartum IUD (fetal deaths occurring during labor).

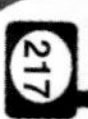

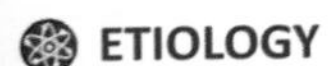

ETIOLOGY

The causes of intrauterine death have been described in **Table 4.16**.

Table 4.16: Causes of intrauterine death

Maternal causes	*Fetal causes*
• Hypertensive disorders • Antepartum hemorrhage • Diabetes • Severe anemia • Hyperpyrexia • Maternal infection • Antiphospholipid syndrome • Placental causes: Placental insufficiency, antepartum hemorrhage, cord accidents, twin-to-twin transfusion syndrome, etc.	• Chromosomal anomalies • Fetal infections • Rh incompatibility • Iatrogenic causes such as external version

DIAGNOSIS

Clinical Presentation

- Absence of fetal movement interpretation by the mother for more than a few hours
- Retrogression of the positive pregnancy changes (breast changes disappear, fundal height becomes smaller than the period of amenorrhea, uterine tone diminishes and the uterus becomes flaccid)
- No fetal heart sounds can be heard
- Fetal head shows egg-shell cracking feeling upon palpation (late sign).

Investigations

- Blood grouping (ABO and Rh) and cross-matching
- *Tests for detecting the underlying cause*: Blood sugar, thyroid function tests, TORCH screening, VDRL, thrombophilia studies, lupus anticoagulant and anticardiolipin antibodies, urine routine microscopy for pus cells and casts
- *Absent fetal heart*: Inability to detect a fetal heartbeat via Doppler
- *Sonography*: Definitive diagnosis is made by observing the lack of fetal cardiac motion during a 10-minute period of careful examination with real-time ultrasound. Late signs are oligohydramnios and collapse of cranial bones

- *X-ray abdomen*: Abdominal X-ray may show presence of Spalding sign (irregular overlapping of the cranial bones); hyperflexion of the spine; crowding of ribs and appearance of gas shadows in the heart and great vessels (Robert's sign)
- *Clotting profile*: Tests, such as blood fibrinogen levels and partial thromboplastin time, may especially be required, if the fetus has been retained for more than 2 weeks.

OBSTETRIC MANAGEMENT

- Reassurance to be provided to the bereaving parents
- Diagnosis and treatment of abnormality, if possible. In most of the cases, spontaneous expulsion occurs within 2 weeks of birth. In cases where spontaneous expulsion does not occur, induction by oxytocin infusion or prostaglandins (PGE2 gel or 25–50 mg of misoprostol) may be required
- Fibrinogen levels to be estimated on a weekly basis. Falling fibrinogen levels to be arrested by controlled infusion of heparin
- Postmortem examination: Examination of the dead baby and placenta needs to be done in order to detect the cause of death. Autopsy and chromosomal analysis for detection of fetal anomalies and dysmorphic features need to be done.

COMPLICATIONS

- Psychological upset
- Infection (typically with anaerobic infections such as *Clostridium welchii*
- Blood coagulation disorder (DIC)
- During labor: Uterine inertia, retained placanta and PPH.

CLINICAL PEARLS

- Deaths due to unexplained cause may occur in 25–35% of the cases
- For all practical purposes, fetal death occurring beyond the period of viability is known as IUD, whereas that occurring before the period of viability is known as an abortion. Stillbirth can be described as intrauterine death during labor
- IUD can be largely prevented by performing antepartum fetal assessment especially in cases with uteroplacental insufficiency
- Dead fetus may undergo aseptic degenerative process called maceration, which is associated with blistering and peeling off of the skin, usually 12–24 hours after death.

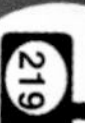

CHAPTER 5

Postnatal Period

1. PUERPERIUM

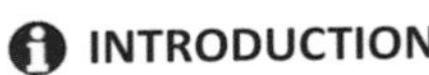

INTRODUCTION

Puerperium is the time period encompassing first few weeks following the birth during which maternal anatomy and physiology revert back to the pre-pregnancy state. This period usually lasts for 4–6 weeks and can be divided into three phases: (1) immediate phase within 24 hours; (2) early phase which lasts up to 7 days and (3) remote phase which may last for about 6 weeks.

ETIOLOGY

The changes occurring during puerperium are related to changes that occur in the various organs (especially uterus, cervix, vagina and breasts) post-delivery.

DIAGNOSIS

Clinical Examination

- *Changes in the vagina and vaginal outlet*: The vaginal outlet, which had transformed itself into a smooth-walled passage, starts returning to its pre-pregnancy state. Vaginal rugae start appearing by 3rd week. Hymen shows tags of tissue which form myrtiform caruncles
- *Cervix and lower uterine segment*: Uterine blood vessels diminish in caliber in the puerperial period. There is also narrowing and thickening of the cervical opening for several weeks following child-birth. The thinned out lower uterine segment contracts and retracts. It eventually gets converted into uterine isthmus. In the immediate postpartum period, the uterus weighs 1,000 gm and is palpable just below the umbilicus. After 1 week, it weighs about 300 gm and has descended into the true pelvis. Nearly 1 month after delivery, the uterus has regained the non-pregnant size of 100 gm

- *After-pains*: Following delivery, the uterus may contract vigorously at irregular intervals giving rise to after-pains, which are milder than uterine contractions during labor
- *Lochia*: Sloughing of the decidual tissue results in vaginal discharge of variable quality (**Table 5.1**). It comprises of erythrocytes, decidual cells, epithelial cells and bacteria. It usually persists for 4–8 weeks after delivery

Table 5.1: Characteristic features of lochia

Type of lochia	*Amount*	*Characteristics*
Lochia rubra	Produced for a few days after delivery (1–4 days)	Bright red in color
Lochia serosa	Produced approximately during 5–9 days after delivery	Pale red/brown/pink in color
Lochia alba	Produced after 10th day of delivery	White or yellowish in color

- *Breasts*: Following delivery, secretion of colostrum, a deep, lemon-yellow liquid occurs from the breasts. This gets converted to mature milk during the ensuing 4 weeks after delivery. The average amount of breast milk produced by the nursing mothers is about 600 mL everyday.

Investigations

Ultrasound examination may help in detection of retained placental bits if any.

MANAGEMENT

- *Patient monitoring*:
  - *Monitoring of vitals*: BP and pulse should be monitored at every 15 minutes for the 1st hour after delivery
  - *Vaginal examination*: Amount of vaginal bleeding must also be monitored
  - *Abdominal examination*: Uterine fundus must be palpated to ensure that the uterus is well-contracted. In case the uterus is relaxed, it must be massaged or the use of uterotonics may be required
  - *Monitoring for the signs of infection*: The women must be monitored for signs of infection such as fever, abdominal pain, foul smelling vaginal discharge, etc.
  - *Ability to void*: The woman must be monitored regarding her ability to void because urinary incontinence can be a common problem for a few hours following delivery

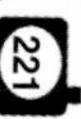

- *Early ambulation*: This helps in reducing problems such as bladder complications, constipation, venous thrombosis and pulmonary embolism
- *Perineal care*: The woman must be instructed to cleanse the vulva from anterior to posterior (vulva to anus). Application of the ice-pack to the perineum, spray of local anesthetic or use of warm sitz bath helps in reducing localized edema and discomfort
- *Dietary restrictions*: There are no dietary restrictions for a woman who has delivered normally. She can be allowed to eat 2 hours after a normal vaginal delivery. In breast feeding mothers, number of calories and protein consumed must be increased. Iron and calcium supplements must be continued for 2 months following delivery
- *Hemoglobin*: Mother's hemoglobin level must be checked on the first postpartum day
- *Testing the eligibility for administration of anti-Rh immunoglobulins*: In case where the baby is Rh positive, anti-Rh immunoglobulins must be administered to the mother
- *Discharge instructions*:
  - *Timing for discharge*: Hospitalization is rarely required for more than 48 hours in cases having normal vaginal delivery and for more than 3–5 days in cases who have had a cesarean section
  - *Patient education*: Before discharge, mother must be educated regarding breast feeding, care of the umblical cord and routine care of the infant
  - *Advice regarding sexual intercourse*: The woman can resume her sexual activities when bright red bleeding from the vagina has ceased, vulva and vagina have healed and the woman is physically comfortable and emotionally ready
  - *Resumption of normal physical activities*: The women who have had a normal vaginal delivery may resume all physical activities upon discharge from the hospital as long as she experiences no pain or discomfort. The woman who has had a cesarean delivery must be called for postpartum visits for stitch removal and then again after 6 weeks of delivery for follow-up. If everything appears normal at the follow-up visit, she can be advised to resume normal activities
  - *Advice regarding contraception*: Due to uncertainty of ovulation amongst the postpartum women, the women must be asked to use some form of contraception as soon as she resumes sexual activity.

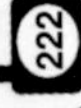

COMPLICATIONS

- *Uterine subinvolution*: This occurs due to the interruption of normal uterine involution. It is characterized by prolongation of lochial discharge production and irregular, profuse bleeding. The management comprises of injection of methergine 0.2 mg at every 3–4 hourly for 24–48 hours. If presence of infection is suspected, antimicrobial therapy can be administered
- *Secondary postpartum hemorrhage*: This is characterized by bleeding occurring 24 hours to 12 weeks after delivery. Curettage may be performed in cases of retained placental tissues. If the uterine cavity is empty on ultrasound examination, administration of oxytocin, methergine and/or prostaglandin analogue may be required
- *Breast engorgement*: Women who do not breast feed may develop breast engorgement. This is associated with breast pain and milk leakage, which may peak at 3–5 days post-delivery. Treatment comprises of the use of a well-fitting brassiere and use of ice packs and oral analgesics for 12–24 hours. Bromocriptine to suppress milk production is no longer used
- *Bladder dysfunction*: Bladder dysfunction is likely to occur in the early puerperium.

CLINICAL PEARLS

- Following child-birth, there is an increased tendency for pelvic organ prolapse and urinary incontinence. This can be reduced by the use of pelvic floor exercises
- Use of OCPs can cause suppression of breast milk; therefore, must be avoided as far as possible
- Breast feeding must be encouraged in all women except those abusing street drugs or alcohol; those having HIV infection or active untreated tuberculosis; those undergoing treatment for breast cancer or those nursing infants with galactosemia.

2. COMPLICATIONS IN THE PUERPERIUM

2.1. PUERPERAL PYREXIA

INTRODUCTION

This is characterized by a rise in temperature of 38° C (100.4° F) or higher in the puerperium. This temperature rise must be observed on two separate

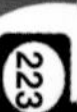

occasions, 24 hours apart, usually within the first 10 days following delivery, excluding the first 24 hours after delivery.

ETIOLOGY

This is usually related to the following factors:

- *Puerperal sepsis*: Uterine infection known as endometritis, which is the commonest of all genital tract infections, can especially occur following cesarean delivery. The microorganisms which are most commonly involved include group A, B and D *Streptococci*, *Enterococcus*, *Staphylococcus aureus*, *S. epidermidis*, gram negative bacteria such as *E. coli*, *Klebsiella*, *Proteus*, etc. Anaerobic infection is commonly present in cases of delivery by cesarean section
- *Other causes*: Besides puerperal sepsis, other causes of puerperal pyrexia are urinary tract infection, mastitis, infection of the cesarean wound, pulmonary infection, thrombophlebitis, etc.

DIAGNOSIS

Symptoms

- *Fever and malaise*: Degree of fever is proportional to the extent of infection and sepsis. Chills may accompany fever
- *Abdominal palpation*: Uterus may be subinvoluted and tender
- *Cesarean wound inspection*: In the presence of infection, the wound may become red and inflamed. There may be a collection of pus, which may eventually result in wound disruption
- *Vaginal examination*: Infected episiotomy may be present. Parametrial tenderness can be elicited. There may be presence of foul smelling lochia.

Investigations

- *Culture and sensitivity*: High vaginal, endocervical swabs and urine analysis for culture and sensitivity are required
- *Blood investigations*: These include performing the tests such as hematocrit (especially hemoglobin estimation), TLC and DLC. Leukocytosis to the extent of 15,000–30,000 cells/μL may be present
- *Pelvic ultrasound*: It helps in detection of any retained placental bits
- *CT or MRI*: Persistent puerperal infection can be evaluated on CT or MRI.

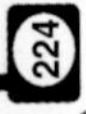

DIFFERENTIAL DIAGNOSIS

Various causes of puerperal sepsis have been described in the "Etiology".

MANAGEMENT

In mild cases, OPD treatment with an oral antibiotic agent may be prescribed. For moderate to severe infection, intravenous therapy with a broad spectrum antibiotic agent may be prescribed. The most commonly used regimen comprises of clindamycin 900 mg and gentamicin 1.5 mg/kg, q 8 hourly.

COMPLICATIONS

- Wound infection/dehiscence
- Necrotizing fasciitis, peritonitis, adnexal infections
- Parametrial phlegmon: This is characterized by parametrial cellulitis and areas of induration or phlegmon within the leaves of broad ligament
- Pelvic thrombophlebitis
- Infection of perineum, vagina and cervix.

CLINICAL PEARLS

- In case of infected episiotomies, sutures must be removed and the infected wound should be debrided daily using povidone iodine solution. Intravenous antibiotics must be started. Secondary closure must be done when the patient is afebrile and there is pink healthy granulation tissue.

2.2. MASTITIS

INTRODUCTION

Mastitis can be defined as the parenchymatous infection of the mammary glands.

ETIOLOGY

The most important causative organism is *S. aureus*, most commonly community-acquired methicillin-resistant *S. aureus* (CA-MRSA).

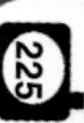

DIAGNOSIS

Symptoms

- Clinical symptoms usually appear by 3rd to 4th weeks of puerperium
- The infection is usually unilateral and is associated with marked breast engorgement and inflammation
- Fever may be associated with chills or rigors
- Hardening and reddening of the breast tissue and intense pain
- Development of abscesses and presence of fluctuation.

Investigations

- *Ultrasound examination*: Ultrasound examination is done to detect the presence of breast abscess
- *Culture and sensitivity*: Culture and sensitivity of the breast milk help in identifying the causative organism.

MANAGEMENT

Treatment mainly comprises of antibiotic treatment after bacterial identification and sensitivity. Infection usually resolves within 48 hours with treatment.

2.3. DEEP VEIN THROMBOSIS (DVT)

INTRODUCTION

Extension of puerperal infection along venous route can result in thrombosis and thrombophlebitis of the affected vein. Thrombosis usually originates as an aggregation of platelets and fibrin on the valves in the veins of the lower extremities (especially calf veins). The thrombus can either break-off and embolize to other veins or cause total occlusion of the veins.

ETIOLOGY

Factors which predispose to the formation of thrombus include:

- Endothelial injury
- Blood stasis and hypercoagulability of blood.

DIAGNOSIS

Clinical Presentation

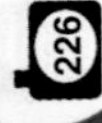

- Pain in the calf muscles, edema of legs
- Rise in the skin temperature

- Difference in the circumference between the affected and the normal leg may be more than 2 cm
- *Homan's sign*: Homan's sign is positive **(Fig. 5.1)**.

Investigations

- *Doppler ultrasound*: This helps in detecting changes in the velocity of blood flow in the femoral veins
- *Duplex Doppler ultrasound*: This is highly sensitive and specific for detection of femoral DVT
- *CT or MRI*
- I^{125} *fibrinogen scanning*: This is not recommended for diagnosis of DVT in pregnancy due to the risk of radiation exposure to the fetus.

MANAGEMENT

- Bed rest with foot elevation above the level of heart
- Analgesics can be used to provide pain relief
- Antimicrobial therapy must be started
- Anticoagulants, such as heparin, low molecular weight heparin and oral anticoagulants, such as warfarin, can also be used
- Knee-length or thigh-length graduated elastic compression stockings help in reducing the risk of thrombosis. Early ambulation also helps in reducing the risk
- Vena cava filters can be used in the cases where anticoagulant therapy is contraindicated.

COMPLICATIONS

- Pulmonary embolism, thrombophlebitis
- Varicose ulceration of leg veins
- Post-thrombotic syndrome (venous stress disorder).

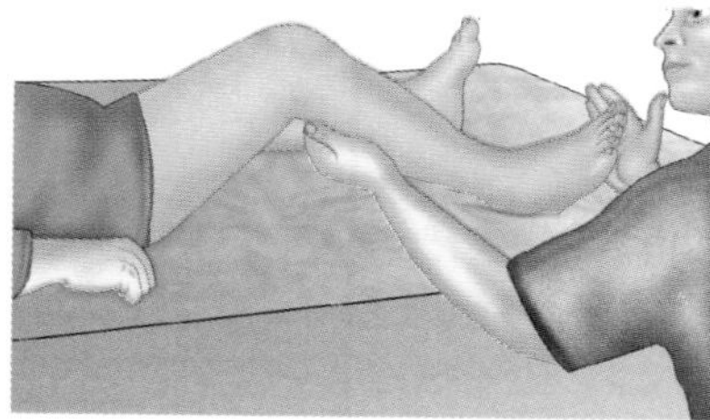

Figure 5.1: Method of eliciting Homan's sign, which is characterized by pain in the calf upon dorsiflexion of the foot

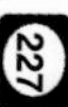

2.4. PULMONARY EMBOLISM

INTRODUCTION

This condition can be characterized by partial or complete blockage of pulmonary vessels resulting in acute respiratory and/or hemodynamic compromise. Acute respiratory consequences of pulmonary embolism include increased alveolar dead space, hypoxemia and hyperventilation. Pulmonary embolism can be either acute (embolus is situated centrally within the vascular lumen and is causing its occlusion) or chronic (embolus is eccentric and contiguous with the vessel wall, thereby reducing the arterial diameter by more than 50%).

ETIOLOGY

See **Figure 5.2**

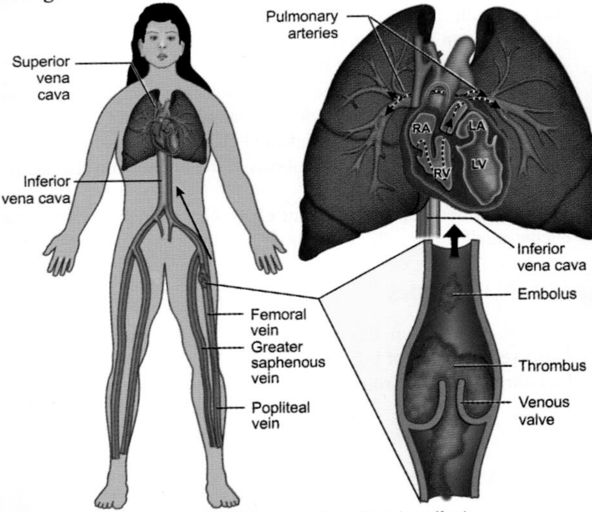

Pulmonary embolism most commonly arises from the calf veins. The venous thromboemboli travel through the right side of the heart to reach the lungs.

Figure 5.2: Pathogenesis of pulmonary embolism

(Abbreviations: RA: Right atrium; RV: Right ventricle; LA: Left atrium; LV: Left ventricle)

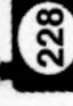

DIAGNOSIS

Symptoms

- Sudden collapse with acute chest pain and air hunger
- Tachypnea, dyspnea, hemoptysis
- Pleuritic chest pain, cough, tachycardia
- Temperature of greater than 37° C.

Investigations

- *X-ray chest*: There may be areas of infraction showing diminished vascular markings, elevation of the dome of diaphragm and pleural effusion
- *ECG*: ECG shows tachycardia and right axis deviation
- *Arterial blood gases*: These may be reduced PO_2 and oxygen saturation
- *Venous perfusion scanning*: These may be diminished perfusion with maintenance of ventilation on ventilation perfusion scanning
- *Pulmonary angiography*: This used to be the most accurate method of diagnosis. Presently the gold standard investigation of choice is CT angiography
- *Doppler ultrasound*: This helps in identifying DVT.

DIFFERENTIAL DIAGNOSIS

It is important to rule out the presence of respiratory abnormalities such as pneumonia and atelectasis.

MANAGEMENT

- *Patient resuscitation*: This comprises of cardiac massage and oxygen therapy
- *Heparin therapy*: Heparin is usually administered in a bolus dose of 5,000 IU, followed by 40,000 IU/day to maintain a clotting time over 12 minutes in the first 48 hours. Thereafter, heparin levels are regulated so as to maintain APTT of twice the normal
- Maintenance of blood pressure using dopamine or adrenaline
- Thrombolytic therapy using streptokinase may be administered
- Tachycardia can be counteracted using digitalis
- *Surgical treatment*: These may include procedures such as vena caval filters, ligation of inferior vena cava and ovarian veins.

COMPLICATIONS

- Pulmonary embolism can be considered as the most important cause of maternal death developed nations, only after sudden cardiac arrest. Death usually occurs due to shock and vagal inhibition
- Recurrent embolism.

CLINICAL PEARLS

- Clinical features are proportional to the size of embolus
- Immediate full anticoagulation is mandatory for all patients suspected to have DVT or pulmonary embolism.

2.5. AMNIOTIC FLUID EMBOLISM

INTRODUCTION

Amniotic fluid embolism is a catastrophic syndrome occurring during labor and delivery or in the immediate postpartum period. This condition occurs when amniotic fluid, fetal cells, hair or other debris enter the maternal circulation via the placental bed of the uterus and trigger an allergic reaction. This reaction then results in cardiorespiratory collapse and DIC.

ETIOLOGY

The pathophysiology of amniotic fluid embolism is presented in **Figure 5.3**.

DIAGNOSIS

The diagnosis of amniotic fluid embolism is one of exclusion and is based on the assessment of symptoms and clinical course, and not on the basis of laboratory or pathology findings.

Symptoms

- Dyspnea
- Non-reassuring fetal status (in case of pregnant women)
- Altered mental status followed by sudden cardiovascular collapse

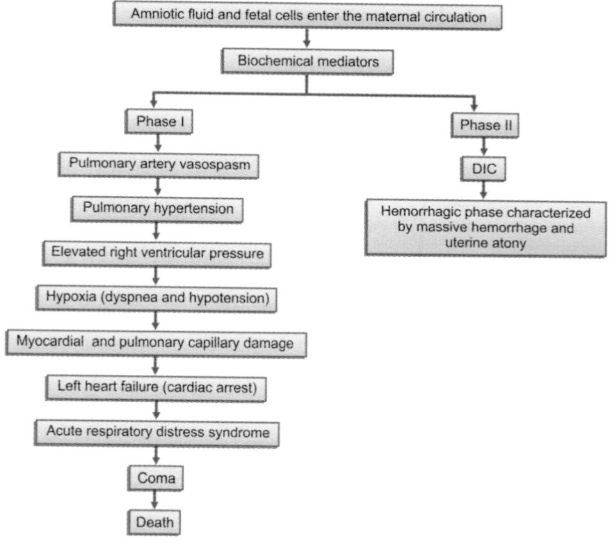

Figure 5.3: Pathophysiology of amniotic fluid embolism

- Profound respiratory failure with deep cyanosis
- Cardiovascular shock
- Convulsions and profound coma
- DIC and maternal death.

Investigations

- *Echocardiography*: This helps in evaluating cardiac function and intravascular volume status
- *Electrocardiography*: This may show a right strain pattern with ST-T changes and tachycardia
- *Complete blood count*: Complete blood count including the coagulation parameters such as PT, APTT, FDP and fibrinogen levels may be required
- *Arterial blood gases*
- *Chest X-ray*
- *Ventilation-perfusion scanning.*

DIFFERENTIAL DIAGNOSIS

See **Table 5.2**

Table 5.2: Differential diagnosis of amniotic fluid embolism

Obstetric causes	*Non-obstetric causes*	*Anesthetic causes*
• Acute hemorrhage (APH, PPH)	• Pulmonary embolism • Air embolism	• High spinal anesthesia • Aspiration
• Placental abruption	• Anaphylaxis	• Local anesthetic toxicity
• Preeclampsia or eclampsia	• Aspiration	• Drug toxicity ($MgSO_4$, etc.)
• Rupture of the uterus	• Aortic dissection	
• Atonicity of the uterus		
• Eclampsia	• Sepsis/septic shock	
• Peripartum cardiomyopathy		

MANAGEMENT

- The goals of management are to restore cardiovascular and pulmonary equilibrium by maintaining the systolic blood pressure > 90 mm Hg; urine output > 25 mL/hour and arterial PO_2 > 60 mm Hg
- In case of uterine atony, efforts must be made to re-establish uterine tone
- Efforts must be made to correct coagulation abnormalities
- Control of the airway is done with tracheal intubation and administration of 100% O_2 with positive pressure ventilation
- Venous access must be maintained with large bore IV catheters
- Infusion of crystalloids must be started to treat hypotension, increase the circulating volume and cardiac output. Dopamine infusion may be started if patient still remains hypotensive
- An immediate cesarean delivery is required in patients who have yet not delivered
- Blood and blood products: This may include use of fresh frozen plasma, platelets, cryoprecipitate, recombinant factor VIIa, etc. Cryoprecipitate must be administered for a fibrinogen level less than 100 mg/dL, and platelet transfusion given for platelet counts less than 20,000/mm^3.

COMPLICATIONS

- High maternal and fetal morbidity and mortality. Various causes of maternal death include sudden cardiac arrest, DIC, acute respiratory distress syndrome, multiple organ failure, etc.

- There may be neurological impairment amongst the mother and fetuses those who survive.

CLINICAL PEARLS

- The main clinical symptom, which should lead the clinician to suspect amniotic fluid embolism, is sudden onset of dyspnea in the face of cardiovascular collapse and DIC
- A multidisciplinary team approach comprising of an obstetrician, anesthesiologist and intensivist is necessary for a successful outcome.

3. EPISIOTOMY AND ITS REPAIR

INTRODUCTION

An episiotomy is a surgical incision, usually made with sterile scissors, which is given through the perineum in order to enlarge the vagina for assisting the process of childbirth. This incision which is believed to guard the muscles of the pelvic floor by protecting them against stretching related to childbirth and delivery. There are two different types of episiotomies depending upon the direction of the surgical incision **(Fig. 5.4)**: (1) the midline episiotomy or (2) the mediolateral episiotomy.

INDICATIONS

According to the current recommendations by the ACOG, an episiotomy must be only performed in the situations, where it is indicated, such as:

- A prophylactic method to spare the strain on the pelvic floor muscles, thereby preventing the occurrence of vaginal tears and lacerations
- Rigidity of perineal muscles, which is responsible for causing an arrest in the natural progress of labor

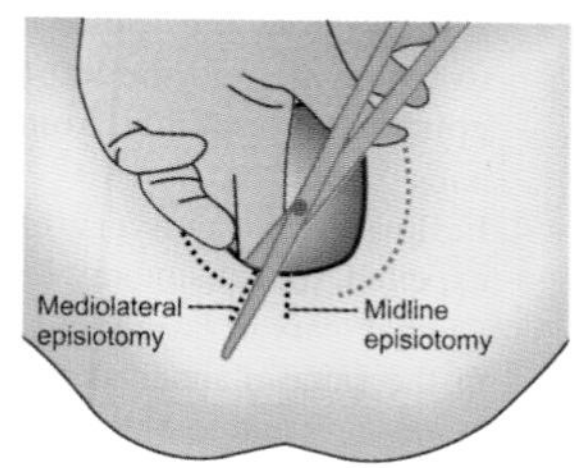

Figure 5.4: Direction of giving different types of episiotomies

- The baby is very big or perineum is short
- In cases where instrumental vaginal delivery is indicated
- Shoulder dystocia
- Breech vaginal delivery
- In cases where a woman has undergone female genital mutilation
- Extremely premature babies in order to prevent compression of fetal head
- To shorten the second stage of labor in cases of high-risk pregnancy (preeclampsia, heart disease, etc.).

SURGICAL MANAGEMENT

Preoperative Preparation

- Under all aseptic precautions after cleaning and draping the perineum, the proposed site of repair is infiltrated with 10 mL of 1% lignocaine solution
- The patient must be placed in lithotomy position, with a good source of light from behind so that the entire genital tract can be inspected for trauma
- Per speculum examination must be performed in order to visualize the cervix and lower genital tract to exclude lacerations.

Steps of Surgery

- Two fingers of the clinician's left hand are placed between the fetal presenting part and the posterior vaginal wall
- The incision is made using a curved scissors at the point when the woman is experiencing uterine contractions; the perineum is being stretched by the maternal presenting part and is at its thinnest
- In case of a mediolateral episiotomy, the cut should be made starting from the center of fourchette extending laterally either to the right or to the left **(Fig. 5.4)**. On the other hand, a median episiotomy extends from the center of fourchette toward the anus
- Following the delivery of the baby after the placenta has been expelled, the episiotomy incision is repaired. In case of presence of vaginal tears or lacerations, their repair is also performed essentially in the same manner as that of the episiotomy in order to achieve hemostasis and to obliterate the dead space **(Figs 5.5A to C)**.

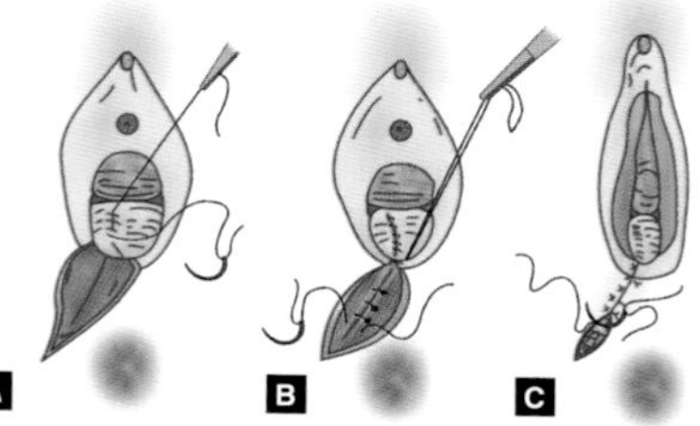

Figures 5.5A to C: Repair of an episiotomy incision: (A) vaginal mucosa being repaired using continuous stitches; (B) muscle layer being repaired using interrupted stitches; (C) skin being repaired using interrupted matrix sutures

Postoperative Care

- If infection is suspected, combinations of broad-spectrum antibiotics can be administered
- Application of an ice-pack or regular use of a warm sitz bath over the stitches may help in reducing pain and inflammation over the site of incision
- The patient must be advised to ambulate around as much as possible and regularly perform pelvic floor exercises
- Use of pain killers, such as paracetamol, may help in providing pain relief
- Immediately following the surgery, the patient must be advised to take liquid diet for a day and then gradually convert to low-residue diet over few days
- Vaginal or rectal examination and sexual intercourse must be avoided for at least 2 weeks following the repair.

COMPLICATIONS

- Bleeding, inflammation, infection and/or swelling at the site of incision
- Pain: While a slight amount of pain which gets relived on taking pain killers can commonly occur, persistent severe pain at the episiotomy site could be an indicator of presence of a large vulvar, paravaginal or ischiorectal hematoma, thereby necessitating a thorough exploration in these cases
- Extension of the episiotomy into third and fourth degree vaginal lacerations or extension into the rectum.

CLINICAL PEARLS

- Any tears or lacerations, if found, must be adequately sutured and repaired
- The prevalence of episiotomy has reduced gradually over the past few years
- The structures which are cut while performing the episiotomy include: posterior vaginal wall; superficial and deep transverse perineal muscles; bulbospongiosus and part of levator ani muscle; fascia covering these muscles; transverse perineal branches of pudendal nerves and vessels and subcutaneous tissues and skin
- While repairing the episiotomy incision, utmost importance must be given toward the maintenance of hemostasis and anatomical restoration without excessive suturing.

4. PERINEAL INJURIES

INTRODUCTION

The perineal injury can be defined as the injury which occurs to the perineum during the process of childbirth and can be classified into the following degrees **(Figs 5.6A to D)**:

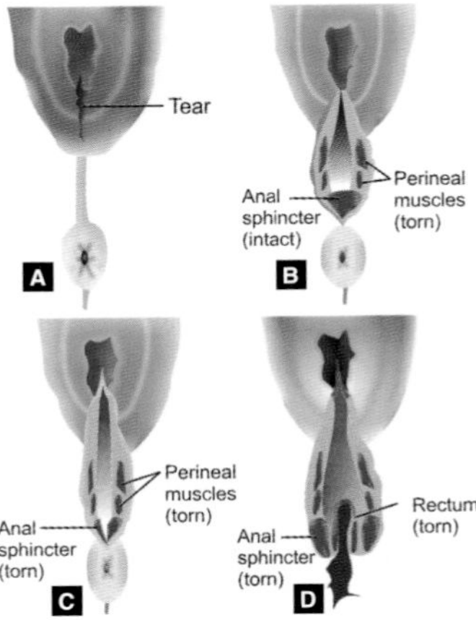

Figures 5.6A to D: (A) First degree perineal tear; (B) second degree perineal tear; (C) third degree perineal tear; (D) fourth degree perineal tear

- *First degree*: Injury to the vaginal mucosa not involving the perineal muscles
- *Second degree*: Injury to the perineum involving the perineal muscles, but not the anal sphincters
- *Third degree*: Injury to the perineum involving the anal sphincter complex (external and internal anal sphincter):
  - *3a*: Less than 50% of external anal sphincter is torn
  - *3b*: More than 50% of external anal sphincter is torn
  - *3c*: Internal anal sphincter also gets involved
- *Fourth degree*: Injury to the perineum involving the anal sphincter complex (external and internal anal sphincters) and rectal mucosa.

SURGICAL MANAGEMENT

Preoperative Preparation

- This is same as that described with episiotomy.

Steps of Surgery

- In case of lacerations, the steps of repair are essentially the same as that of an episiotomy repair except in the cases of third degree and fourth degree lacerations where there might be an extension up to the anal sphincters and rectal mucosa respectively. In case of fourth degree laceration, it is important to approximate the torn edges of the anorectal mucosa with the fine absorbable 3-0 or 4-0 chromic catgut or vicryl sutures in a running or an interrupted manner
- Approximation of the anorectal mucosa and submucosa is done using 3-0 or 4-0 chromic catgut or vicryl sutures in a running or an interrupted manner **(Fig. 5.7A)**
- The superior extent of the anterior anal laceration is identified and sutures are placed through the submucosa of the anorectum starting above the apex of the tear and extending down until the anal verge **(Fig. 5.7B)**
- Finally, the torn edges of the anal sphincter are isolated, approximated and sutured together with 3 or 4 interrupted stitches
- Following the repair of internal anal sphincters, the torn edges of external anal sphincters are identified and grasped with Allis clamp. The repair of these sphincters can be performed either using end-to-end repair **(Figs 5.7C to F)** or the overlap method.

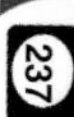

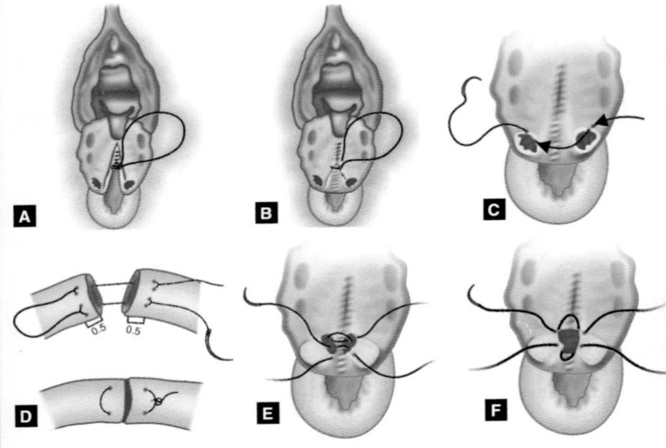

Figures 5.7A to F: Repair of anal sphincters: (A) approximation of anorectal mucosa and submucosa using continuous sutures; (B) second layer of sutures placed through the rectal muscularis; (C) end-to-end approximation of the external anal sphincter. Sutures being placed through the posterior wall of external anal sphincters (these would be tied in the end); (D) close-up view of the external anal sphincters showing end-to-end approximation; (E) end-to-end sutures taken through the interior of external anal sphincter (shown in whitish blue); (F) approximation of the anterior wall of external anal sphincter

Postoperative Care

- In case of fourth degree tears where the injury has extended until the rectal mucosa, the patient should be prescribed stool softeners for about a week or two
- Rest of the steps are same as those described with an episiotomy.

COMPLICATIONS

- Postpartum hemorrhage
- Infection
- Extension of tears resulting in the involvement of internal and external anal sphincters, fecal incontinence.

CLINICAL PEARLS

- Perineal injuries can be considered as the commonest cause of traumatic postpartum hemorrhage
- Gross injury to the perineum in the form of third and fourth degree tears occur invariably as a result of mismanaged second stage of labor
- Perineal tears should be immediately repaired following delivery of the placenta.

5. MANUAL REMOVAL OF PLACENTA

INTRODUCTION

In normal cases, the mean time from delivery until placental expulsion is approximately 8–9 minutes. In majority of patients, the placenta may have completely separated within a few minutes after the delivery of baby. It may however not be able to deliver outside the uterine cavity. In these cases, manual removal of the placenta may be required. In presence of continuing bleeding, the obstetrician must immediately proceed with the removal. Even in the absence of any continuing bleeding, the surgeon must not wait for more than half an hour before attempting manual removal of placenta.

ETIOLOGY

Possible causes of placental adhesion, when it remains undelivered outside the uterine cavity are enumerated in **Figure 5.8**. In case of simple adherent placenta, manual removal of the placenta is the most suitable option to facilitate the placental delivery. However, in cases of pathologically adherent placenta (placenta accreta, increta or percreta) **(Fig. 5.9)**, it may not be possible to find the correct cleavage plane between the placenta and the uterine musculature and, therefore, it may become impossible to manually remove the placenta.

DIAGNOSIS

Clinical Presentation

- No signs of placental separation are observed even after half an hour of the delivery of the baby
- Bleeding through the cervical os may be present.

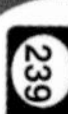

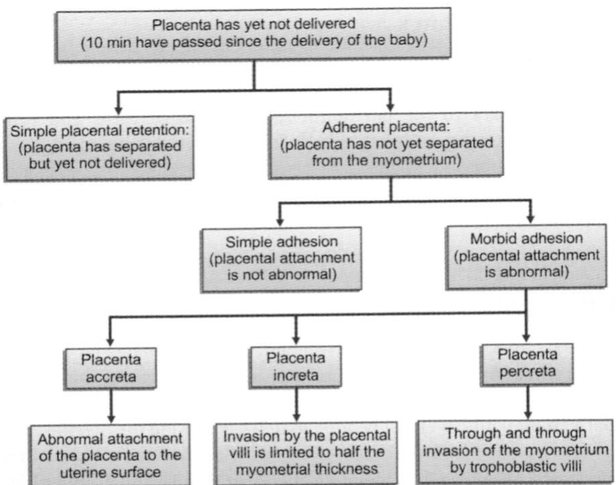

Figure 5.8: Possible causes of placental adhesion when it remains undelivered

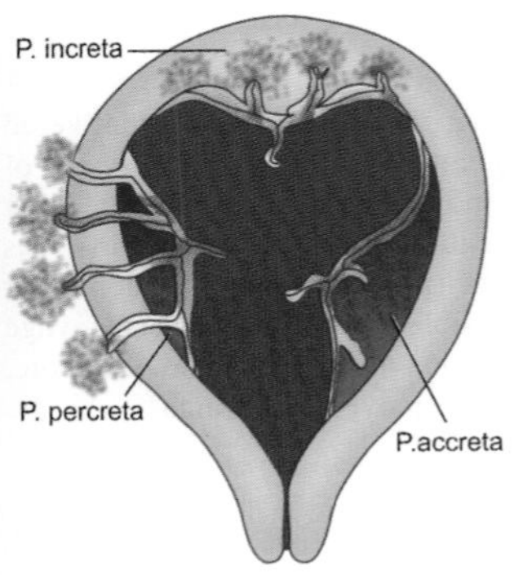

Figure 5.9: Different types of abnormally adherent placenta

Investigations

- *Ultrasonography*: The various sonographic criteria for the detection of morbidly adherent placenta are as follows:

- Absence of a normal, hypodense retroplacental myometric zone
- A reduced surface area between uterine serosa and urinary bladder
- The presence of focal exophytic masses with the same echogenicity as placenta beyond the uterine serosa
- Presence of unusual, prominent, lacunar vascular spaces within the placental parenchyma

- *Color Doppler*: Color flow Doppler serves as a useful investigation in making a prenatal diagnosis of morbidly adherent placenta because Doppler sonography can help in detection of abnormal vascularization of the myometrium **(Fig. 5.10)**
- *Magnetic resonance imaging*: MRI is often used as an adjunct to sonography in cases of strong clinical suspicion of placenta accreta.

SURGICAL MANAGEMENT

Preoperative Preparation

- *Anesthesia*: The procedure of manual placental removal must be performed under adequate anesthesia (either general or regional)

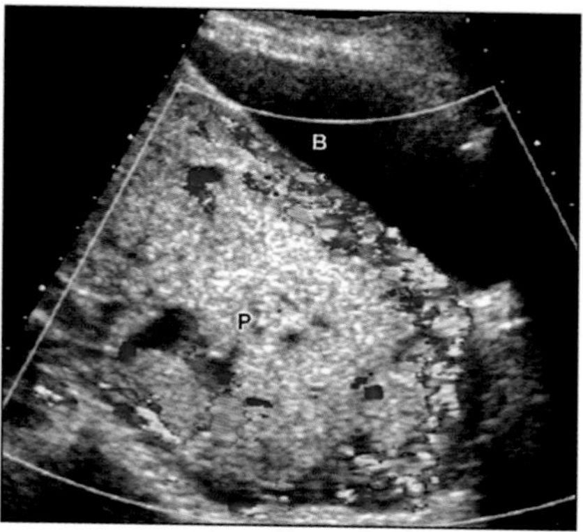

Figure 5.10: Color Doppler scanning at 27 weeks gestation in a case of placenta percreta demonstrating prominent placental vessels extending across the myometrium into the bladder wall (*Abbreviations*: B: Bladder; P: Placenta)

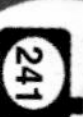

- *Patient position*: The patient must be placed in lithotomy position for manual removal procedure
- *Bladder catheterization*: The bladder must be catheterized before attempting the manual placental removal
- *Monitoring of vitals*: Maternal vital signs must be assessed and, if unstable, immediate steps must be taken to bring them under control
- *Immediate resuscitation*: Four units of blood must be arranged especially if woman is having PPH. Two wide-bore IV cannulae must be inserted and immediate resuscitation with crystalloids started
- *Antibiotics*: A broad-spectrum antibiotic must be administered to the patient
- *Informed consent*: An informed consent must be taken from the patient before starting the procedure
- *Cleaning and draping*: Under all aseptic precautions, vulva and vagina must be swabbed with antiseptic solution and the patient cleaned and draped with sterile towels.

Steps of Surgery

The steps of surgery are described in **Figure 5.11** and are as follows:

- One of the surgeon's hands must be placed over the patient's abdomen in order to steady the fundus

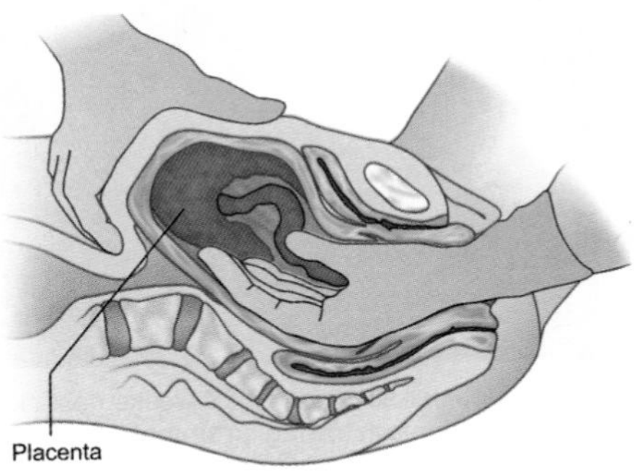

Figure 5.11: Procedure of manual removal of the placenta

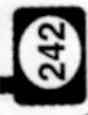

- At the same time, the surgeon's right hand, smeared with antibiotics, is introduced inside the vagina in a cone-shaped manner
- It is then passed into the uterine cavity along the course of the umbilical cord. As soon as the lower placental margin is reached, the ulnar border of the hand is used to gradually separate the placenta from the uterine wall
- The placental tissue is gradually separated by using the sideways slicing movements of the fingers. Once the placenta has separated, it can be grasped with the help of the entire hand and gradually taken out. The abdominal hand helps in stabilizing the uterine fundus and in guiding the movements of the fingers inside the uterine cavity until the placenta has completely separated out
- Once the entire placenta has been separated, it should be withdrawn out with the help of gentle traction. Before withdrawing the hand, the surgeon must also look for any possible placental remnants or damage to the uterine wall
- Before withdrawing the hand from vagina, bimanual compression of the uterus must be done until it becomes firm.

Postoperative Care

- Postoperatively, charting of the following parameters must be done: vital signs; input-output charting; evidence of fresh bleeding; etc.
- In order to achieve sustained uterine contractions even after surgery, infusion of oxytocics must be continued
- Intramuscular methergine or ergometrine 0.5 mg must be administered following completion of the procedure
- Blood transfusion may be required depending upon the patient's condition
- Broad spectrum antibiotics must be administered to the patient.

COMPLICATIONS

- Abnormally adherent placenta can result in severe bleeding, which may become life-threatening and may even require cesarean hysterectomy
- Manual removal of placenta can result in complications such as perforation or uterine rupture; incomplete placental removal; hemorrhage; infection; secondary PPH; etc.

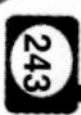

CLINICAL PEARLS

- In patients with placenta previa the incidence of placenta accreta appears to correlate with the number of previous cesarean deliveries
- Ergometrine or syntometrine must be avoided for retained placenta because they may cause tonic uterine contractions, which may further delay expulsion.

6. THE NEWBORN INFANT

6.1. CARE OF A NEWBORN

INTRODUCTION

Examination of a baby allows the midwife or pediatrician or the obstetrician to assess and monitor the baby's condition and promptly provide appropriate care and treatment as soon as possible. Every new born must be examined thoroughly within 24 hours of the birth.

DIAGNOSIS

General Physical Examination

- *Vital signs*: Normal respiratory rate in a newborn child varies between 30–60 breaths/minute, whereas the pulse rate varies between 100–160 beats/minute. Normal range of blood pressure in a newborn child is 45–60 mm Hg systolic and 25–40 mm Hg diastolic. Baby's temperature is recorded through rectal, oral or axillary route
- *Skin color*: A normal baby is usually pink in color. Pallor may be due to anemia, birth asphyxia or shock. Cyanosis or bluish discoloration of the skin may be indicative of cardiorespiratory dysfunction. Yellowish discoloration of the baby's skin, nail beds or the sclera could be indicative of jaundice (bilirubin levels > 5 mg /dL)
- *Congenital anomalies*: There should be no major visible abnormality such as cleft lip and palate; congenital heart disease; etc.
- *Infant's weight*: There is 7–10% weight loss during 1st week of life. Weight gain begins from 2nd week onwards
- *Infant's length*: Crown-foot length is 48–53 cm. Normal weekly gain in length is 0.8–1 cm for the first 8–12 weeks of life

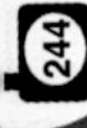

- *Dermatological changes*: Various types of non-pathological skin rashes which may be present in the newborn child include, milia; Mongolian spots; erythema toxicum; capillary hemangiomas or stork bites; etc. They are usually of no significance and usually disappear with time. Some pathological skin changes include port-wine stain, strawberry naevus, etc.
- *Examination of the head*: The head circumference is measured with a paper tape. Head circumference on average is 33–38 cm and increases by 0.5–0.8 cm/week. The head fontanelles and sutures are palpated. Bulging fontanelles may be due to the increased intracranial pressure, meningitis or hydrocephalus. Depressed fontanelles are seen with dehydration. The baby's head must also be examined for the presence of any abnormal swellings such as caput succedaneum, cephalohematoma, chignon, molding, etc.
- *Neck*: Neck is checked for movements, and presence of abnormal swellings such as goiter, thyroglossal cysts, sternomastoid hematoma, etc. and abnormal shortening (indicative of Turner's syndrome)
- *Eyes*: The eyes are checked with an ophthalmoscope for abnormalities such as cataracts, retinoblastoma and corneal opacities. The eyes must be checked of any abnormal or sticky discharge which could be indicative of infection
- *Face and mouth*: Face of the newborn is evaluated for various dysmorphic features such as hypertelorism (eyes widely separated) or low set ears (trisomy 9, 18, triploidy) or the facial nerve injury. Mouth is checked for cleft palate or lip, deciduous teeth, lingual frenulum (tongue-tie), macroglossia or oral thrush (candidal infection). Excessive drooling from the mouth could be indicative of condition such as esophageal atresia
- *Chest*: Breathing and chest wall movements are observed for the signs of respiratory distress. Presence of wheeze or crepitations must be noted. While examining the chest, the breasts of the new born are also evaluated. They may sometimes be enlarged under the effect of maternal estrogen
- *Heart*: Heart is examined for rate, rhythm, and the quality of heart sounds and presence of any murmurs. Presence of murmurs in the newborn child could be indicative of congenital heart disease
- *Abdomen*: On palpating the abdomen, the liver normally extends 1–2 cm below the costal margin; the spleen tip may be palpable, as may be the kidney on the left side. Any intra-abdominal masses

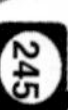

may require further investigations. Umbilicus is examined for any discharge, redness or infection and presence of any hernia. The cut end of the cord must also be inspected for the number of umbilical arteries and veins

- *Genitalia*: Genitalia should be examined carefully before gender assignment. Anus and rectum are checked to rule out imperforation and their position. A normal baby must pass meconium within 48 hours of the birth
- *Limbs*: Extremities, spine and joints must be examined for abnormalities such as syndactyly (fusion of the digits), polydactyly (multiple digits), simian crease (Down syndrome), talipes equinovarus and hip dislocation (Ortolani and Barlow maneuvers)
- *Nervous system*: The baby must be examined for any irritability, abnormal muscle tone, reflexes, cranial and peripheral nerves
- *General fetal characteristics*: These may vary based on the gestational age **(Table 5.3)**.

Table 5.3: Fetal characteristics based on the period of gestation

	Preterm	*Term*	*Post-term*
Breast nodule	$\leq$ 2 mm	2–4 mm	4–7 mm
Scalp hair	Fine hair	Fuzzy, fine hair	Coarse hair
Ear lobe	No cartilage	Moderate amount of cartilage	Thick cartilage, resulting in a stiff ear lobe
Testes and scrotum	Partially descended testes; small scrotum with few rugae		Fully descended testes with normal sized scrotum having prominent rugae

Investigations

Hematological findings: Normal hematological parameters in a newborn child are RBC count: 6–8 million; Hb:18–20 gm%; WBC: 10,000–17,000/cumm; Platelets: 35,000/cumm; sedimentation rate—markedly elevated

MANAGEMENT

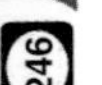

- Immediately following birth, the baby must be placed on a cot where neutral thermal condition is being maintained. Hypothermia

must be avoided. The baby must be dried immediately after birth and must be covered from head to toe with a pre-warmed towel. Early breast feeding must be encouraged

- Routine baby bath must be delayed until the baby is able to maintain the body temperature and breast feeding has been started. The excessive blood, vernix, blood or meconium must be wiped off from the baby's skin using sterile moist swabs, following which the skin is dried using a soft towel
- Daily cleansing of the umbilical cord stump with spirit and antibiotic powder must be done
- Single dose of vitamin K (0.5–1 mg) is given to all newborn babies within 6 hours of birth. This helps in preventing bleeding due to the deficiency of vitamin K
- Hepatitis B vaccine is administered at birth.

COMPLICATIONS

The important danger signs, which require medical attention, include the following:

- Not feeding well, reduced activity
- Tachypnea (> 60 breaths/minute)
- Grunting or moaning
- Convulsions or floppy or stiff baby
- Temperature greater than 37.5°C or less than 35.5°C
- Blood or pus coming out from the umbilical stump.

CLINICAL PEARLS

- Babies become clinically jaundiced when the bilirubin levels exceed 80–120 μmol/L. Jaundice starting within 24 hours of birth usually results from hemolysis
- Presence of hydrocele, vaginal bleeding or mastitis in the neonate during the 1st week of life is no cause of concern and usually disappears on its own
- A neonate which has delivered vaginally, has a gestational age greater than 38 weeks, is a singleton birth having birth weight appropriate for gestational age, has normal vitals, has passed stools and urine, feeds successfully and is normal on general physical examination, can be discharged by 48 hours of birth

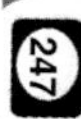

6.2. ASPHYXIA NEONATORUM

INTRODUCTION

This condition occurs due to non-establishment of satisfactory pulmonary respiration at birth. If allowed to progress, this condition can result in hypoxia, hypercarbia and metabolic acidosis.

ETIOLOGY

Continuation of intrauterine hypoxia: The main cause for asphyxia neonatorum includes perinatal asphyxia and fetal distress linked to many causes before birth (**Table 5.4**).

Table 5.4: Causes of fetal distress

Antepartum	*Intrapartum*
Abruption placenta	Uterine rupture/scar dehiscence
Oxytocin induction	Oxytocin induction: strong uterine contractions
Strong hypertonic uterine contractions	Operative vaginal delivery due to vacuum or forceps application
Placental insufficiency (preeclampsia, IUGR, etc.)	Cord around the neck and cord compression
Hypertensive disorders of pregnancy	Cord prolapse
Maternal hypotension (supine position, epidural anesthesia)	Prolonged second stage of labor
Chorioamnionitis	Abnormal uterine contractions (dystocia)
Postmaturity	

Postnatal factors: These include pulmonary, cardiovascular and neurological abnormalities in the neonate.

Following the birth of the baby, when the placental oxygen supply is interrupted, the fetus attempts to breathe. In case, these attempts fail to inflate the lung with air, the baby develops hypoxia, which if continued ultimately results in the depression of respiratory center.

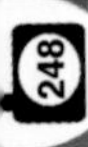

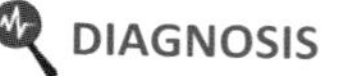

DIAGNOSIS

Clinical Presentation

- *Evaluation of APGAR score*: **A**ctivity, **p**ulse, **g**rimace, **a**ppearance and **r**espiration (APGAR) score **(Table 5.5)** helps in the assessment of fetal condition and is usually calculated at 1, 5 and 15 minutes of birth. Persistence of APGAR score of 0–3 for greater than 5 minutes after birth may be associated with neonatal asphyxia
- Neurological manifestations such as hypotonia, coma, seizures, etc.
- Multiorgan dysfunction.

Table 5.5: APGAR score

Signs	*0*	*1*	*2*	*Component of acronym*
Color	Blue, pale	Acrocyanosis: body pink, extremities blue	Complete pink	**A**ppearance
Heart rate	Absent	Slow (below 100 BPM)	Over 100 BPM	**P**ulse
Reflex irritability	No response	Grimace/ feeble cry	Strong cry, cough or sneeze	**G**rimace
Muscle tone	Flaccid	Flexion of extremities	Active body movements	**A**ctivity
Breathing	Apnea	Slow, irregular	Good, crying	**R**espiratory effort

Total score: 10; No depression/normal: 7–10; Mild depression: 4–6; Severe depression: 0–3

Investigations

- *Antepartum/intrapartum tests of fetal surveillance*: These tests, such as nonstress test, contraction stress test, biophysical profile, electronic fetal monitoring (both external and internal), may be abnormal
- *Fetal blood pH sampling*: Metabolic acidosis (< 7.2)
- *Fetal blood lactate sampling*: Presence of lactic acidosis (> 4.8 mmol/L).

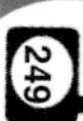

MANAGEMENT

Neonatal Management

Most babies, even those born apnoeic, will resuscitate themselves given a clear airway. However, the basic approach to resuscitation is **A**irway, **B**reathing and **C**irculation, with the following initial actions:

- Get extra help and start the clock
- *Thermoregulation*: The baby should be dried, wrapped and kept warm, which help in avoiding hypothermia. The aim should be to maintain the axillary temperature of 36.5° C. After placing the infant in a heated environment, suctioning of the mouth and nose using a bulb syringe must be performed
- Further steps of management depend upon the APGAR score:
  - *APGAR score between 7 and 10*: These are healthy babies and they should be kept warm and given to their mothers
  - *APGAR score between 4 and 6*: This may be associated with irregular or inadequate breathing, slow heart rate (< 100 beats/minute), blue color, normal or reduced tone. Tactile stimulation in the form of slapping of the soles of feet or rubbing the back may also be given. The clinician must perform an immediate suction of the oropharynx and nasopharynx. If the baby responds, then no further resuscitation is needed. If there is no response, the clinician must progress to lung inflation. Oxygen by bag and mask ventilation **(Fig. 5.12)** at a pressure of 30–40 cm of H_2O must be given. Once the lung have inflated and the heart rate has increased or if the chest has been seen to move in response to passive inflation, then ventilation should be continued at a rate of 30–40/minute. Ventilatory support must be continued until regular breathing is established
  - *APGAR score of < 4*: This may be associated with absent breathing, slow or absent heart rate (< 100 beats/minute), blue or pale and/or floppy baby. The airway must be opened and then the lungs inflated. While most babies can be resuscitated using mask inflation, tracheal intubation **(Figs 5.13A and B)** remains the gold standard of airway management. It is especially required in cases where direct tracheal suctioning is required (in case of meconium aspiration); effective bag and mask ventilation cannot be provided; chest compressions

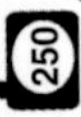

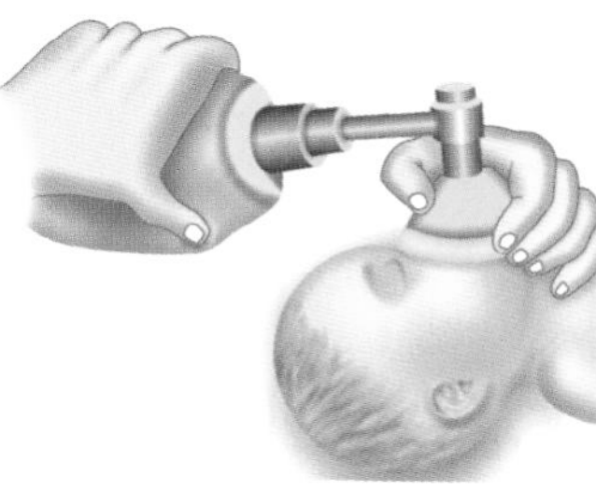

Figure 5.12: Bag and mask ventilation

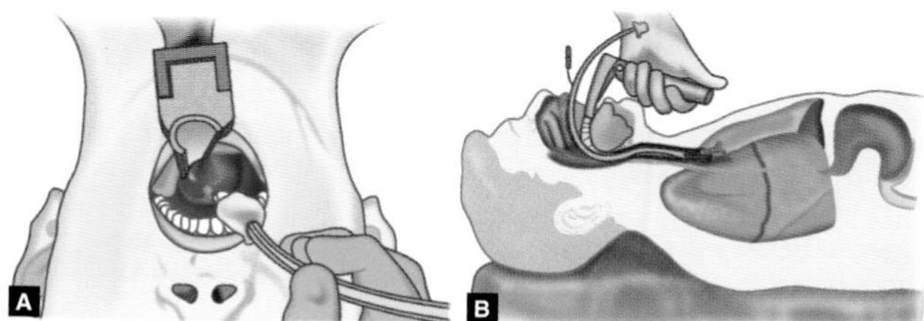

Figures 5.13A and B: (A) Tracheal intubation; (B) Magnified view of endotracheal intubation

are performed; endotracheal intubation is required or there is prolonged requirement for assisted ventilation

- Once the lungs have inflated, reassessment of heart rate response directs further resuscitation. If the heart rate remains slow (< 60 beats/minute) even after the lungs have been aerated, chest compressions must be started. The most effective technique of giving chest compressions comprises of encircling the chest with both hands, so that the fingers lie behind the baby and the thumbs are opposed on the sternum just below the inter-nipple line **(Figs 5.14A and B)** and the chest is compressed by one-third of its depth. Current recommendation is to perform three compressions for each ventilation breath (3:1 ratio). Once the heart rate increases above 60 beats/minute and the chest is seen rising, chest compression can be discontinued. If after adequate lung inflation and chest compressions the heart rate has not responded, drug therapy as described in **Table 5.6** should be considered.

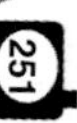

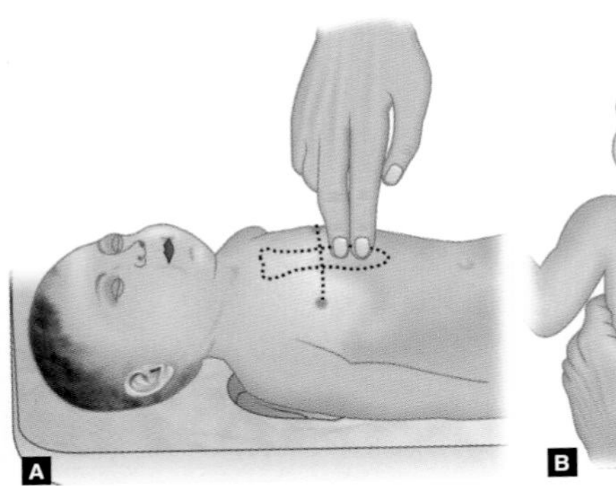

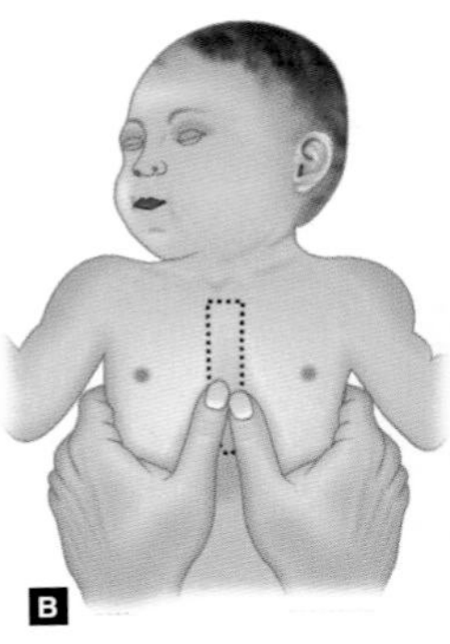

Figures 5.14A and B: Infant chest compression: (A) two finger compression; (B) chest encircling technique

Table 5.6: Drugs to be used for neonatal resuscitation

Drug	*Indication*	*Dosage*
Adrenaline (epinephrine)	Profound unresponsive bradycardia or circulatory standstill	10 µg/kg (0·1 mL/kg 1:10,000) adrenaline may be given intravenously Further doses of 10–30 µg/kg may be tried at 3–5 minute intervals if there is no response
Bicarbonate	Metabolic acidosis	1–2 mmol/kg (2 mL/kg of 4·2% solution) may be used to raise the pH
Dextrose	Hypoglycemia	A slow bolus of 5 mL/kg of 10% dextrose is administered intravenously, followed by secure intravenous dextrose infusion at a rate of 100 mL/kg/day
Fluid	Hypovolemia	Volume expansion, initially with 10 mL/kg of normal saline
Naloxone	Alleviation of effects of maternal opiates	

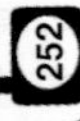

COMPLICATIONS

- *Neurological damage*: Neurological deprivation of the oxygen supply to the brain can result in neurological damage, cerebral edema, seizures, cerebral palsy, hypoxic ischemic encephalopathy, etc.
- *Cardiovascular complications*: Hypotension, cardiac failure
- *Renal complications*: Acute cortical necrosis, renal failure
- Impaired liver function tests
- *Gastrointestinal complications*: Ulcers and necrotizing enterocolitis
- *Lungs*: Persistent pulmonary hypertension.

CLINICAL PEARLS

- Careful antepartum and intrapartum fetal surveillance helps in preventing asphyxia and thereby avoiding the development of fetal distress
- Usually, the first indication of success of neonatal resuscitation is an increase in heart rate.

7. POSTPARTUM HEMORRHAGE

INTRODUCTION

According to the World Health Organization, postpartum hemorrhage (PPH) can be defined as excessive blood loss per vaginum (> 500 mL in case of normal vaginal delivery or > 1,000 mL following a cesarean section) from the time period extending within 24 hours of delivery and lasting until the end of the puerperium. The ACOG has defined PPH as a decrease in hematocrit by 10% or requirement of blood transfusion 24 hours after the delivery. The WHO has classified PPH into two: (1) primary PPH and (2) secondary PPH.

Primary (PPH) can be defined as blood loss, estimated to be greater than 500 mL, occurring from the genital tract, within 24 hours of delivery. Secondary PPH, on the other hand, can be defined as abnormal bleeding from the genital tract, occurring 24 hours after delivery until 6 weeks postpartum.

ETIOLOGY

The mnemonic "4 Ts" (tone, trauma, tissue and thrombin) help in describing the four important causes of PPH, which are enumerated in **Table 5.7**.

Table 5.7: Causes of PPH	
Cause	*Description*
Tone: Atonic uterus (commonest cause)	Overdistension of uterus, induction of labor, prolonged/precipitate labor, anesthesia (use of halogenated drugs like halothane), analgesia, grand multiparity, etc.
Trauma: Cervical, vaginal and perineal lacerations, pelvic hematomas, uterine inversion, ruptured uterus	Large episiotomy and extensions, tears and lacerations of perineum, vagina or cervix, pelvic hematomas, uterine inversion, ruptured uterus, etc.
Tissue: Retained tissue (placental fragments), invasive placenta	
Thrombin: Coagulopathies	Drugs (e.g. aspirin, heparin, warfarin, alcohol, chemotherapy); liver diseases; severe vitamin K deficiency; Von Willebrand's disease; hemophilia; DIC; etc.

DIAGNOSIS

General Physical Examination

Features of shock, such as hypotension and tachycardia, may be present.

Abdominal Examination

On abdominal palpation, the uterus may appear to be atonic.

Per Speculum Examination

- Bleeding through the cervical os may be observed
- Tears or lacerations of the genital tract (particularly vagina and cervix) which may be responsible for bleeding may be visualized.

Investigations

- Complete blood count with peripheral smear
- *Coagulation profile*: Platelet count, PT, APTT, thrombin time, etc.
- Urinalysis (for hematuria)
- *High vaginal swab*: To rule out infection (especially gonorrhea, chlamydia, etc.)
- *Transabdominal or transvaginal ultrasound*: Ultrasound examination may especially be required if retained products of conception are suspected.

MANAGEMENT

According to the guidelines by the Scottish Executive Committee of the RCOG, the immediate management in case with PPH comprises of steps which are enumerated in **Box 5.1**, all of which may be required to be undertaken simultaneously. Next step of management depends on whether the placenta has delivered **(Fig. 5.15)** or not **(Fig. 5.16)**.

Placenta has delivered
Abdominal palpation
Uterus soft and flabby (atonic PPH)
Uterus hard and contracted
Oxytocics, fundal massage
Explore the cervix, vagina and vulva
Uterus still remains atonic
Bimanual uterine compression
Uterine tamponade
Vaginal or vulval hematoma
Vaginal or cervical tears
No lesions
Uterus atonic
Consider surgical procedures:
Uterine artery/ ovarian artery ligation
Internal iliac artery ligation
B-lynch brace sutures
Angiographic embolization
Repair
Manual exploration of uterus
Up to 4 cm and stable
4 cm or larger and expanding
Nothing works
Hysterectomy
Ice packs and observation
Incise, drain and pack
Retained placental bits or clots
Uterine rupture
Uterine inversion
No cause found
Remove
Resuscitation/ urgent laparotomy
Resuscitation/ replace uterus
Seek consultant advice, observation, stabilize mother, repeat algorithm

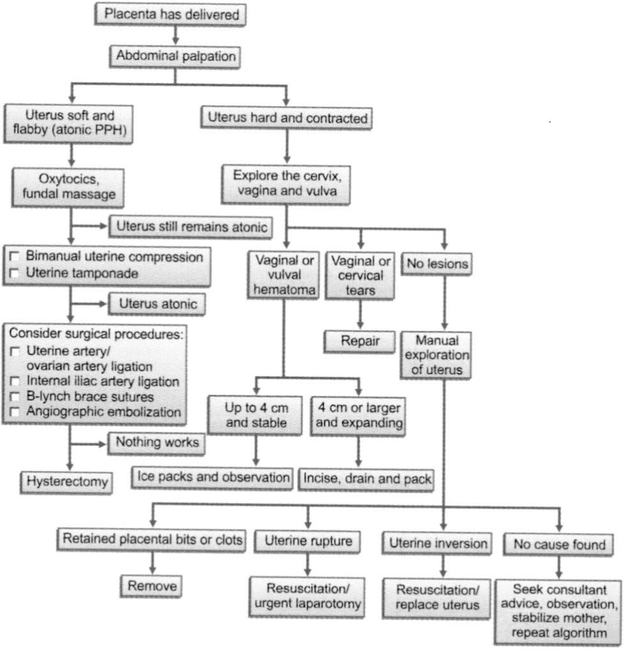

Figure 5.15: Management of a case of PPH where placenta has delivered

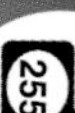

Box 5.1: Steps involved in the immediate management of patients with PPH

- Communicate (call for additional staff to manage the obstetric emergency)
- Resuscitation of the patient (evaluation of ABC: **A**irway, **B**reathing and **C**irculation)
- Blood to be sent for typing and cross-matching. Blood transfusion can be considered in these cases
- Administration of oxygen via a face mask
- Establishment of intravenous access and infusion of crystalloids
- Identifying and treating the underlying cause of bleeding.

Surgical management becomes necessary if the uterus remains atonic and flabby despite of conservative or medical management. Some such surgical procedures are as follows:

- Application of aortal compression at the time of surgery
- Brace sutures of uterus (B lynch compression sutures) **(Fig. 5.17)**
- Uterine artery or utero-ovarian artery ligation **(Fig. 5.18)**
- Bilateral ligation of internal iliac (hypogastric arteries) **(Fig. 5.19)**
- Angiographic embolization
- Hysterectomy (as a last option if nothing seems to work).

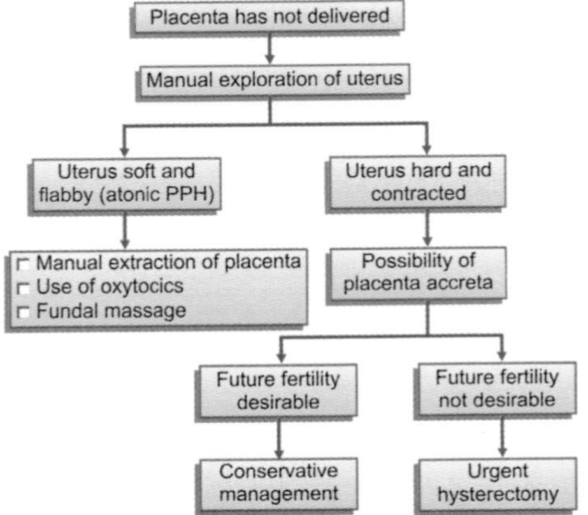

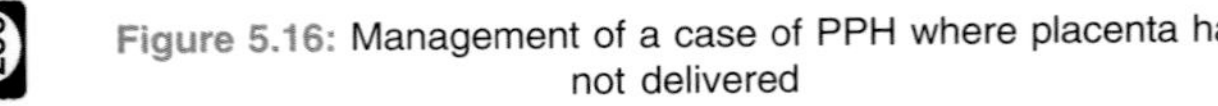
Figure 5.16: Management of a case of PPH where placenta has not delivered

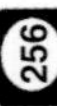

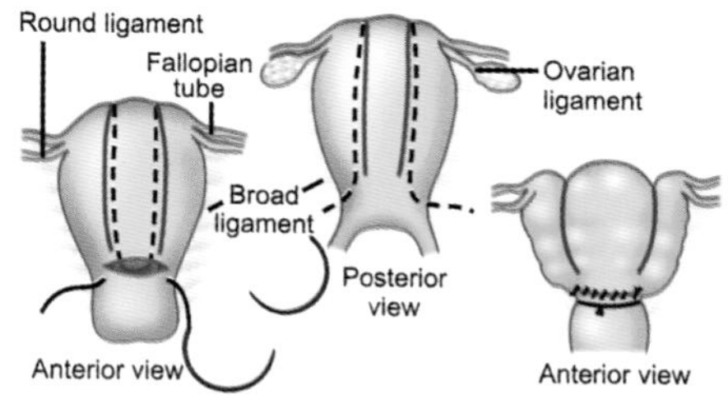

Figure 5.17: B-lynch suture

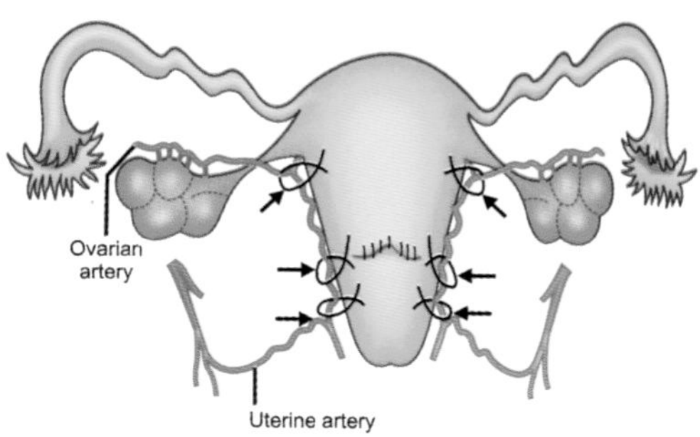

Figure 5.18: Various sites of uterine artery ligation

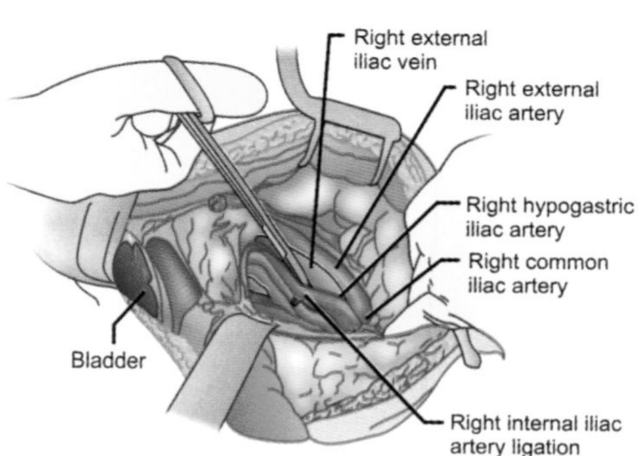

Figure 5.19: Internal iliac artery ligation

COMPLICATIONS

PPH is one of the important causes of maternal morbidity and mortality. Some of the complications are as follows:

- Blood loss resulting in shock, DIC
- Septicemia and death
- Renal failure
- Puerperal sepsis; failure of lactation
- Blood transfusion reaction; thromboembolism; Sheehan's syndrome; hypovolemic shock; puerperal shock and multiple organ failure associated with circulatory collapse and decreased organ perfusion.

CLINICAL PEARLS

- The most important step which must routinely be used in the third stage for prevention of PPH is the active management of third stage of labor which comprises of the following steps:
  - Administration of a uterotonic drug, usually 0.25 mg of methergine or ergometrine 0.2 mg soon after the delivery of the anterior shoulder and/or oxytocin 10 IU within 1 minute of birth of the baby
  - Clamping the cord as soon as it stops pulsating
  - Uterine massage
  - Controlled cord traction or Brandt-Andrews maneuver to deliver the placenta **(Fig. 5.20)**.

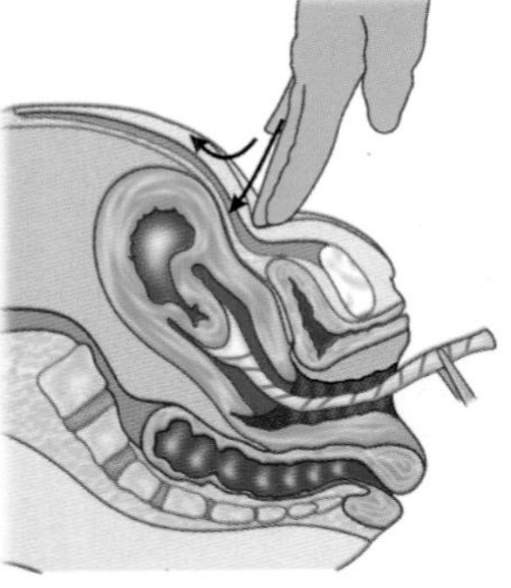

Figure 5.20: Method of controlled cord traction. This involves applying firm traction on the umbilical cord with one hand and suprapubic counter pressure with the other hand

- Some of the signs of placental separation are as follows: appearance of a suprapubic bulge due to hardening and contracting of uterus; sudden gush of blood; a rise in the height of the uterus (as observed over the abdomen) due to the passage of placenta to the lower uterine segment and irreversible cord lengthening.

8. UTERINE RUPTURE

INTRODUCTION

Uterine rupture is defined as a disruption of the uterine muscle extending to and involving the uterine serosa. At times, there may be disruption of the uterine muscle with extension to the bladder or broad ligament. The uterine rupture can be of two types:

1. *Complete rupture*: Complete rupture describes a full-thickness defect of the uterine wall and serosa, resulting in direct communication between the uterine and the peritoneal cavity.
2. *Incomplete rupture*: Incomplete rupture is also known as uterine dehiscence and describes partial separation of the previous cesarean in association with minimal bleeding, with the peritoneum and fetal membranes remaining intact.

ETIOLOGY

Causes during pregnancy: With intact uterus, the causes may include perforating mole, multiparity, congenital uterine malformations, abruption placentae, etc. With the history of scarred uterus, the various causes may be previous history of cesarean delivery, hysterotomy, uterine surgery, etc.

Causes during labor: During labor the various causes may be similar to that during pregnancy, with the following exceptions:

- Obstructive labor is an important cause of spontaneous rupture
- Forceful delivery in the form of internal version or manual removal may sometimes be responsible.

Disintegration of the scar is one of the most disastrous complications associated with VBAC. The reported incidence of scar rupture for all pregnancies is 0.05% and commonly occurs during labor. The exact risk of scar rupture depends upon the type of uterine incision, given at the time of previous cesarean, with the previous history of classical scar or a T-shaped incision being associated with almost 10% risk.

DIAGNOSIS

Clinical Presentation

Symptoms of impending scar rupture during labor include the following:

- Dull suprapubic pain or severe abdominal pain, especially if persisting in between the uterine contractions
- Slight vaginal bleeding or hematuria
- Bladder tenesmus or frequent desire to pass urine
- Unexplained maternal tachycardia
- Maternal hypotension
- Abnormal fetal heart rate pattern (e.g. fetal bradycardia, which may be preceded by variable and/or late decelerations)
- Scar tenderness
- Chest pain or shoulder tip pain or sudden onset of shortness of breath
- Onset of unexpected antepartum or postpartum hemorrhage
- On vaginal examination, there may be a failure of normal descent of the presenting part and the presenting part may remain high up. There may also be a sudden loss of station of the presenting part. All this may result in poor progress of labor.

Investigations

- *Assessment of scar integrity*: In order to identify the previous cesarean scars, which are likely to give way during VBAC, the following investigations can be done:
  - *Ultrasound imaging*: Ultrasound examination for visualization of scar defects and measurement of scar thickness must be done at approximately 37 weeks of gestation because this is the time when a defective scar is likely to be thinnest
  - *Manual exploration*: Manual exploration of placenta to check scar integrity is especially useful, in case of continuing postpartum hemorrhage and in case of other third stage problems.

MANAGEMENT

When uterine rupture is diagnosed or strongly suspected, surgery is necessary. Immediate steps must be taken to resuscitate the patient. While in the previous days, most cases of uterine rupture were managed with hysterectomy, nowadays most cases are managed by controlling the bleeding surgically and repairing the defect. If future fertility is desirable and the rent in the uterus appears to be repairable, repair of the rupture site must be performed. If future fertility is not desirable or the uterine

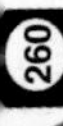

rent appears to be unrepairable (multiple rents with ragged margins, injury to the iliac vessels, etc.), hysterectomy should be performed.

COMPLICATIONS

- Massive postpartum hemorrhage
- Hypovolemic shock
- Increased maternal mortality and morbidity.

CLINICAL PEARLS

- The identification or suspicion of uterine rupture is a medical emergency and must be followed by an immediate and urgent laparotomy to save the patient's life
- Due to the risk of rupture recurrence in subsequent pregnancies, a repeat cesarean section may be required for future pregnancies
- Several factors, which are indicative of a weak scar, include the following: improper hemostasis at the time of surgery; imperfect coaptation of uterine margins at the time of surgery; extension of the angles of uterine incision; infection during healing; implantation of the placenta at the site of incision; etc.

9. UTERINE INVERSION

INTRODUCTION

Uterine inversion during the acute postpartum period is a relatively rare complication in which the uterus is turned inside out either partially or completely. The uterine endometrium with or without attached placenta may be visible. Uterine inversion can be classified as follows **(Figs 5.21A to C)**:

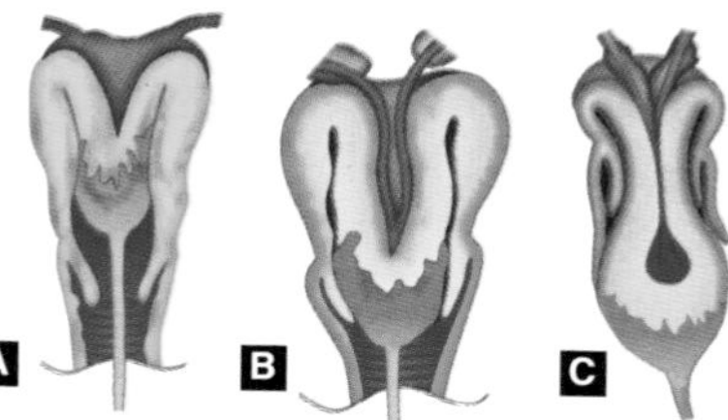

Figures 5.21A to C: Degrees of uterine inversion (A) first degree; (B) second degree and (C) third degree

- *First degree*: Dimpling of the uterine fundus which remains well above the level of internal os
- *Second degree*: Uterine fundus passes through the cervix, but lies insides the vagina
- *Third degree (complete)*: The uterus protrudes completely out of the vaginal introitus. The uterine endometrium with or without the attached placenta may be visible
- In terms of onset of the inversion, it can be classified as acute, subacute and chronic.

ETIOLOGY

The exact etiology behind uterus inversion remains unclear. The most likely factors include the following:

- Spontaneous prolapse is commonly associated with a sharp rise in intra-abdominal pressure accompanied with uterine atony
- Strong traction on the umbilical cord, particularly when the placenta is in a fundal location, during the third stage of labor
- Placenta accreta, particularly involving the uterine fundus
- Short umbilical cord
- Antepartum use of magnesium sulfate or oxytocin
- Iatrogenic causes: Mismanaged third stage of labor, pulling the cord, Crede's method of placental delivery, application of fundal pressure in an atonic uterus.

DIAGNOSIS

Symptoms

- Severe hypotension with shock
- Acute pain in the lower abdomen with bearing down sensation.

Abdominal Examination

- Absence of uterine fundus or presence of an obvious defect of the fundus upon abdominal palpation.

Bimanual Examination

This helps in conforming the diagnosis and degree of prolapse

- Profuse bleeding through the cervical os
- Palpation of the inverted fundus at the cervical os or vaginal introitus

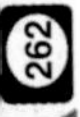

- In cases of incomplete inversion, the fundal wall may be palpated in the lower uterine segment and cervix.

Imaging Studies

- *Ultrasound*: On transverse scans, a hyperechoic mass in the vagina with a central hypoechoic H-shaped cavity may be visualized. A depressed longitudinal groove, extending from the uterine fundus to the center of the inverted part may be observed on longitudinal scans
- *Magnetic resonance imaging*: Appearance of the uterus is similar to that found in sonographic imaging; however, MRI findings are much more accurate.

CONSERVATIVE MANAGEMENT

- *Treatment of shock*: This may include blood transfusion
- *Manual manipulation of the uterus (Johnson's maneuver)*: This consists of pushing the inverted fundus through the cervical ring with pressure directed toward the umbilicus **(Figs 5.22A to C)**:
  - The part which inverted last must be replaced first by applying firm pressure with the fingers
  - Counter-pressure must be applied by the hand placed over the abdomen
  - Following the replacement, hand must remain inside the vagina until the uterus is contracted
  - Following uterine replacement, the vagina must be packed with antiseptic roller gauze and the foot end of the bed must be elevated

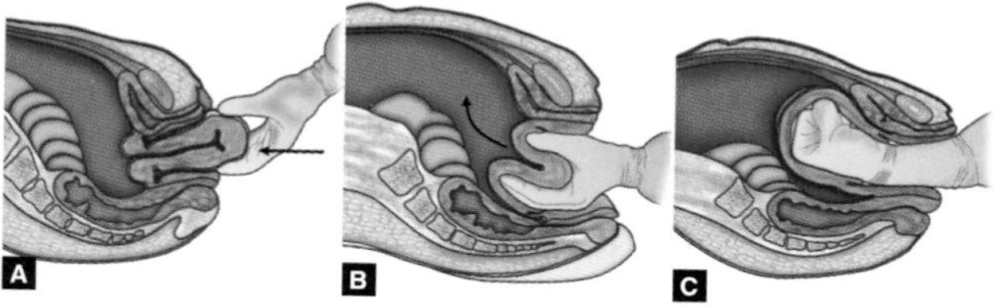

Figures 5.22A to C: Reduction of uterine inversion using Johnson's method: (A) the protruding fundus is grasped with fingers directed toward the posterior fornix; (B and C) the uterus is returned to position by pushing it through by steady application of pressure towards the umbilicus

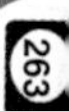

- *Use of pharmacologic agents*: Most commonly used uterine relaxants comprise of magnesium sulfate or terbutaline. In extreme cases intravenous nitroglycerine or general anesthetic agent, such as halothane, can also be used
- Use of oxytocic agents must be withheld if the diagnosis of uterine inversion is made
- *O'Sullivan's method*: Use of hydrostatic pressure to correct the inversion.

SURGICAL MANAGEMENT

Surgical intervention may be required if conservative management is unsuccessful.

- *Huntington procedure*: A laparotomy is performed to locate the cup of the uterus. Gentle traction is applied in an upward direction after placing the clamps in the cup of the inversion below the cervical ring. Repeated clamping and traction must be continued until the inversion is corrected
- *Haultain procedure*: An incision is made in the posterior portion of the inversion ring through the abdomen, to increase the size of the ring and allow repositioning of the uterus.

COMPLICATIONS

- Postpartum hemorrhage and shock
- Maternal death
- Pulmonary embolism
- Untreated cases may develop infection and/or sloughing.

CLINICAL PEARLS

- Uterine inversion can be a life-threatening obstetric complication, which must be treated like an obstetric emergency
- The best prognosis is achieved by prompt recognition of the condition and immediate attempts to correct the inversion.

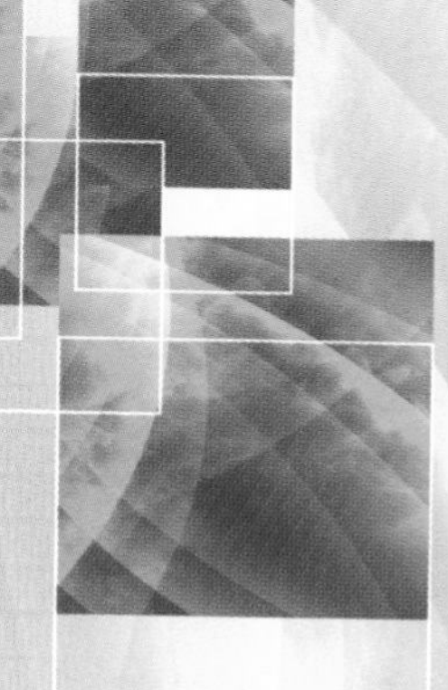

Section II

GYNECOLOGY

- General Gynecology
- Abnormalities of Menstruation
- Gynecological Oncology
- Gynecological Surgery
- Disorders of the Uterus
- Gynecological Infections
- Infertility
- Disorders of Ovaries and Fallopian Tubes
- Urogynecology
- Contraception

CHAPTER 6

General Gynecology

1. GYNECOLOGICAL EXAMINATION

INTRODUCTION

There are many aspects to women's health which are related to gynecological care. Some gynecological problems commonly encountered in clinical practice include abnormal menstrual bleeding, abdominal mass, gynecological cancers, pelvic pain, infertility, etc. For being able to diagnose the abnormal gynecological complaints, it is important for the clinician to be able to take history, and perform a normal gynecological examination **(Box 6.1)**, following which the management plan **(Box 6.2)** is decided.

Box 6.1: Conducting a normal gynecological examination

Diagnosis

History

The history must be taken in a nonjudgmental, sensitive and thorough manner. Importance must be given toward maintenance of patient-physician relationship. The following points need to be asked while taking history:

- *Pain*: Exact site of pain, nature of pain (whether burning, gnawing, throbbing, aching or excruciating in nature), intensity of pain (mild, moderate or severe), aggravating and relieving factors for pain, radiation of pain (to the inner aspect of the thighs, etc.) and relationship of other factors with pain such as menstruation (dysmenorrhea), coital activity (dyspareunia), micturition (dysuria), defecation (dyschezia), posture and movement needs to be determined
- Infertility or amenorrhea
- *Hirsutism*: Refer to the coming-up fragments
- Vaginal discharge
- *Past medical history*: Past history of medical illnesses, such as hypertension, hepatitis, diabetes mellitus, cancer, heart disease, pulmonary disease and thyroid disease, needs to be taken
- *Family history*: Certain gynecological cancers (e.g. ovary, uterus and breast) have a genetic predisposition

Contd...

Contd...

- *Marital and sexual history*: Details of the woman's marital life including her age at the time of marriage, how long she has been married and sexual history need to be asked
- *Obstetric History*: Details of every pregnancy conceived irrespective of their ultimate outcome need to be recorded
- *History of previous surgery*: The patient should be asked about any surgery she has undergone in the past, the reason for undergoing that surgery, particularly of abdominal or pelvic origin, type of incision (laparoscopy or laparotomy) and any history of postoperative complications
- *Previous gynecological history*: History of prior gynecologic problems including abnormalities in Pap smear, bleeding problems, sexually transmitted diseases, etc. also needs to be taken
- *Menstrual history*: The following details need to be recorded: age of menarche; date of last menstrual period; cycle length, whether regular or irregular; number of days the bleeding takes place; amount of bleeding (in terms of pads soaked) and presence of any associated symptoms such as cramps, bloating or headaches.

General Physical Examination

- *Vital signs*: Patient's vitals signs, such as temperature, blood pressure, pulse, respiratory rate, height and weight, need to be taken
- *Breasts examination*: Examination of the breasts should be carried out in three positions: with patient's hands on her hips (to accentuate the pectoral muscles), with her arms raised and then in supine position
- *Anemia, dehydration*: Excessive blood loss may result in the development of anemia
- *Signs suggestive of hyperandrogenemia*: Signs suggestive of hyperandrogenemia, such as hirsutism (presence of facial hair), deepening of voice, etc., may be related to the presence of androgen secreting tumors or chronic anovulatory states (polycystic ovarian disease)
- *Neck examination*: Local examination of the neck may reveal enlargement of thyroid gland or lymph nodes of the neck. Neck examination should also involve palpation of cervical and supraclavicular lymph nodes
- *Thyroid examination*: It is important to examine the thyroid gland because menstrual abnormalities may be commonly associated with thyroid dysfunction.

Abdominal Examination

- *Abdominal mass*: If an abdominal mass is felt on abdominal palpation, location of the mass in relation to the various abdominal quadrants needs to be determined. Other features of the mass which need to be determined include shape of the mass (round, oval, irregular, etc.); its

Contd...

Contd...

size (in cm); its consistency (hard, jirm, rubbery, soft or fluctuant); margins (well-defined or irregular); mobility (free or fixed to the adjacent tissues); tenderness on palpation and presence of guarding, rigidity and rebound tenderness of the lower abdomen

- *Presence of ascites*: Ascites is commonly associated with malignant tumors and sometimes with benign conditions such as tubercular peritonitis and Pseudomeig's syndrome. Presence of ascites is detected by two tests: (1) Fluid thrill and (2) shifting dullness. Dullness in the flanks upon percussion and shifting dullness indicates the presence of free fluid in the peritoneal cavity.

Pelvic Examination

The patient must be described the procedure of pelvic examination and her informed consent be taken before proceeding with the examination. The full dorsal position with the knees flexed is the most commonly employed position used for gynecological examination in clinical practice. Pelvic examination comprises of the following: examination of the external genitalia, a per speculum examination, bimanual vaginal examination and a per rectal examination (if required). Following the per speculum examination, which is performed using a Cusko's or a Sim's speculum **(Fig. 6.1)**, a bimanual vaginal examination must be performed. First one and then two fingers are inserted into the vaginal introitus following which a bimanual vaginal examination is done. Cervical shape, size, position, mobility, consistency and tenderness caused by pressure or movement need to be assessed. In clinical scenario, the vaginal examination **(Fig. 6.2A)** is immediately followed by a bimanual examination **(Fig. 6.2B)** without removing fingers from the vaginal introitus. While the fingers of the examiner's right hand are still inside the vaginal introitus, the palm of his or her left hand is placed over the abdomen. To feel the uterus, the vaginal fingers should move the cervix as far backward as possible to rotate the fundus downward and forward. The abdominal hand is then placed just below the umbilicus and gradually moved lower until the fundus is caught and pressed against the fingers in the anterior fornix. The following points are noted on bimanual examination: size of the uterus; its position (anteverted or retroverted); mobility, (restricted mobility or fixed uterus). If there is a mass felt, its relation to the uterus is noted, like whether the mass is felt separate to the uterus or is continuous with it.

Investigations

- *Ultrasound examination*: Ultrasound for the diagnosis of gynecological pathology is primarily done by two ways: (1) transvaginal and (2) transabdominal ultrasound. Recently Doppler ultrasound is also increasingly being used. Tranvaginal examination provides images with much better resolution as compared to transabdominal examination. The normal uterine endometrium as visualized by TVS is shown in **Figures 6.3A and B and 6.4**

Contd...

Contd...

- *CT examination*: CT examination is usually indicated in the presence of malignancy. CT examination may also help in delineating enlarged lymph nodes and other retroperitoneal pathologies
- *MRI examination*: MRI examination helps in identification of soft tissue planes and diagnosis of adenomyosis, Müllerian defects such as vaginal agenesis and uterine didelphys, ureteral stones and urethral obstruction
- *Hysterosalpingography*: HSG is a radiological procedure which involves injection of a radiopaque material into uterine cavity through cervical canal, followed by fluoroscopy with image intensification in order to investigate shape of the uterine cavity and the shape and patency of the fallopian tubes
- *Pap smear (papanicolaou test)*: Refer to Chapter 8 for details.

Box 6.2: Devising a management plan in case of a gynecological complaint

Gynecological Management

Gynecological diagnosis is made after careful analysis of the positive findings related to the history, clinical examination and various investigations. After ascertaining the diagnosis, the next step is to establish the severity of the disease. In case of malignancy, the cancer staging must be done. Treatment is decided based on diagnosis and severity of the disease. The duty of the gynecologist does not end once the treatment has been dispensed; the duty of the clinician is also to assess the patient's response to the treatment by calling her for follow-up visits.

CLINICAL PEARLS

- As far as possible a per vaginal examination must be avoided in virginal women
- The "three line sign" appearance of the proliferative phase endometrium on TVS is formed by the central hyerechoic reflection representing the endometrial cavity and the additional hyperchoic reflections representing the thin developing layers of the endometrium.

2. NORMAL GYNECOLOGICAL ANATOMY

This fragment would cover external genital organs **(Box 6.3)**, internal genital organs **(Box 6.4)**, blood vessels, nerves and lymph nodes of pelvis **(Box 6.5)** and anatomy of the abdominal wall **(Box 6.6)**.

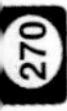

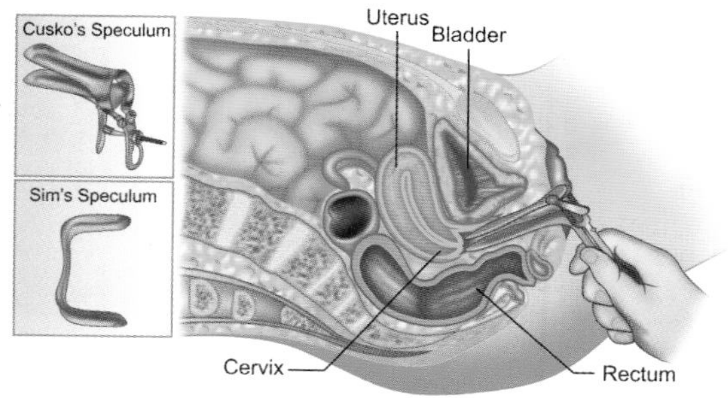

Figure 6.1: Per speculum examination

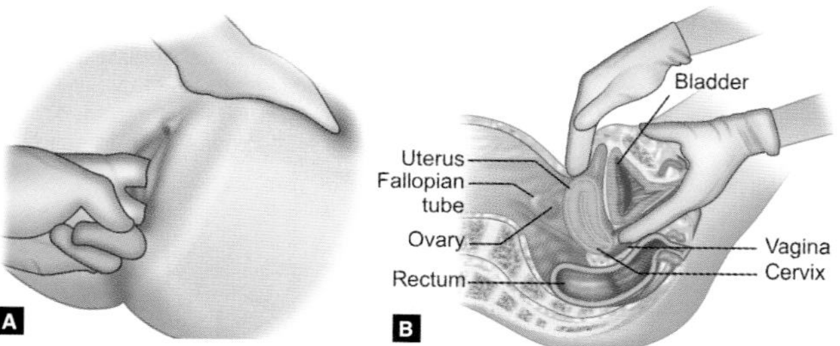

Figures 6.2A and B: (A) Two finger vaginal examination, performed by inserting two fingers of right hand inside the vagina; (B) bimanual vaginal examination performed with the palm of left hand over the abdomen and the fingers of right hand still inside the vagina

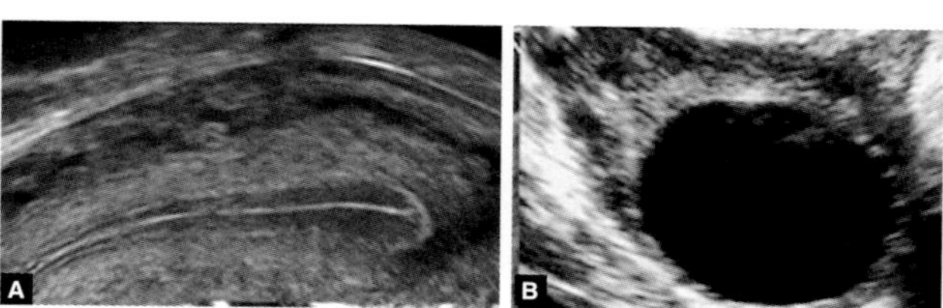

Figures 6.3A and B: (A) TVS of the uterus in the proliferative phase, showing presence of a well defined "three line sign"; (B) ovary showing presence of a dominant follicle

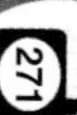

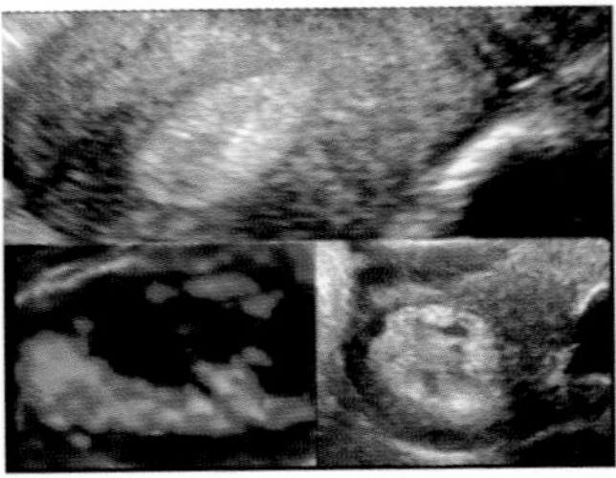

Figure 6.4: TVS in the luteal phase showing uniformly hyper-echogenic endometrium. The total double layer thickness in the luteal phase ranges from 4 mm to 12 mm with an average of 7.5 mm; two small pictures in the bottom half show corpus luteum which appears as an echogenic structure within the ovary with prominent peripheral vascularization

Box 6.3: External genital organs

External genital organs

The external genital organs include mons pubis, labia majora, labia minora, Bartholin'sglands, and clitoris **(Fig. 6.5)**. An ill-defined area containing these external genital organs along with the perineum is known as the vulva. The external genital organs have three main functions: (1) enabling sperm to enter the body; (2) protecting the internal genital organs from infectious organisms and (3) provision of sexual pleasure.

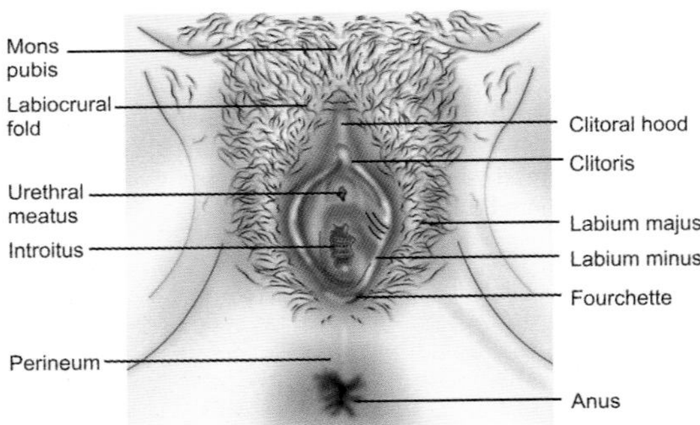

Figure 6.5: Female external genital organs

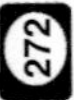

Box 6.4: Female internal genitalia

Female Internal Genitalia

The internal genital organs form the genital tract. This pathway consists of the following **(Figs 6.6A and B)**:

a. *Vagina*: Where sperms are deposited
b. *Uterus*: Where the embryo develops into a fetus
c. *Fallopian tubes (oviducts)*: Where the fertilization of sperm with egg occurs
d. *Ovaries*: Which produce and release eggs
   - *Hymen*: At the beginning of the tract, just inside the opening of the vagina, is the hymen, a mucous membrane. In virgins, the hymen usually encircles the vaginal opening like a tight ring, but it may completely cover the opening
   - *Vagina*: The vagina is the main female organ of sexual intercourse. It also acts as the passageway for transportation of sperms and for the expulsion of the menstrual blood. It also helps in the delivery of the baby. The vaginal portion of the cervix projects into the upper part of the vagina, resulting in the formation of anterior, posterior and lateral fornices. The vaginal mucosa is lined by stratified squamous epithelium. There are no glands in the vagina and the vaginal secretions are mainly derived from the mucus discharge of the cervix and transudation through the vaginal epithelium. The vaginal secretions during the reproductive life are acidic due to the presence of lactic acid
   - *Fallopian tubes*: Also known as the oviduct or the uterine tube, each fallopian tube is about 2–3 inches long and extends from the upper edge of the uterus toward the ovaries. The two fallopian tubes normally extend laterally from the uterine cornua and open into the peritoneal cavity near the ovaries by flaring into a funnel shaped structure, infundibulum having finger-like projections (fimbriae). When an oocyte is released from an ovary, the fimbriae guide it toward the infundibulum of the fallopian tube. The fallopian tubes are lined with tiny hair-like projections (cilia), which along with the muscles of the tube's wall help in propelling an oocyte downward into the uterine cavity where it ultimately implants in the form of a blastocyst. Starting from the lateral to medial side, the fallopian tube can be divided into four parts: (1) infundibulum; (2) ampulla; (3) isthmus and (4) the uterine part (which opens via the uterine ostium into the uterine cavity)
   - *Ovaries*: The ovaries are almond-shaped, pearl-colored, female gonads responsible for producing the oocytes (female gametes or the germ cells). The developing oocytes are contained in the fluid-filled cavities called follicles in the wall of the ovaries. Each ovary is suspended by a short fold of peritoneum known as the mesovarium, which arises from the broad ligament

Contd...

Contd...

A baby girl is born with oocytes in her ovaries. No new oocytes develop after birth. Between 16 and 20 weeks of gestation, the ovaries of a female fetus contain 6–7 million oocytes. Most of these oocytes gradually die away, leaving about 1–2 million oocytes to be present at birth. At puberty, only about 300,000 oocytes remain, of which only a small percentage mature into eggs. The many thousands of oocytes that do not mature undergo degeneration. Degeneration is usually complete by the time, the woman attains menopause

- *Uterus*: The uterus is a thick-walled, muscular, pear-shaped organ located in the middle of the pelvis, in which the development of fetus and embryo occurs. The adult uterus comprises of two main parts: (1) body (uterine corpus) and (2) cervix. The non-gravid uterus lies in the lesser pelvis, with its body lying on the urinary bladder and cervix between the urinary bladder and the rectum. The uterus is anchored in its position by several ligaments. The adult uterus is usually anteverted and anteflexed so that its mass lies over the bladder. The cervix is composed of two parts: (1) supravaginal part (between the uterine isthmus and the vagina) and (2) the vaginal part (which protrudes into the vagina), also known as ectocervix or portiovaginalis. The wall of the body of uterus comprises of three layers: (1) parametrium (the serosa or the outer serous coat); (2) myometrium (the middle coat of smooth muscles) and (3) endometrium (the inner mucous coat).

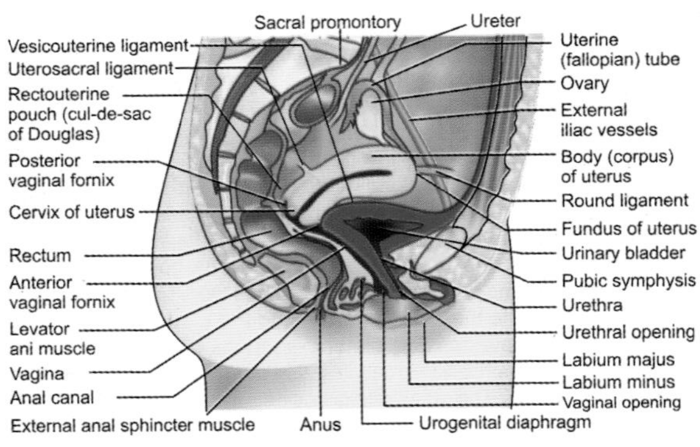

Figure 6.6A: Midsagittal section of female pelvis

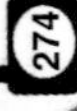

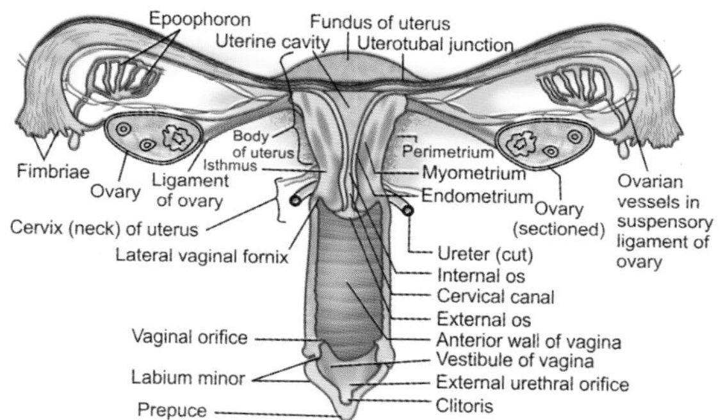

Figure 6.6B: Female internal genital organs

Box 6.5: Blood vessels, nerves and lymph nodes of pelvis

Blood Supply of the Pelvis

- The blood supply to the pelvis is mainly by the internal iliac artery, also known as the hypogastric artery **(Fig. 6.7)**, which is branch of the common iliac artery at the level of sacroiliac joint
- *Blood supply to the uterus*: Blood supply to the uterus is mainly by the uterine arteries (branch of internal iliac arteries) with the collateral supply from ovarian arteries **(Fig. 6.8)**
- *Blood supply to the vagina*: The arteries supplying the superior part of vagina derive from the uterine artery. The arteries supplying the middle and inferior parts of vagina are derived from the vaginal and internal pudental arteries respectivly
- *Arteries of the vulva and perineum*: The vulva and perineum is supplied by the branches from internal pudental artery, which is a branch of internal iliac artery. This branch ends in the form of the dorsal artery of clitoris, which supplies the clitoris and the vestibule.

Lymph Nodes of Pelvis

- Lymph nodes of the pelvic region, which drain the female genital organs, comprise of the following groups: lumbar; inferior mesenteric; common iliac; internal iliac; external iliac; superficial inguinal; deep inguinal; sacral and pararectal groups. The cervix drains primarily into the external and internal iliac group of lymph nodes, whereas body of the uterus drains mainly into the external iliac and lumbar nodes.

Nerve Supply to Pelvis

- *Pelvic nerves*: The pelvis is innervated mainly by sacral and coccygeal spinal nerves and the pelvic part of autonomic nervous system.

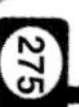

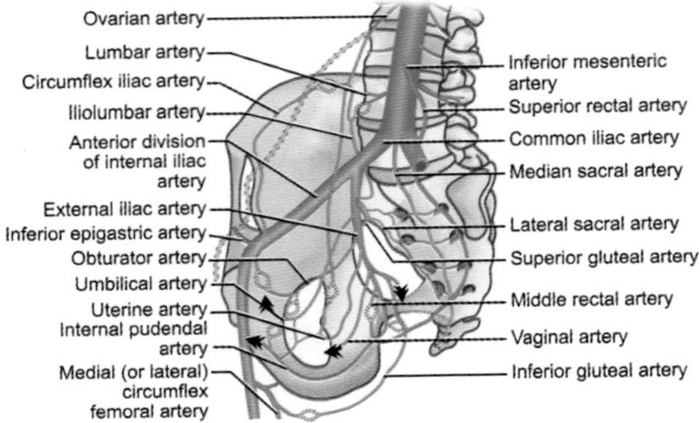

Figure 6.7: Blood supply to the pelvis

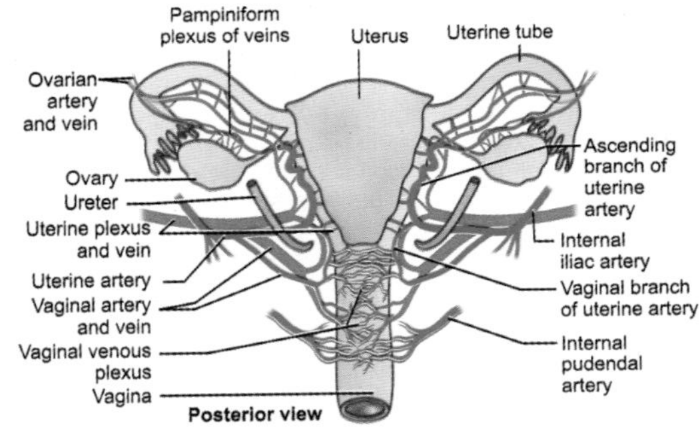

Figure 6.8: Blood supply to internal genital organs

Box 6.6: Anatomy of the abdominal wall

Muscles of the Abdominal Wall

- The musculature of the abdominal wall is composed of two muscle groups. One group, comprising of the flat muscles, consists of three muscles: (1) external oblique; (2) internal oblique and (3) transverses abdominis. The second group is composed of two muscles that run vertically and comprise of the muscles, rectus abdominis and the pyramidalis

Contd...

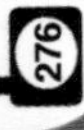

Contd...

- *Rectus sheath*: The rectus sheath is formed by the conjoined aponeuroses of flat abdominal muscles. It is formed by the decussation and interweaving of the aponeurosis of these muscles. The aponeurosis of external oblique muscle contributes to the formation of the anterior wall of the sheath throughout its length. A concentric line, "arcuate line" lies midway between the umbilicus and pubis symphysis and demarcates the transition between the aponeurotic posterior wall of the sheath covering the superior three-fourths of the rectus and the transversalis fascia covering the inferior quarter. Throughout the length of the sheath, the fibers of the anterior and posterior layer of the sheath interlace in the anterior median line to form the complex linea alba. The composition of the rectus sheath above and below the arcuate line is described in **Figure 6.9**

Vessels of the Abdominal Wall

- The primary blood supply to the abdominal wall is from the superficial and deep blood vessels. The main blood vessels supplying the anterolateral abdominal wall are as follows:
  - Superior epigastric vessels and the branches of musculophrenic artery
  - Inferior epigastric and deep circumflex iliac arteries
  - Superficial circumflex iliac and superficial epigastric arteries
  - Posterior intercostal vessels of the 11th intercostal space and the anterior branches of the subcostal vessels

The blood supply of the anterior abdominal wall is demonstrated in **Figure 6.10**.

CLINICAL PEARLS

- The posterior vaginal fornix is the deepest and the posterior vaginal wall the longest in comparison to the anterior or lateral walls
- Ampulla is the widest and the largest part of the tube, which lies medial to the infundibulum. Fertilization of the oocyte usually occurs in the ampulla
- Uterine artery assumes important role at the time of pregnancy because it supplies maternal circulation to the placenta during this time.

3. MENSTRUAL CYCLE

Box 6.7 describes the events of a normal menstrual cycle. Interplay of various hormones, involved in the pathogenesis of a normal menstrual cycle is described in **Box 6.8**.

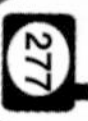

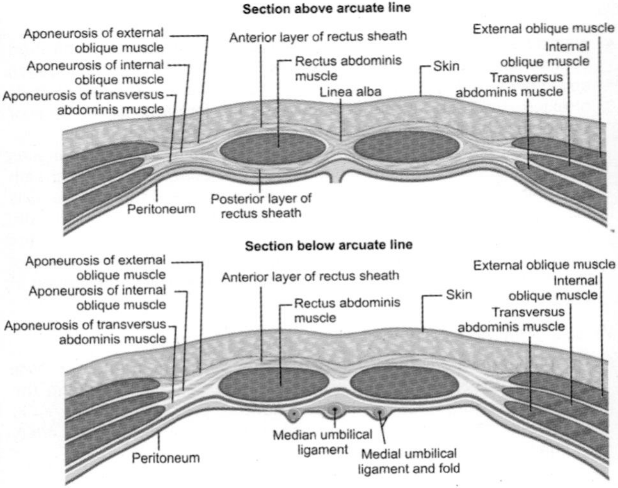

Section above arcuate line
Aponeurosis of external oblique muscle
Aponeurosis of internal oblique muscle
Aponeurosis of transversus abdominis muscle
Anterior layer of rectus sheath
Rectus abdominis muscle
Linea alba
Skin
External oblique muscle
Internal oblique muscle
Transversus abdominis muscle
Peritoneum
Posterior layer of rectus sheath
Section below arcuate line
Aponeurosis of external oblique muscle
Aponeurosis of internal oblique muscle
Aponeurosis of transversus abdominis muscle
Anterior layer of rectus sheath
Rectus abdominis muscle
Skin
External oblique muscle
Internal oblique muscle
Transversus abdominis muscle
Peritoneum
Median umbilical ligament
Medial umbilical ligament and fold

Figure 6.9: The rectus sheath

Internal thoracic artery
Musculophrenic artery
Superior epigastric artery
10th posterior intercostal artery
External oblique
11th posterior intercostal artery
Internal oblique
Subcostal artery
Inferior epigastric artery
Deep circumflex iliac artery
Superficial epigastric artery
Superficial circumflex iliac artery
External iliac artery
Femoral artery

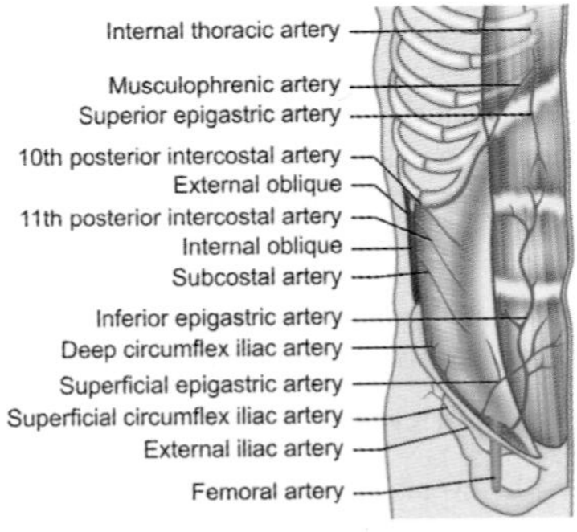

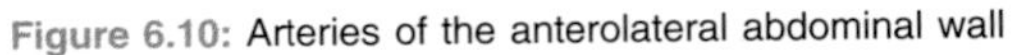

Figure 6.10: Arteries of the anterolateral abdominal wall

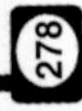

Box 6.7: Events of a normal menstrual cycle

- The events of the normal menstrual cycle are shown in **Figure 6.11**. The menstrual phase usually lasts for 5 days and involves disintegration and sloughing of the functionalis layer of the endometrium. Interplay of various prostaglandins (e.g. prostaglandin F2-alpha and prostaglandin E2) is involved in regulation of menstrual cycle. A typical menstrual cycle comprises of 28 days. Ovulation occurs in the middle of the menstrual cycle, i.e. day 14 of a typical cycle. The first 14 days of the cycle, before the menstruation occurs form the proliferative phase, while the next 14 days of the cycle form the secretory phase
- *Follicular (proliferative phase)*: During this phase of normal menstrual cycle, there is an increase in the blood levels of the hormone estrogen and maturation of the dominant follicle takes place. The following changes take place during the proliferative phase:
  - The functional and the basal layers of endometrium become well defined. The proliferation mainly occurs in the functional layer
  - The glands become elongated and slightly sinuous and the columnar epithelium lining them becomes taller
  - There is an increase in ciliated and microvillous cells in the endometrial glands
  - In initial phase, the spiral vessels are uncoiled and unbranched. However, soon the growth of the straight vessels occurs then they start becoming more coiled and spiraled
- *Ovulation*: Ovulation occurs at the mid-point of menstrual cycle. The events preceding ovulation are as follows: estrogen production peaks (must be > 200 pg/mL for more than 24 hours) and is responsible for triggering the FSH and LH surge. FSH is responsible for further development of primary follicles. Of these 15–20 primary follicles which start developing, only 1 follicle eventually develops near the surface of the ovary to the stage of full maturity. The other oocytes, which are not destined to ovulate, die and get converted into fibrous tissue, the corpus atreticum. Rupture of the dominant ovarian follicle follows, resulting in ovulation
- *The secretory (luteal) phase*: Following the process of ovulation, the ruptured ovarian follicle gets converted into corpus luteum (CL); the main hormone produced by CL being progesterone. The endometrium during this phase gets transformed for implantation of conceptus in anticipation of pregnancy. If pregnancy occurs, the rising levels of hCG stimulate and rescue the endometrium. In case the pregnancy does not occur, the CL undergoes regression. As a result, the levels of estrogen and progesterone rapidly decline causing withdrawal of functional support of endometrium. This results in menstrual bleeding, marking the end of one endometrial cycle and the beginning of the other. Some characteristic features of this stage are:

Contd...

Contd...

- There is production of progesterone and less potent estrogens by the corpus luteum. This phase extends from day 15 to day 28 of the typical cycle
- During this phase, the functionalis layer of the endometrium increases in thickness, stroma becomes edematous and the glands become tortuous with dilated lumen and stored glycogen
- The most characteristic feature of this phase is development of subnuclear vacoulation in the glandular epithelial cells. In this, the glycogen filled vacuoles develop between the nuclei and the basement membrane (by the day 17–18). This is the first evidence that ovulation has taken place
- The endometrium measures about 8–10 mm in the secretory phase
- The secretory phase reaches its peak activity by the 22nd day of the cycle after which no growth occurs. The glands become crenated and tortuous to assume a characteristic corkscrew shaped appearance. The cork-screw pattern of the glands becomes saw-toothed in the later part of secretory phase
- The stroma of the functional layer further becomes edematous during this phase. The functional layer of the endometrium can be divided into two layers: superficial or compact layer and deep spongy layer. The spiral vessels further become dense and deeply coiled.

Box 6.8: Role of various hormones in regulation of menstrual cycle

- Initial follicular development is independent of hormonal influence. **Figure 6.12** illustrates the levels of different hormones during various phases of menstrual cycle. However, soon FSH takes control and stimulates a cohort of follicles encouraging them to develop into preantral stage. FSH causes aromatization of the androgens present in the theca cells into estrogen in the granulosa cells. Out of the various follicles, only one single follicle is destined to develop into a dominant follicle, which eventually undergoes ovulation **(Fig. 6.13)**. Estrogen exerts a negative feedback effect on FSH as a result of which growth of all the follicles except dominant follicle is inhibited. While causing a decline in FHS levels, the mid-follicular rise in estradiol levels exert a positive feedback influence on LH secretion. The presence of LH in the follicle prior to ovulation is important for optimal follicular development which ultimately results in the formation of a healthy oocyte. A surge of LH takes place just prior to ovulation. LH initiates luteinization and progesterone production in the granulosa layer
- Ovulation occurs about 10–12 hours after the LH peak and 24–36 hours after the peak estradiol levels have been attained. The onset of LH surge is the most reliable indicator of impending ovulation

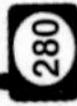

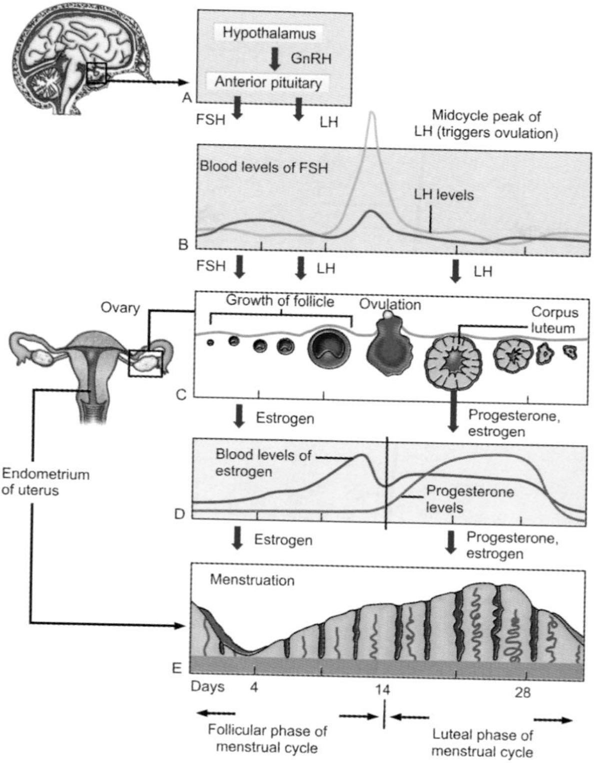

Hypothalamus
GnRH
Anterior pituitary
A
FSH
LH
Midcycle peak of LH (triggers ovulation)
Blood levels of FSH
LH levels
B
FSH
LH
LH
Ovary
Growth of follicle
Ovulation
Corpus luteum
C
Estrogen
Progesterone, estrogen
Endometrium of uterus
Blood levels of estrogen
Progesterone levels
D
Estrogen
Progesterone, estrogen
Menstruation
E
Days 4 14 28
Follicular phase of menstrual cycle
Luteal phase of menstrual cycle

Figure 6.11: Events in a normal menstrual cycle

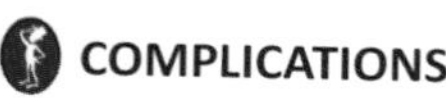

COMPLICATIONS

For various abnormalities of menstrual cycle please refer to Chapter 7.

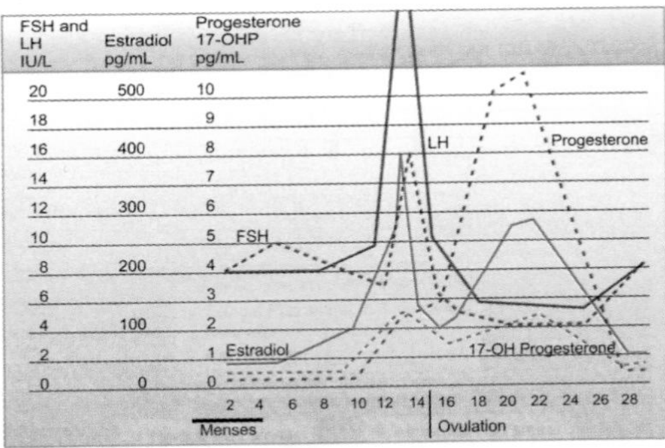

Figure 6.12: Levels of various hormones during various phases of menstrual cycle

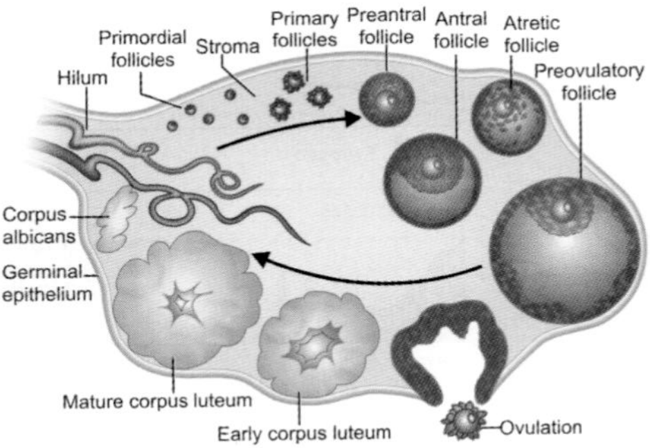

Figure 6.13: Changes in ovarian follicles during various phases of menstrual cycle

CLINICAL PEARLS

- Initial follicular development is independent of hormonal influence
- Insulin like growth factors (IGF I and IGF II) are also involved in the pathogenesis of normal menstrual cycle. The most abundant IGF in human follicles is IGF II

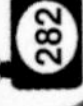

- Inhibin B secreted by granulosa cells of the ovary helps in suppressing pituitary FSH production. On the other hand, activin originating in both pituitary and granulosa cells augments FSH production.

4. ADOLESCENT AND PEDIATRIC GYNECOLOGY

4.1. PUBERTY

INTRODUCTION

Puberty is the process of physical changes which cause transformation of the child's body into that of an adult, capable of reproduction. It can be defined as progression from appearance of sexual characteristics to sexual, reproductive and mental maturity. Before puberty, body differences between boys and girls are almost entirely restricted to the genitalia. During puberty, there is development of secondary sexual characteristics which lead to development of major differences in size, shape, composition and function in many body structures and systems.

ETIOLOGY

Puberty is initiated as a result of hormone signals sent from the brain to the gonads (the ovaries and testes). The hormal signals are responsible for stimulating the growth and function of a variety of organs such as brain, bones, muscles, skin, breast and sex organs. The principal hormone involved in the males is testosterone, while that in females is estradiol. Interaction of various hormones secreted through the hypothalamus-pituitary-ovarian axis and other endocrine organs such as adrenals and thyroid glands, plays a role. Other factors, such as genetic, environmental (nutrition, emotional stress and childhood illnesses), etc., may also play a role.

DIAGNOSIS

Clinical Presentation

The process of puberty typically begins by the age of 10 or 11 years in girls and by the age of 12 or 13 years in boys. During the period of puberty, there are anatomical (development of secondary sexual and genital organs), physical, endocrinological, psychological and emotional changes. The sequence of occurance of pubertal changes is as follows: physical growth **(Fig. 6.14)** followed by development of secondary sexual characters and thelarche (by 10–12 years). Pubarche occurs after approximately 1 year and lastly there is development of ovaries and genital organs followed by occurance of menarche.

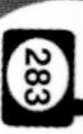

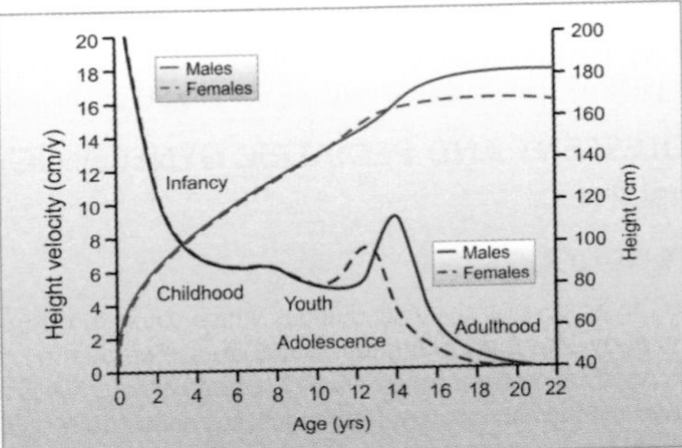

Figure 6.14: Changes in height in both girls and boys at the time of puberty

- *Thelarche*: This refers to the breast development and occurs at the average age of 10.5 years. The first physical sign of puberty in girls is appearance of a firm, tender lump under the center of the areola in one or both the breasts
- *Pubarche*: The next noticeable change of puberty is development of pubic hair, usually occurring within a few months of thelarche
- *Menarche*: This refers to the occurance of first menstrual bleeding and typically occurs about 2 years after thelarche. The average age of menarche in girls is 11.75 years
- *Vagina, uterus, ovaries*: The mucosal surface of the vagina also responds to the increasing levels of estogen, changing from a thin, bright red prepubertal vaginal mucosa to a thicker, dull-pink color post-puberty. There also occurs keratinization of skin and transformation of the vaginal epithelium into a multilayered squamous epithelim under the influence of estrogen. Vaginal epithelium turns acidic with the appearance of Doderlein's bacilli. There is development of labia majora with deposition of fat. Rapid growth of the uterus occurs so that the prepubertal uterus to cervix ratio changes from 1:1 to 2:1 or 3:1. There is also enlargement of ovaries and occurance of ovulation
- *Body shape, fat distribution and physical development*: There is an increase in the girl's height and weight, which is usually completed by 14 years of age. There is broadening of the lower half of the pelvis

and hips, thereby resulting in a wider birth canal. Fat deposition occurs in a typical female distribution in the areas of breasts, hips, buttocks, thighs, upper arms and pubis

Physical Examination

- *Breast enlargement*: This may initially be unilateral or asymmetric. Gradually, the breast diameter increases, the areola darkens and thickens, and the nipple becomes more prominent. Tanner's stage of breast and pubic hair development has been described in Chapter 12
- *Examination of the external genitalia*: This may reveal presence of pubic hair, or enlargement of the clitoris. The vaginal mucosa, which is a deep-red color in prepubertal girls, becomes pastel-pink in appearance as estrogen exposure increases

Investigations

X-ray of the non-dominant hand, elbow and knees is done in order to assess the bone age.

MANAGEMENT

Sex education: Although puberty is a natural physiological process, sex education regarding the pubertal changes helps in allaying stress and anxiety from the minds of young girls. Young girls need to be educated about sex and sexually transmiited diseases. In case of possibility of sexual intercourse at young age, contraception (barrier methods, initially) must be prescribed. Extra nutrition (especially proteins, iron and calcium) may be required to support their growth.

COMPLICATIONS

Some commonly occurring gynecological problems during this period are:

- Precocious puberty
- Delayed puberty
- Menstrual abnormalities
- Dysmenorrhea
- Vaginal discharge
- Teenage or unwanted pregnancies
- Cryptomenorrhea (occurance of menstruation without any external flow of blood, e.g. in cases of imperforate hymen).

CLINICAL PEARLS

- While puberty refers to an individual's sexual and physical maturation rather than the psychosocial and cultural aspects of development, adolescence is the period of psychological and social transition between childhood and adulthood
- Although the growth and maturation of graafian follicles occur at the time of puberty, ovulation may not occur as late as 1–2 years after menarche. Due to this, menstrual periods largely remain anovular and may be irregular, prolonged, scanty or excessive
- Occurance of menstruation before the development of secondary sexual characteristics can be considered as abnormal and is usually due to the feminizing ovarian tumors or the malignancy of the genital tract.

4.2. PRECOCIOUS PUBERTY

INTRODUCTION

Precocious puberty refers to the appearance of physical and hormonal signs of pubertal development at an earlier age than is considered normal. Puberty is considered precocious in case there is develoment of secondary sexual characteristics in girls younger than 8 years **(Fig. 6.15)** or there is onset of menses before the age of 10 years (chronological age). For boys, onset of puberty before the age of 9 years is considered precocious.

ETIOLOGY

Precocious puberty can be of two types: (1) central precocious puberty (CPP) (constitutional/true/complete precocious puberty), which is gonadotropin-dependent and (2) precocious pseudopuberty, which is gonadotropin-independent. CPP is characterized by premature activation of the entire hypothalamic-pituitary-gonadal axis, with the full spectrum

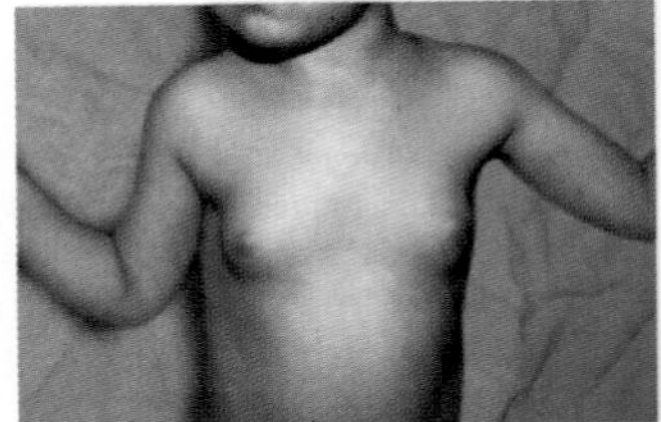

Figure 6.15: Precocious breast development in a 7-year old girl

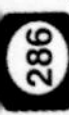

of physical and hormonal changes of puberty. On the other hand, precocious pseudopuberty may be associated with the following causes:

- Congenital adrenal hyperplasia (CAH)
- Human chorionic gonadotropin secreting tumors
- Tumors of the adrenal gland, ovary or testis
  McCune-Albright's syndrome
- Exposure to exogeneous sex steroid hormones.

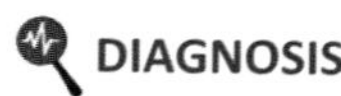

DIAGNOSIS

Clinical Presentation

The diagnosis is made with the help of a careful history and physical examination in conjunction with the use of radiologic and laboratory evaluations. The clinician must differentiate CPP from precocious pseudopuberty at the time of examination. In CPP, the secondary sexual characteristics appear in a chronological order, and eventually regular menstrual cycles are established. Due to exposure to estrogens, there is an initial spurt of height followed by premature closure of epiphysis due to which the ultimate height remains stunted.

Investigations

- *Sex steroid levels*: Serum estradiol levels that exceed 20 pg/mL usually indicate puberty, but the levels may frequently vary. Moreover, the levels of adrenal androgens [e.g. dehydroepiandrosterone (DHEA), dehydroepiandrosterone sulfate (DHEAS)] are usually elevated in boys and girls with premature pubarche
- *Gonadotropins*: Gonadotropin levels (LH and FSH) may be raised in cases of CPP
- *Thyroid function tests*: Thyroid tests are not a routine requirement in the evaluation of precocious puberty
- *Imaging studies*: These include radiography of the hand and wrist in order to determine bone age. If bone age is within 1 year of chronological age, puberty has not started (e.g. a 2-year old girl with premature thelarche) or the duration of the pubertal process has been relatively brief. If bone age is advanced by 2 years or more, puberty likely has been present for a year or more or is progressing more rapidly
- Radiography of the pituitary fossa, CT scan or MRI, etc. may be indicated to look for a tumor or a hamartoma, especially if the hormonal studies indicate a diagnosis of CPP. Pelvic ultrasonography is essential

when precocious pseudopuberty is suspected in girls (based on examination or hormone levels) in order to detect an ovarian tumor or cyst.

SURGICAL MANAGEMENT

When CPP is caused by a CNS tumor other than a hamartoma, surgical resection may be attempted. Radiation therapy is often indicated if surgical resection is incomplete.

MEDICAL MANAGEMENT

- *Gonadotropin-releasing hormone analog*: Continuous administration of LHRH and GnRH agonists provides negative feedback and results in decreased levels of LH and FSH 2–4 weeks after initiating treatment. GnRH analogues in the dosage of 100 μg intransally BD for 6 months can be used to suppress menstruation because the young girls might not be capable of managing menstrual hygiene.

COMPLICATIONS

- Rapid bone maturation can cause linear growth to cease too early and can result in an ultimate short adult stature
- The early appearance of breasts or menses in girls and increased libido in boys can cause emotional distress for some children
- Children with precocious puberty may be stressed, may become withdrawn, may exhibit behavioral problems (such as poor self-esteem and higher anxiety, irritability or withdrawal) and may have difficulty adjusting to wearing and changing pads.

CLINICAL PEARLS

- A history of early puberty in a parent or sibling is relevant and decreases the likelihood that early puberty has an organic cause
- Future reproductive capacity is usually not compromised in cases of true precocious puberty.

4.3. DELAYED PUBERTY

INTRODUCTION

Delayed puberty in girls can be defined as no occurance of breast development by 13 years, or no menarche by 3 years after breast development or by the age of 16 years. In boys, delayed puberty can be defined as no testicular enlargement by 14 years, or delay in development for 5 years or more after onset of genitalia enlargement.

ETIOLOGY

Some likely causes for delayed puberty are as follows:

- Variation of normal (constitutional delay)
- Pituitary hypothalamic inadequacy
- Prolonged high level of physical exertion or stress, e.g. athlete, belly dancer, etc.
- Systemic diseases, e.g. inflammatory bowel disease, chronic renal failure, etc.
- Undernutrition, e.g. anorexia nervosa
- Hypothalamic defects and diseases, e.g. Kallmann's syndrome
- Pituitary defects and diseases, e.g. hypopituitarism
- Gonadal defects and diseases, e.g. Turner's syndrome, premature ovarian failure, Klinefelter's syndrome
- Irradiation, chemotherapy or trauma to the hypothalamus and/or pituitary
- Hormonal imbalances, and endocrine disorders, e.g. hypothyroidism, Cushing's syndrome, CAH
- Genetic abnormalities, e.g. cystic fibrosis, Biedl-Bardet's syndrome, etc.
- Brain tumors, e.g. craniopharyngioma, prolactinoma, germinoma, etc.

DIAGNOSIS

Investigations

- *Radiology*: An X-ray of the hand to assess bone age helps in revealing whether the child has reached a stage of physical maturation at which puberty should be occurring. Visible secondary sexual development usually begins when girls achieve a bone age of 10.5–11 years
- *Gonadotropin levels*: Measurement of gonadotropin levels helps in revealing if the cause is due to the defect of the gonads (elevated gonadotropin levels) or due to the deficiency of the sex steroids (reduced gonadotropin levels).

MANAGEMENT

- If on radiological assessment, bone age is less than the chronological age, wait and watch policy must be adopted. Most of these girls eventually develop secondary sexual characteristics and menarche

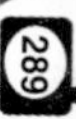

- The treatment most commonly involves administration of testosterone or related compounds to boys and estrogens to girls in extreme cases. Pubertal delay due to gonadotropin deficiency may be treated with testosterone replacement or hCG. Growth hormone can also be sometimes prescribed.

COMPLICATIONS

Delayed puberty may cause anxiety or stress to the girls as well as her parents.

CLINICAL PEARLS

- A delay of two standard deviations has been proposed as a standard
- If no obvious cause of delayed puberty can be detected, reassurance and prediction of puberty based on bone age work in most cases.

5. SEX AND INTERSEXUALITY

INTRODUCTION

Intersexuality refers to individuals whose biological sex cannot be classified as clearly male or female. The intersex disorders are now termed as the disorders of sexual development (DSD) and are due to the presence of intermediate or atypical combinations of physical features which distinguish male and female genders from each other. In a normal individual, sexual differentiation involves the following aspects: gonadal development; genital development and behavioral differentiation, and has been described in details in Chapter 1 (fragment of embryology).

ETIOLOGY

Intersexuality commonly occurs due to the abnormal development of chromosomal, gonadal or anatomical sex (e.g. masculinization of female or partial or incomplete masculinization in a male). Some of these are as follows:

Disorders of Gender Identity Associated with Normal Constitution of Sex Chromosomes

- *Female pseudohermaphroditism*: Female pseudohermaphrodites have a chromosomal sex of a female, but have external genitalia of a male. This can occur due to adrenogenital syndrome (associated with excessive testosterone production), etc.

- *Male pseudohermaphroditism*: Male pseudohermaphrodites have chromosomal sex of a male, but have external genitalia of a female. This can occur due to causes such as primary gonadal deficit, testicular regression syndrome, leydig cell agenesis, defects in testosterone synthesis, deficiency of 17-γ-hydroxylase, defect in Müllerian inhibiting system, end organ defects such as androgen insensitivity syndrome (testicular feminization), incomplete androgen insensitivity syndrome (Reifenstein's syndrome); disorders of testosterone metabolism such as 5-γ-reductase deficiency

Disorders of Gender Identity Associated with Abnormal Constitution of Sex Chromosomes

- *Infrequently associated with ambiguous genitalia*: Klinefelter's syndrome, Turner's syndrome, pure gonadal dysgenesis, etc.
- *Frequently associated with ambiguous genitalia*: Mixed gonadal dysgenesis, true hermaphroditism [an individual containing both male gonadal tissue (testes) and female gonadal tissue (ovaries)]
- *Hormonal influences*: Excessive exposure to androgens (e.g. virilizing tumors of ovaries, etc.) can cause masculinization of female external genitalia. Presence of estrogens in males can cause gynecomastia.

DIAGNOSIS

General Physical Examination

- An intersex individual may have biological characteristics of both male and the female sexes. Signs of feminism in male include hypospadias (opening of urethra below the phallus), underdevelopment of the phallus, split scrotum and undescended testicles. Signs of masculinization in females include, hypertrophy of phallus, fusion of labia, hirsutism, etc.
- *External anatomical sex*: This is determined from features such as body contours, development of musculature, bone (pelvis), distribution of hair on the face, chest, etc., breast development and appearance of external genitalia
- *Internal anatomical sex*: Presence of internal genitalia, such as uterus, fallopian tubes and ovary, is an evidence of the individual being a female
- *Gonadal sex*: This is evident on the biopsy of the gonadal structure
- *Psychological sex*: This is determined by one's behavior, speech, dress and sexual inclination.

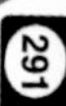

Investigations

- *Genetic/chromosomal or nuclear screening*: study of buccal smear (presence of barr bodies), skin biopsy or a neutrophil examination (drumstick-like projection)
- *Examination of external genitalia*: Detailed examination of external genitalia preferably under general anesthesia must be performed
- *Gonadal biopsy*: This helps in identifying either male or female genitalia and may also reveal the presence of degenerated testis or streak gonads
- *Imaging studies*: This includes ultrasound examination, which may help in identifying ovarian neoplasms and adrenal tumors. Magnetic resonance imaging to check for suspected adrenal neoplasms, radiography of pituitary fossa and the skeleton may be also performed in some cases. Intravenous pyelography may be done to check for any renal anomalies
- *Hormone estimation*: This includes determination of the serum levels of hormones such as estrogens, 17-ketosteroids and testosterone, and 17-hydroxyprogesterone in urine
- Serum electrolyte levels
- Psychological assessment of the patient's sexuality.

SURGICAL MANAGEMENT

Surgical management of intersex can be categorized into one of the following two:

- *Restoration of functionality (or potential functionality)*
- *Enhancement surgery*: Enhancement surgery to enable the individual to identify with a particular sex, e.g., breast enlargement surgery, may be required in some cases.

CLINICAL PEARLS

- Presence of one barr body suggests presence of two X-chromosomes
- Treatment should be best deferred until puberty when the pragmatic sex of the individual becomes apparent.

6. AMBIGUOUS GENITALIA

INTRODUCTION

Ambiguous genitalia refer to sexual anatomy of external genitalia, which cannot be classified as typically female or male.

ETIOLOGY

Ambiguous genitalia occur due to variation in any of the processes of development of sexual organs. Some important causes are:

- *Virilization*: This could be due to adrogenital syndrome which causes hyperplasia of adrenal cortex and can be of two types: (1) congenital or intrauterine and androgenital syndrome (deficiency of 21 hydroxylase) and (2) postnatal androgenital syndrome (due to excessive production of ACTH from a basophil adenoma of anterior pituitary). Other causes of virilization include virilizing tumors and conditions of ovary (arrhenoblastoma, hilus cell tumor, PCOS, hyperthecosis, etc.)
- *Exposure to maternal androgens*: Virilization of a female fetus may occur if progestational agents or androgens are used during the first trimester of pregnancy.

DIAGNOSIS

Clinical Presentation

- A family history of genital ambiguity, infertility or unexpected changes at puberty may suggest a genetically transmitted trait
- *Physical examination*: Virilism may be associated with hirsutism, male appearance and breast atrophy
- *External genitalia examination*:
  - External genitalia may show a feminine appearance with larger-than-average clitoris (clitoral hypertrophy) and partially fused labia, giving appearance of scrotum or
  - External genitalia may appear masculine with a smaller-than-average penis that is open along the underside (hypospadic). The scrotum may be empty without the presence of testicles
  - The position of urethral meatus must be noted
- *Gonadal examination*: Documentation of palpable gonads is important
- *Rectal examination*: Rectal examination may reveal the cervix and uterus, confirming internal Müllerian structures.

Investigations

Logical work-up in infants with ambiguous genitalia includes the following:

- Chromosomal analysis
- Endocrine screening

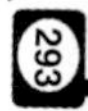

- Serum chemistry or electrolyte tests
- Androgen-receptor levels
- 5-alpha reductase type II levels
- Imaging studies: Renal or bladder ultrasonography can be performed at the bedside in the neonatal ICU. Ultrasonography usually allows visualization of a neonate's adrenal glands, which may be enlarged and show a cribriform appearance in infants with CAH. Ultrasonography also helps in identifying Müllerian structures. CT scanning and MRI are usually not indicated but may help identify internal anatomy.

MANAGEMENT

- *Exploratory laparotomy or gonadal biopsy*: Open exploration may help to identify internal duct anatomy and allow gonadal tissue to be obtained for histologic characterization
- *Diagnostic laparoscopy or gonadal biopsy*: Laparoscopic examination under general anesthesia may allow rapid identification and delineation of the internal duct anatomy. Biopsy of gonads may also be performed laparoscopically
- *Male pseudohermaphroditism*: These individuals look like females and are therefore reared as women and must be continued to be reared as such. In cases of complete androgen insensitivity, gonadectomy (removal of undescended testis) must be performed after completion of puberty due to high chances of development of malignancy in an undescended male gonad. However, in cases of incomplete androgen insensitivity, earlier surgery may be required to prevent hirsutism and/or virilization at the time of puberty. Administration of estrogens near puberty helps in the growth of breasts. Surgical correction of external genitalia and creation of an artificial vagina is required for sexual functioning
- *Female pseudohermaphroditism*: In cases of congenital adrenogenital syndrome, administration of synthetic cortisone or synthetic corticosteroids (glucocorticoids, hydrocortisone, etc.) may help to control the excessive production of ACTH and may also help in restoring menstruation. Restoration of external genitalia to a feminine pattern can be done by plastic surgery. McIndoe's vaginoplasty to create an artificial vagina can be considered if the patient is engaged and married.

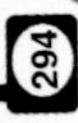

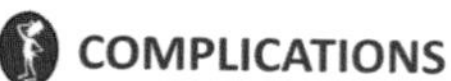

COMPLICATIONS

In the cases where nonfunctional testes are present (e.g. androgen insensitivity syndrome), there is a risk of development of malignancy later in life.

CLINICAL PEARLS

- Congenial adrenal hyperplasia is the most common cause of ambiguous genitalia in the newborn
- As convention, surgery (vaginoplasty) is best performed at birth.

7. HIRSUTISM

INTRODUCTION

This can be defined as distribution of excessive hair (which is coarse and dark) in a male pattern in a female, i.e. presence of hair over the upper lip, chin, chest, lower abdomen, back and thighs. Hirsutism associated with male characteristics, such as temporal baldness, hoarse voice, clitoromegaly, etc., as well as features of defeminization, such as amenorrhea and breast atrophy, is known as virlization.

ETIOLOGY

Most of the cases of hirsutism are associated with high levels of male sex hormones—androgens. Some of the possible causes for this include:

- *Ovarian causes*: Polycystic ovarian disease, hyperthecosis, masculinizing ovarian tumors (arrhenoblastomas, hilus cell tumors, etc.)
- *Adrenal causes*: CAH, Cushing's syndrome, adrenal tumors
- *Drugs*: Androgens (anabolic steroids), progestogens with androgenic effects, drugs such as minoxidil, danazol, phenytoin, diazoxide, etc.

In many cases of hirsutism, no underlying cause may be detected.

DIAGNOSIS

General Physical Examination

There may be presence of excessive coarse, dark hair in male-pattern, i.e. over the abdomen, breasts and upper lip. If hirsutism is caused by high levels of androgens, symptoms associated with hyperandrogenism, such as irregular menstrual periods, acne, loss of feminine body shape and other

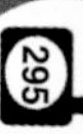

signs of masculinization such as deepening of voice, male pattern baldness, etc., may be present. Symptoms associated with the specific cause may include:

- *Cushing's syndrome*: Some signs and symptoms may include, obesity, especially around the abdominal region, hypertension, diabetes, thinning of skin, striae in the abdominal region, etc.
- *PCOS*: This may present with oligomenorrhea, obesity, hirsutism, infertility, etc.
- *Masculinizing ovarian tumors*: Features of defeminization, such as breast atrophy and amenorrhea, may be present. Bimanual pelvic examination is required for detection of a pelvic mass.

Investigations

- *Imaging*: Imaging modalities such as ultrasound and MRI may be indicated to locate the ovarian or adrenal tumor. Ultrasound features related to PCOS are described in Chapter 13. A CT scan often helps in the diagnosis of a pituitary tumor, especially hyperprolactinoma
- *Hormonal studies*: CAH occurs due to the deficiency of 21 hydroxylase. In these cases, the levels of 17-hydroxyprogesterone may be raised to greater than 8 ng/mL. Other tests include determination of levels of testosterone, DHEAS, thyroid hormones, LH:FSH ratio, testosterone levels, sex hormone binding globulins, and prolactin
- *Dexamethasone suppression test*: This involves administration of 1 mg of dexamethasone at night and study of single plasma cortisol levels in the morning. The levels should be less than 100 μgm
- *Hyperprolactinomas*: In these cases, there may be a presence of a pituitary tumor and prolactin levels are greater than 100 ng/mL.

MANAGEMENT

- *Treatment of the cause*: Removal of ovarian or adrenal tumors
- *Dexamethasone*: This must be administered in the dosage of 0.25–0.5 mg daily at night in case of adrenal hyperplasia. Combined oral contraceptive pills (not containing androgenic progestogens) may be required, in addition, to suppress androgen production
- *Antiandrogens*: Antiandrogens such as spironolactone (100–200 mg daily) and cyproterone acetate (a potent progestogen)
- *Weight reduction*: This helps in elevating the levels of sex hormone binding globulins which bind with free testosterone.
- *Cosmetic methods*: These may include agents such as bleaching, waxing, shaving, laser, electrolysis, etc.

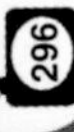

CLINICAL PEARLS

- New agents being tried for the treatment of hirsutism include flutamide and finasteride.

8. MENOPAUSE AND HORMONE REPLACEMENT THERAPY

INTRODUCTION

Menopause can be defined as the cessation of ovarian function resulting in permanent amenorrhea (lasting for at least 1 year). Climacteric (perimenopause) is the phase of waning ovarian activity and may begin 2–3 years before menopause and may continue 2–5 years after it. The onset of menopause involves physical, sexual and psychological adjustments. Menopause normally occurs between the age of 45 and 50 years, with the average being about 47 years.

Hormone replacement therapy (HRT) refers to a woman taking supplements of hormones such as estrogen alone or estrogen in combination with progesterone (progestin in its synthetic form).

ETIOLOGY

Menopause occurs due to decline in ovarian activity. There is failure of ovulation, failure of formation of corpus luteum and failure of secretion of progesterone by the ovaries. Estrogenic activity is reduced and there occurs endometrial atrophy, resulting in amenorrhea. Initially, there is a rebound increase in the secretion of FSH and LH by the anterior pituitary. However, with further advancing years, the gonadotropic activity of pituitary glands also cease and a fall in FSH levels eventually occurs **(Fig. 6.16)**.

HRT is not prescribed to all menopausal women. It must be slectively prescribed to women who are at high risk for menopausal abnormalities. Indications for the use of HRT are as follows:

- *Menopausal and postmenopausal patients*: Symptomatic patients suffering from vasomotor, urinary symptoms or symptoms related to genital atrophy such as dryness, itching, dysuria, dyspareunia, etc. Individuals at high risk for cardiovascular diseases, osteoporosis, Alzeimer's disease, etc. may also require HRT. Estrogen exerts a cardioprotective effect by maintaining high levels of HDL and lowering the levels of LDL
- *Premature Menopause*: Women suffering from premature menopause, such as premature ovarian failure, or those who have undergone surgical oophorectomy.

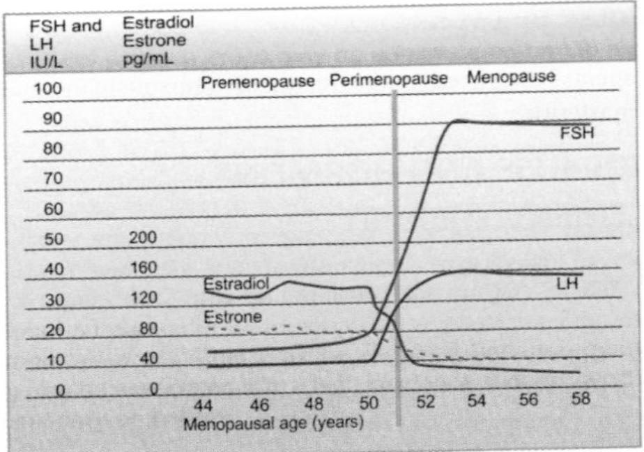

Figure 6.16: Changes in the levels of various hormones at the time of menopause

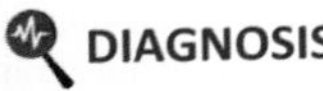

DIAGNOSIS

Clinical Presentation

Anatomical changes: Anatomical changes occuring during menopause include atrophy and retrogression of the genital organs. Moreover, there are aberrations in the endocrine balance maintained during the child-bearing period.

Symptoms

Nearly 60–70% of women remain asymptomatic; others may experience symptoms such as:

- *Vaginal dryness*: Signs and symptoms of vaginal dryness include dryness, itching, burning, pain or light bleeding with sexual intercouse, urinary frequency or urgency
- *Cessation of periods*: This could be a sudden cessation or gradual diminution in the amount of blood loss for each successive menstrual period, until the menstrual flow eventually ceases
- *Hot flashes*: Hot flashes and sweating commonly occur as a result of vasomotor disturbances and may occur in nearly 85% of women. These may be preceded by a headache
- *Osteoporosis*: There is likely to be reduction in bone mineral mass, resulting in osteopenia and/or osteoporosis, which may predispose to fracture development

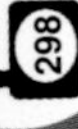

- *Mental symptoms*: Mental depression may occur due to disturbed sleep and inabity to cope up with the body changes. There may also be irritability and loss of concentration. Pseudocyesis (fear of pregnancy) and cancer phobia may develop in some women
- *Neurological symptoms*: These may include paresthesias (sensation of pins and needles)
- *Libido*: Although many women experience reduced libido, some women may also experience an increase in libido due to riddance of menstruation and fear of pregnancy
- *Urinary symptoms*: These may include symptoms such as dysuria, stress and urge incontinence and recurrent vaginal infections. Genital symptoms, such as dryness of vagina, dyspareunia, genital prolapse and urinary and/or fecal incontinence may also occur
- *Long-term effects*: In the long term, menopause is likely to result in complications such as arthritis, osteoporosis, fracture, cerebrovascular accidents, ischemic heart disease, myocardial infraction, atherosclerosis, stroke, skin changes, Alzheimer's disease, etc.

General Physical Examination

- *Vulva*: Atrophic changes in vulva are natural sequelae of estrogen deficiency characterized by loss of normal architecture and thinning of the skin. Vulvar atrophy may occur
- *Vagina*: There may be loss of thick keratinized mucosa and reduction in the amount of glycogen produced by the vaginal epithelium. These changes are clinically visible in the form of thinning of the vaginal walls, loss of rugae, narrowing of the vaginal orifice and dyspareunia. There may be thinning of the skin of labia minora and vestibule, and reduction in the amount of fat in labia majora. There is also reduction of pubic hair. Red patches around the urethra and introitus caused by senile vulvulitis may occur
- *Uterus*: There is reduction in the size of the fundus relative to the cervix, a decrease in myometrial thickness, and thinning of the endometrium. Laxity of the pelvic cellular tissues and ligaments predispose to the development of uterovaginal prolapse
- *Ovaries*: The postmenopausal ovary decreases in size even during use of HRT and should not be palpable by routine pelvic examination. Any enlargement of the ovary should be considered as malignancy until proven otherwise.

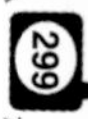

Investigations

Prior to the initiation of HRT, the following investigations need to be performed:

- *History and physical examination*: A complete history and physical examination including blood pressure measurement, assessment of breasts, pelvic and rectal examination must be done
- *Routine investigations*: These include estimation of blood sugar, lipid profile, electrocardiogram, mammography, Pap smear and pelvic ultrasound
- *Endometrial sampling and/or biopsy*: This may be required in cases with high-risk factors for endometrial cancer (e.g. morbid obesity, diabetes), history of abnormal uterine bleeding, history of polycystic ovary disease or prior use of estrogenic medications
- *Dual energy X-ray absorpitometry*: This helps in determining the level of osteopenia and osteoporosis and the propensity for fracture development
- *Hormone levels*: Measurement of levels of estrogen and FSH help in deciding the requirement for HRT.

MANAGEMENT

- *Counseling*: This involves explaining the normal menopause-related changes to the patient, giving her advice related to contraception, and asking her to eat a well-balanced nutritious diet (rich in vitamin A, C, D and E). She must be advised to do weight-bearing exercises, which may help to prevent or delay osteoporosis
- *Antidepressants or antianxiety agents*: These may be prescribed to relieve the woman of her anxiety and depression
- *Hormone replacement therapy*: There are three routes of estrogen administration available: (1) oral; (2) transdermal and (3) vaginal. HRT can be taken in the form of a pill, patch, gel, vaginal cream or slow-releasing suppository which can be placed in the vagina. Non-hormonal alternatives, such as black cohosh, soy or isoflavones, red clover, vitamin E, etc., can also be used.

Typical HRT Schedules

- *Conjugated estrogen and progesterone*: Natural equine conjugated estrogen must be prescribed in the dosage of 0.625 mg for days 1–25 each month and progestogen, such as medroxyprogesterone acetate

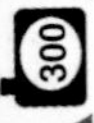

(5–10 mg), duphaston (5–10 mg) or primolut N (2.5 mg) must also be administered daily for days 13–25 each month in order to prevent endometrial hyperplasia and/or cancer. No hormones are given during the remainder of the month. Instead of conjugated estrogens, alternative estrogen preparations include ethinylestradiol (0.01 mg), micronized estrogen (1–2 mg) or evalon (1–2 gm). Most patients demonstrate withdrawal bleeding during the hormone-free interval. These hormones can also be prescribed continuously. Many patients may have irregular bleeding but 95% are likely to become amenorrheic within 1 year

- *Vaginal cream*: Use of estrogen vaginal cream (evalon) in the dosage of 1–2 gm everyday for days 10–12 each month, for a period of 3–6 months until the symptoms disappear
- *Treatment of hot flashes*: Low doses of certain antidepressants (selective serotonin reuptake inhibitors) and serotonin and norepinephrine reuptake inhibitors (SNRIs), such as venlafaxine, paroxetine, fluoxetine, etc., may decrease hot flashes. Drugs, such as Gabapentin (Neurontin) and Clonidine, (antihypertensive medication), can be used for the treatment of hot flashes
- *Transdermal skin patches*: Their use help in avoiding first pass effect and liver metabolism. The estraderm patch contains about 3–4 mg of estradiol which is released at the rate of 50-g daily. Hormonal implants and mirena also have been recently introduced in HRT
- *Osteoporosis treatment*: Medicines, such as bisphosphonates (etidronate, tiludronate, etc.), hormones, such as estrogen, and selective estrogen receptor modulators (e.g. raloxifene) play a role in osteoporosis treatment
- *Tibolone*: This is a synthetic derivative of 19 nortestosterone, which has weak estrogenic, progestogenic and androgenic action. In the dosage of 2.5 mg daily, tibolone is cardioprotective, helps in improving bone resorption and relieving vasomotor symptoms. This drug may however cause irregular bleeding in nearly 15% of individuals.

COMPLICATIONS

Use of HRT may be associated with the following complications:

- According to Women's Health Initiative (2002), women who use HRT may be at a higher risk for breast cancer, blood clots, heart attacks and strokes. Nevertheless, many clinicians believe that short-term use of HRT for controling menopausal symptoms is still safe for most women. Women with a past history of heart disease or blood clots are at the highest risk and most likely must not be prescribed HRT

- Endometrial hyperplasia
- Breast cancer
- Thromboembolism
- Hypertension.

Absolute contraindications to HRT include undiagnosed genital bleeding, active intrinsic liver disease, active thromboembolic disease, recent myocardial infarction, estrogen dependent tumors, history of estrogen-related thromboembolism, breast cancer, uterine cancer or a family history of cancer.

CLINICAL PEARLS

- There is 50% reduction in androgen production and 66% reduction in estrogen production at the time of menopause. Estrogen levels may become as low as 10–20 pg/mL
- Continuous bleeding, menorrhagia or irregular bleeding during the perimenopausal or menopausal period must be considered as abnormal and warrant investigations to rule out any potential malignancies
- Chronic vulvar puritis or irritation which does not respond to estrogen therapy must be fully evaluated to rule out underlying malignancy
- In order to reduce the inherent risks of hormone therapy, lowest effective dose of HRT must be used for the shortest amount of time needed to treat symptoms.

9. INJURIES OF THE FEMALE GENITAL TRACT

INTRODUCTION

A genital injury can be defined as injury occuring to the genitals or perineum. Genital injuries can be very painful and can bleed heavily. It can affect the reproductive organs as well as the bladder and urethra. The amount of damage can range from minimal to severe.

ETIOLOGY

Injury to the genitals can occur due to the following causes:

- *Obstetric causes*: Most injuries to the genital tract occur during childbirth and delivery, especially in cases of abnormal labor and/or obstetric manipulation
- *Rape or sexual assault*: Violent intercourse or an alleged rape in young girls is a frequent cause of injury to the genital tract

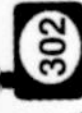

- *Vaginal atrophy*: Forceful penetration in postmenopausal women having vaginal atrophy is another important cause of injury to the genital tract
- Zipper injury
- *Malformations*: Presence of malformations, such as imperforate hymen, presence of vaginal septum, etc., may be responsible for producing injury with unintentional causes of trauma (e.g. sexual intercourse)
- *Trauma*: Vulvar injuries due to direct trauma (e.g. falling astride sharp objects, etc.)
- *Criminal abortion*: Insertion of foreign bodies in the vagina for attempting criminal abortion
- *Female genital mutilation*: In some regions of the world, injuries to the genital tract can occur as a result of female genital mutilation
- *Placement of foreign bodies in the vagina*: Young girls (usually < 4 years of age) may insert foreign objects into the vagina as part of a developmentally normal exploration of the body
- *Perforation of uterus*: This can occur during the procedures such as suction evacuation, dilatation and curettage, transcervical resection of endometrium, etc. An important injury occurring as a result of home delivery by untrained midwives is rupture uterus.

DIAGNOSIS

- A per speculum examination must be conducted to examine the vaginal walls fornices and the cervix in order to check for any associated injuries. Anesthesia may be required to perform a thorough examination and repair of severe injuries
- Information about the nature of the object, which has caused injury, must be obtained; sharp objects may have penetrated adjacent to the organs
- In case of insertion of a foreign body, there may be persistent and malodorous discharge from the vagina.

MANAGEMENT

- If the patient has urinary retention, bladder may be catheterized
- The area of injury must thoroughly be cleaned with soap, water and antiseptic solution. Lacerations must be irrigated with saline
- Hemostasis must be maintained and bleeding vessels must be ligated. All devitalized tissues must be excised

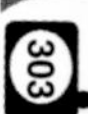

- All deep lacerations must be repaired with absorbable sutures without tension and the skin be repaired with non-absorbable sutures
- A laparotomy with complete exploration of the genital and gastrointestinal tract may be required, if the peritoneum has been penetrated
- *Hematomas*: Small hematomas respond to bed rest, seitz bath, hot fomentation and magnesium sulfate ointment. For large hematomas, incision of the swelling under general anesthesia for evacuation of clots may be required
- *Rape*: All the alleged cases of rape must be treated like medico-legal cases and police must also be informed. A dose of penicillin should be administered in order to protect the patient against bacterial infection (especially sexually transmitted diseases). The patient can be protected against pregnancy by using emergency contraception. Psychological counseling must be arranged
- *Foreign bodies*: The foreign body in the vagina must be removed on a per speculum examination followed by application of local antiseptic douches. Uterine foreign bodies must be removed under anesthesia and antibiotics be prescribed based on culture and sensitivity
- *Perforation*: In case of perforation, antibiotics need to be prescribed. If signs of peritoneal infection are present, laparotomy may be required.

COMPLICATIONS

- Extensive hemorrhage: This may result in the development of shock. There may be the development of subsequent anemia and local infection
- Hematoma in the parametrium
- Rectovaginal fistula
- Fibrosis and atresia of vaginal or cervical lacerations can result in dyspareunia or even apareunia
- Injury to the cervix may result in cervical incompetence or cervical stenosis.

CLINICAL PEARLS

- An important cause of vulvovaginal hematoma is inadequate hemostasis during repair of an episiotomy or a perineal tear.

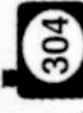

10. TUBERCULOSIS OF THE GENITAL TRACT

INTRODUCTION

Tubercular infection of the genital tract first affects the fallopian tubes resulting in pelvic inflammatory disease. Later, it spreads downward causing uterine synechiae and Asherman's syndrome. Cervical and vulvar lesions are rare.

ETIOLOGY

Infection of genital tract with *Mycobacterium tuberculosis* is always secondary to a focus elsewhere in the body. In nearly 50% of cases, the primary focus is the lungs; whereas in nearly 40% of the cases, it is lymph nodes. Spread through the blood stream is the most common mode of spread of infection.

DIAGNOSIS

Clinical Presentation

- *Infertility*: Infertility due to tubal factor may be the only complaint in 35–60% of individuals. There may or may not be an associated blockage of the tubes
- *Asymptomatic*: There may be no symptoms in nearly 11% of cases
- *Past history of tuberculosis*: Past history of tuberculosis or contact with a tubercular patient may be present in nearly 50% of cases
- *Menstrual disorders*: This may include disorders such as menorrhagia, secondary amenorrhea, oligomenorrhea, postmenopausal bleeding, puberty menorrhagia, etc.
- *Pain*: Pain is a rare symptom, unless there is development of tubercular peritonitis or a tubo-ovarian abscess, with tender, fixed pelvic mass or a history of recurrent subacute PID
- *Vaginal discharge*: This could present as blood-stained discharge or leucorrhoea and/or painful ulcers
- *Abdominal mass*: There may be the following clinical presentations: immobile tumor mass associated with menstrual abnormalities; fixed uterus; encysted ascites; matted intestinal mass; pyometra; tubo-ovarian mass; etc.
- *Fistula formation*: There may be persistant fistula formation following surgery for abscess
- Ectopic pregnancy.

General Physical Examination

The patient may appear healthy and there may not be any evidence of active primary focus. Fever may be absent.

Pelvic Examination

- No significant finding may be detected on pelvic examination
- Frozen pelvis: Pelvic masses are matted together and fixed to the pelvis. This usually presents as a painless pelvic mass.

Abdominal Examination

- Abdomen may appear doughy in case of peritoneal tuberculosis
- Tubercular encysted cyst may present as an immobile, tender mass
- The abdomen may appear typanitic on percussion
- There may be a pelvic adnexal mass, which may be fixed and immobile.

Investigations

- Complete blood count (Hb, TLC, DLC, ESR)
- Search for primary focus on X-ray chest and bone, and sputum and urine culture and sensitivity
- Microscopy, histopathological examination, culture and guinea pig innoculation: Specimen is commonly obtained by D and C. This should be performed in the late premenstrual phase because tubercles are present in the superficial layers, which may be shed during menstruation. Histopathological examination may demonstrate granulomatous epitheloid changes, with langhans giant cells showing central caseation
- PCR analysis: This is a very sensitive method which gives rapid results and can detect as few as 10 bacilli/mL
- Other major advances: These include DNA probes; ribosomal RNA based probes; isothermal amplification technique; etc.
- Ultrasonography: Ultrasound examination can detect abnormalities such as ascites or loculated fluid, adnexal mass, peritoneal thickening, omental thickening and endometrial involvement
- Hysterosalpingography: Findings suggestive of tubercular salpingitis, if HSG is done in an asymptomatic woman include the following (**Fig. 6.17**):
  - Lead pipe appearance of the tubes
  - Beading and variations in the filling density

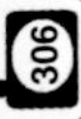

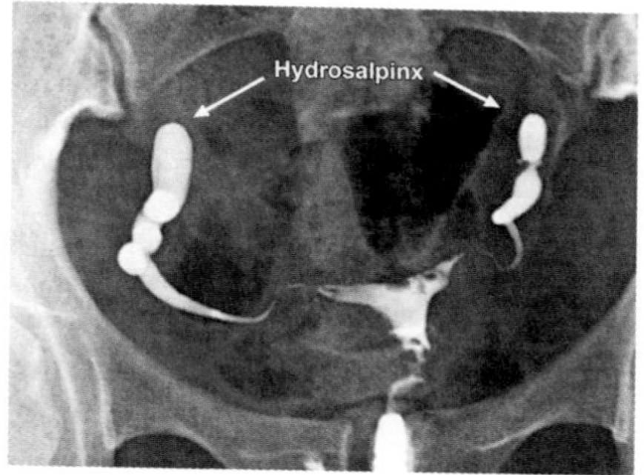

Figure 6.17: Hysterosalpingogram in an asymptomatic patient (later diagnosed as genital tuberculosis) showing lead pipe like appearance of fallopian tubes and bilateral tubal obstruction along with bilateral hydrosalpinx

  - Tobacco pouch appearance
  - Calcification of tube and jagged fluffiness of the tubal outline
  - Cornual block
  - Distorted uterine contour
  - Vascular or lymphatic intravasation of the dye
- Diagnostic laparoscopy: This may show features such as tubercular lesions, thickening of the fallopian tubes, hydrosalpinx, pyosalpinx or tubo-ovarian abscess.

DIFFERENTIAL DIAGNOSIS

- Ovarian cyst
- Pelvic inflammatory disease
- Ectopic pregnancy
- Carcinoma cervix
- Intrauterine pregnancy
- Puberty menorrhagia and postmenopausal bleeding.

MEDICAL MANAGEMENT

- Treatment mainly comprises of chemotherapy with antitubercular therapy. The most commonly used antitubercular drugs include

isoniazid (5–10 mg/kg body weight); rifampicin (10 mg/kg body weight); pyrazinamide (25–30 mg/kg body weight); ethambutol (15 mg/kg body weight) and streptomycin (12–18 mg/kg body weight, intramuscularly) everyday. The newer drugs which are now being used include capreomycin, kanamycin, ethionamide, para-aminosalicyclic acid, cycloserine, etc.

- Most commonly used treatment regimen involves an intensive phase for the first 2–3 months where four drugs (isoniazid; rifampicin; pyrazinamide and ethambutol) are given either daily or thrice weekly. This phase is followed by the treatment in the continuation phase where two drugs, either isoniazid or rifampicin, are administered for 4 months, or isoniazid and pyrazinamide are administered for 6 months.

SURGICAL MANAGEMENT

Surgical treatment may be indicated for the following conditions:

- Progression of disease or presence of persistent active lesion
- Persistence of a large inflammatory masses, i.e. pyosalpinx and pyometra
- Persistence of symptoms such as fistula, pain, menorrhagia, etc.
- Chemotherapy may cause restoration of fertility in nearly 10% of cases.
- IVF-ET offers the best chance of successful pregnancy outcome up to 40%.

COMPLICATIONS

- Infertility
- Ectopic pregnancy
- Menstrual disorders.

CLINICAL PEARLS

- Genital tuberculosis is very common in India, but largely remains silent and often goes unnoticed
- Fallopian tubes are involved in nearly 90% of cases of genital tuberculosis
- PID not responding to standard antibiotic therapy is suggestive of tubercular infection
- Tuberculosis is a descending infection from the fallopian tubes and the cornual ends are the first to get affected.

CHAPTER 7

Abnormalities of Menstruation

1. DYSFUNCTIONAL UTERINE BLEEDING

INTRODUCTION

Dysfunctional uterine bleeding (DUB), defined as abnormal bleeding not caused by pelvic pathology, medications, pregnancy or systemic disease, is the most common cause of abnormal uterine bleeding. In these cases, no obvious structural (pelvic or adnexal or extragenital) cause of bleeding can be demonstrated on clinical examination or laboratory evaluation.

ETIOLOGY

Imbalance between the levels of various hormones involved in the menstrual cycle could be responsible for producing irregular bleeding related to DUB. Dysfunctional bleeding could be related to estrogen withdrawal, estrogen breakthrough, progesterone withdrawal and progesterone breakthrough. DUB can be of two types: anovulatory and ovulatory type, of which the anovulatory causes account for nearly 80% cases.

- *Anovulatory DUB*: Anovulatory dysfunctional uterine bleeding is related to disturbances of the hypothalamic-pituitary ovarian axis that causes anovulation, thereby resulting in irregular, prolonged and sometimes heavy menstrual bleeding
- *Ovulatory DUB*: Ovulatory dysfunctional bleeding may include menstrual abnormalities like polymenorrhea, oligomenorrhea, premenstrual spotting (Mittelschmerz syndrome), hypomenorrhea and menorrhagia.

DIAGNOSIS

Symptoms

- *Intermenstrual intervals*: Intermenstrual intervals between the episodes of bleeding may be shortened due to prolongation of the duration of bleeding

- *Number of days bleeding occurs*: Number of days when the bleeding occurs, may be increased
- *Cycle regularity*: Cycles may lose their regularity because of irregular episodes of bleeding
- *Volume of bleeding*: Volume of bleeding may be heavy
- *Duration of the bleeding episode*: Duration of the bleeding episode may be prolonged.

General Physical Examination

Signs related to excessive blood loss (tachycardia, hypotension), may be evident on the general physical examination.

Pelvic Examination

- Pelvic examination must not be done in young girls presenting with the history of menorrhagia, who are not sexually active. However, it may be useful in women belonging to reproductive age group, presenting with DUB
- Gynecologic examination helps in excluding the various conditions described in **Box 7.1**, which may be responsible for producing abnormal bleeding.

Investigations

Various investigations, which must be considered in cases of DUB, are tabulated in **Table 7.1**.

Table 7.1: Laboratory investigations to be considered in the cases of DUB

Test	*Indication (to rule out)*
Urine pregnancy test	Bleeding due to pregnancy related complications such as threatened abortion, incomplete abortion or ectopic pregnancy
CBC with platelet count	Anemia and coagulation defects
PT/aPTT	Coagulation abnormalities
Pap smear	Cervical cancer
Liver and/or renal function tests	Hepatic and renal diseases
TSH	Thyroid disease
Prolactin levels	Pituitary adenoma

Contd...

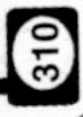

Contd...

Test	*Indication (to rule out)*
LH, FSH and androgen levels	Polycystic ovary disease
Endometrial biopsy/endometrial aspiration/fractional curettage	To rule out endometrial cancer
Imaging studies (transabdominal and transvaginal sonography)	Evaluation of endometrial thickness, uterine shape, size and contour and adnexae and helps in ruling out different pelvic pathology (leiomyomas, endometriosis, etc.)
Basal body temperature charting	A sustained rise in basal temperature of 0.3–0.6°C in the mid-cycle helps in ruling out anovulation
Serum progesterone levels	Values greater than 3 ng/ml in the mid-luteal phase rule out anovulation

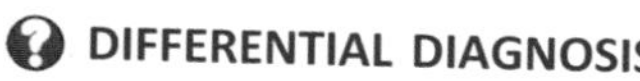

DIFFERENTIAL DIAGNOSIS

The various conditions, which must be ruled out in order to establish the diagnosis of DUB are listed in **Box 7.1**. Exclusion of endometrial cancer is very important in the cases of abnormal bleeding amongst perimenopausal women.

Box 7.1: Differential diagnosis of DUB

Postmenopausal women

- Cervical cancer, cervicitis, atrophic vaginitis, endometrial atrophy
- Submucous fibroids, endometrial hyperplasia and endometrial polyps
- Hormone replacement therapy (HRT).

Premenopausal women

- *Complications of pregnancy*
- *Infection, trauma*: Cervicitis, PID, endometritis, laceration, abrasion, foreign body, IUCD
- *Benign pelvic pathology*: Cervical polyp, endometrial polyp, leiomyoma, adenomyosis, etc.
- *Malignancy, neoplasm*: Cervical, endometrial or ovarian malignancy
- *Premalignant lesions*: Cervical lesions, endometrial hyperplasia
- *Trauma*: Foreign bodies, abrasions, lacerations, sexual abuse or assault
- *Medications/iatrogenic*: Intrauterine device, hormones (oral contraceptives, estrogen, progesterone)
- *Systemic diseases*: Hepatic disease, renal disease, coagulopathy, thrombocytopenia, von Willebrand's disease, leukemia.

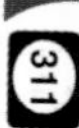

MEDICAL MANAGEMENT

- The treatment of moderate to severe DUB or that uncontrolled by clinical observation mainly comprises of medical therapy **(Table 7.2)**
- For severe bleeding, intravenous estrogen therapy (2.4 mg) conjugated equine estrogens every 4 hours until bleeding subsides or for 24 hours can be very effective

Table 7.2: Summary of medical treatment used for controlling DUB

Age group	*Treatment*	*Comments*
Premenopausal (adolescents and women belonging to reproductive age groups)	Oral contraceptives	Low-dose (34 μg) monophasic or triphasic oral contraceptives can regulate cycles, at the same time providing contraception
	Progestogens	If contraception is not required, medroxyprogesterone acetate can be used to regulate cycles
	Clomiphene citrate, 50–150 mg per day on days 4th to 9th of the cycle	Clomiphene citrate can induce ovulation in a woman with anovulatory cycles, who desires pregnancy
Perimenopausal	Medroxyprogesterone, 10 mg/day for 10 days	May use monthly to regulate bleeding patterns
	Oral contraceptives	Oral contraceptive pills can be continued until a woman has reached menopause and then HRT may be started
Postmenopausal women (receiving HRT)	Cyclic HRT	HRT (cyclic or combined continuous) may be initiated in postmenopausal women
	Continuous combined HRT	Clinician may increase the estrogen dose for 1–3 months to stabilize the endometrium

- For patients with severe bleeding, who are also anemic and whose lifestyle is compromised by persistence of irregular bleeding, D&C may be sometimes used to help in temporarily stopping the bleeding
- Nonsteroidal anti-inflammatory drugs (NSAIDs) are some of the most commonly used drugs, which may help in bringing out nearly 24–34% reduction in the menstrual blood flow.

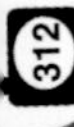

SURGICAL MANAGEMENT

- Surgical procedure, which is commonly used in cases of DUB include endometrial ablation
- These can be used in patients who are unresponsive to medical therapy, those who have completed their families or those with severe DUB
- Transcervical resection procedure mainly involves the destruction of a thin endometrial layer with help of wire loop, which helps in controlling the amount of bleeding (**Figs 7.1A and B**).

COMPLICATIONS

- Severe anemia
- Infertility (due to anovulatory DUB)
- Social consequences: adverse effect on school/work performance
- Chronic pelvic pain (resulting from infection due to prolonged use of tampons)
- Depression
- Hemorrhagic shock (rarely due to massive bleeding)
- Side effects related to endometrial ablation: Uterine perforation, fluid overload, hemorrhage, infection, etc.

CLINICAL PEARLS

- All perimenopausal patients with persistent abnormal uterine bleeding should be evaluated with endometrial studies in order to exclude the presence of endometrial hyperplasia or carcinoma
- Endometrial aspiration is a commonly used method of endometrial sampling, which can be performed as an outpatient procedure without any anesthetic requirements.

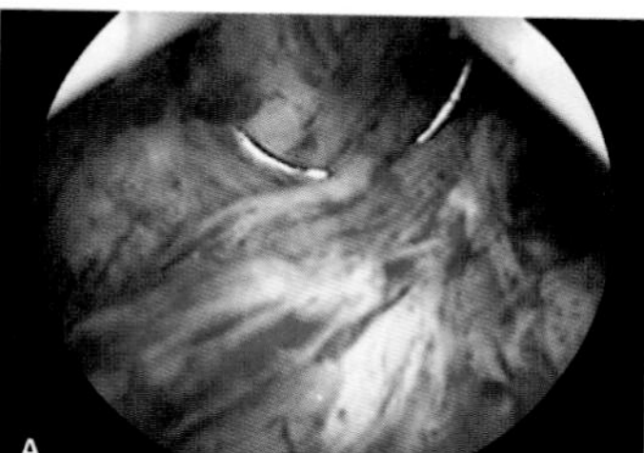

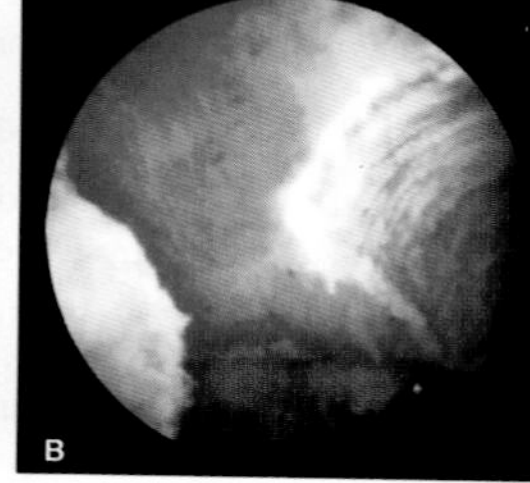

Figures 7.1A and B: Transcervical resection of the endometrium: (A) wire loop touching the endometrial surface; (B) wire loop resecting out the endometrium

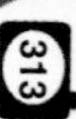

2. MENORRHAGIA

INTRODUCTION

- A normal menstrual cycle lasts for about 4–6 days, has a volume of approximately 30–80 ml, and comes at the interval of 24–34 days
- Any deviation from this trend can be defined as abnormal uterine bleeding (AUB)
- Menorrhagia can be defined as abnormal uterine bleeding, which is associated with prolonged or excessive blood loss of greater than 80 mL at regular intervals.

ETIOLOGY

- Abnormalities of coagulation
- Consumption of anticoagulants (warfarin)
- Periods soon after menarche
- Periods immediately before menopause
- Endometrial infection (acute or chronic inflammatory disease)
- Intrauterine contraceptive device (IUCD)
- Leiomyomas (fibroid) in the uterus.

DIAGNOSIS

Symptoms

- Intermenstrual intervals between the episodes of bleeding may be shortened due to prolongation of the duration of bleeding
- Number of days when the bleeding occurs is increased
- Cycles remain regular despite of prolonged or excessive blood flow
- Volume of blood loss may be heavy
- Duration of the bleeding episode may be prolonged.

General Physical Examination

Signs related to excessive blood loss (tachycardia, hypotension) may be evident on the general physical examination.

Pelvic Examination

- Gynecologic examination includes inspection of the vagina and cervix for presence of visible lesions [polyps, erosions, tears, malignancy, pregnancy related complications (expulsion of products of conception) or infection]

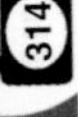

- On vaginal and bimanual examination the size, shape, position and firmness of the uterus should also be examined.

Investigations

- *Uterine imaging*: Uterine imaging (both TAS and TVS) forms an important investigation modality. Transvaginal ultrasound is especially indicated in the women at high risk for endometrial cancer. If the endometrial stripe on ultrasound examination is greater than or equal to 4 mm, endometrial sampling should be performed to rule out the presence of endometrial cancer
- *Hysteroscopy:* Hysteroscopy with biopsy can be regarded as the "gold standard" investigation for the diagnosis of menorrhagia. Hysteroscopy allows for direct visualization of the endometrial cavity along with the facility for directed biopsy.

DIFFERENTIAL DIAGNOSIS

Differential diagnosis of menorrhagia is given in **Box 7.2**.

Box 7.2: Differential diagnosis of menorrhagia

Pregnancy complications
- Ectopic pregnancy
- Incomplete abortion
- Miscarriage
- Threatened abortion.

Gynecological causes
- Cervical ectropion/erosion
- Cervical neoplasia/polyp
- Cervical or vaginal trauma
- Condylomata
- Atrophic vaginitis
- Foreign bodies in the vagina
- Pelvic inflammatory disease
- Endometritis.

Systemic causes
- Tuberculosis
- Hypothyroidism.

CONSERVATIVE MANAGEMENT

This comprises of patient reassurance, maintenance of a menstrual calendar and correction of anemia using iron preparations.

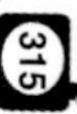

MEDICAL MANAGEMENT

Medical treatment is the option of choice in young women (< 20 years of age) presenting with menorrhagia. Medical treatment with conjugated estrogens is also indicated in cases of acute, heavy and uncontrollable bleeding. Various other medical modalities include the following:

- *Hormonal therapy*: These include oral contraceptive pills, progesterone only pills, injections of depo Provera or progesterone releasing intrauterine system
- *Hemostatic agents*: Hemostatic agents such as tranexamic acid, ethamsylate, etc. can also be used
- *NSAIDS:* These are the most commonly used medicines.

SURGICAL MANAGEMENT

- Surgical options used for treatment of AUB can be of two types: uterine conservative surgery (endometrial ablation) and hysterectomy
- Endometrial ablative techniques are sometimes used in cases of DUB as an alternative to hysterectomy
- The main advantage of hysterectomy is that it helps in providing complete cure and it ensures the removal of any missed underlying pathology
- Treatment options for uterine fibroids have been discussed in details in the fragment on uterine fibroids.

COMPLICATIONS

Complications associated with menorrhagia are similar to those described with DUB in the previous fragment.

CLINICAL PEARLS

- Menorrhagia related with menarche and menopause may settle spontaneously on its own
- Besides menorrhagia, other types of abnormal uterine bleeding include polymenorrhea, oligomenorrhea, intermenstrual bleeding, menometrorrhagia, metrorrhagia, hypomenorrhea, etc.
    - Polymenorrhea can be defined as episodes of regular bleeding at intervals of less than 21 days
    - Oligomenorrhea is infrequent menstruation at intervals greater than every 34 days

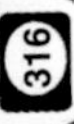

- Intermenstrual bleeding is defined as episodes of uterine bleeding of varying amounts (spotting) occurring between the regular menstrual periods
- Menometrorrhagia is combination of both menorrhagia and metrorrhagia, associated with prolonged or excessive bleeding (> 80 ml) at irregular intervals
- Metrorrhagia is defined as irregular, frequent uterine bleeding of varying amounts, but not excessive, at irregular intervals
- Hypomenorrhea is scanty menstruation.

3. LEIOMYOMA

INTRODUCTION

Uterine leiomyomas (uterine myomas, fibromyomas or fibroids) are well-circumscribed benign tumors developing from uterine myometrium, most commonly encountered amongst women of reproductive age group (30–44 years). A typical myoma is a pale, firm, rubbery, well-circumscribed mass distinct from neighboring tissues and has a whorled appearance due to presence of interlacing fibers of myometrial muscle, surrounded by a connective tissue capsule **(Fig. 7.2)**.

There are three types of fibroids **(Fig. 7.3)**. Of the different types of fibroids, the commonest are intramural or interstitial fibroids, (which are present within the uterine myometrium), followed by submucousal fibroids (which grow beneath the uterine endometrial lining) and subserosal fibroids, (which grow beneath the uterine serosa).

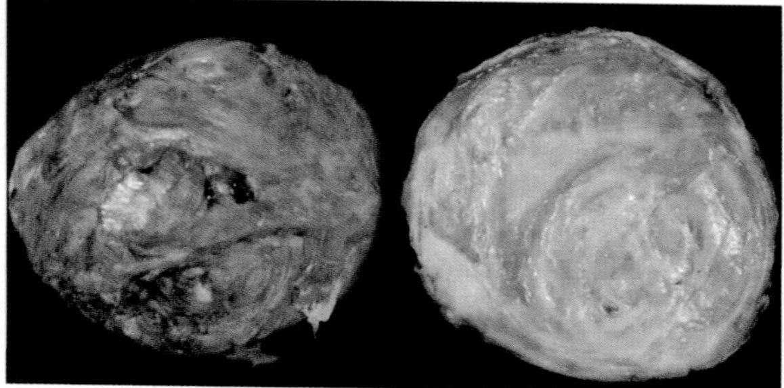

Figure 7.2: Appearance of fibroid

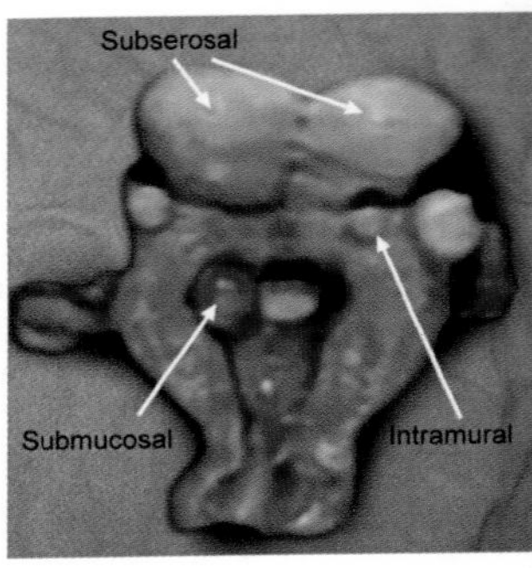

Figure 7.3: Types of fibroid

ETIOLOGY

Various risk factors which can result in the development of fibroids are as follows:

- *Heredity*: Patient with a positive family history of fibroid, especially in the first degree relatives (mother or sister) is especially at an increased risk of developing fibroids
- *Race*: Black women are more likely to have fibroids than the women of other racial groups
- *High estrogen levels*: Some factors, which may be responsible for an increased risk of fibroids related to hyperestrogenism, are as follows:
  - Exposure to OCPs at the age of 13–16 years
  - Obesity increases the risk probably due to higher levels of endogenous estrogens
  - Child bearing during the reproductive years (24–29) provides greatest protection against myoma development by producing amenorrhea (thereby reduced estrogen levels) during pregnancy
- *Pelvic inflammatory disease*: There is a positive association between fibroids and PID.

DIAGNOSIS

Symptoms

- *Menorrhagia*: The main symptom attributable to leiomyomas is menorrhagia. The blood loss is usually heaviest on day 2nd or 3rd of the menstrual periods

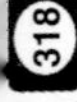

- *Anemia*: Excessive bleeding, if remains untreated over a long period of time, can result in the development of anemia
- *Other symptoms*: These may include symptoms such as urinary symptoms, low backache, rectal tenesmus and constipation
- *Abdominal pain*: Fibroids are usually not painful
- *Infertility*: Uterine fibroids could be responsible for infertility by interfering with the implantation of the fertilized ovum, by distorting the endometrial cavity and by causing disturbances of ovulation.

Abdominal Examination

- In case of a large fibroid, the mass may be palpable per abdomen and usually appears to be arising from the pelvis, i.e. it may be difficult to get below the mass
- It is usually well-defined, having a firm consistency and a smooth surface
- It is usually movable from side to side, but not from above downwards
- The mass is nearly always dull to percussion.

Pelvic Examination

- Presence of an enlarged, irregularly shaped, non-tender, mobile uterus with firm consistency on bimanual examination is suggestive of fibroids in women aged 30–40 years
- The tumor is found to either replace the uterus or be attached to the cervix.

Investigations

The following investigations are required in a patient presenting with leiomyomas:

- *Complete blood count along with platelet count and a peripheral smear*: To rule out anemia and coangulation disorder
- *Ultrasound examination*: Ultrasound examination (both TVS and TAS) has become the investigation of choice for diagnosing myomas. Ultrasound examination can help in assessing the size, location and number of uterine fibroids **(Figs 7.4 to 7.6)**
- *MRI*: Though the use of MRI is not routinely recommended due to its high cost, it is useful in mapping the size and location of leiomyomas and in accurately identifying adenomyosis
- *Ruling out presence of malignancy*: In case the patient has risk factors for endometrial cancer or she is in the perimenopausal age group or gives history of intermenstrual and postcoital bleeding, endometrial biopsy and Pap smear are required to rule out carcinoma endometrium and carcinoma cervix respectively.

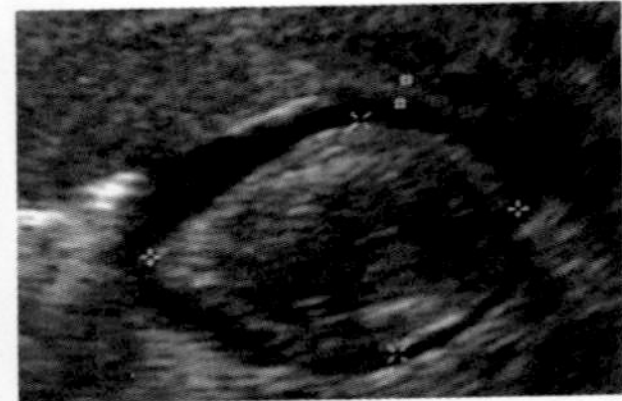

Figure 7.4: Visualization of intracavitary fibroids on saline infusion sonography

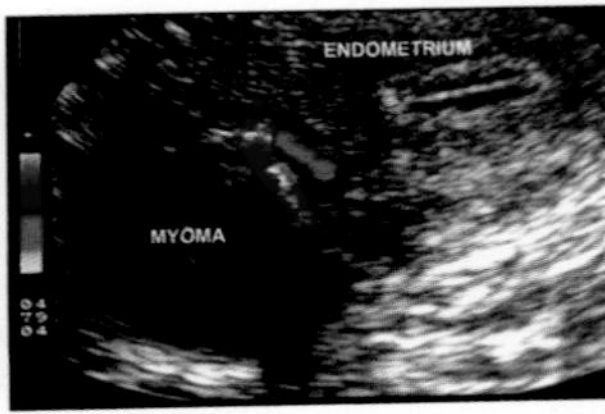

Figure 7.5: Color Doppler shows presence of subserosal fibroids with peripheral vascularization

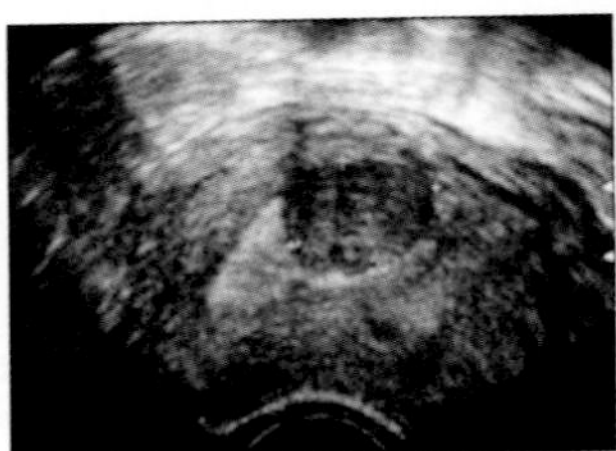

Figure 7.6: Submucous fibroid protruding inside the endometrial cavity

DIFFERENTIAL DIAGNOSIS

- The various causes of menorrhagia, which need to be excluded, have been described previously in the fragment on menorrhagia
- Various causes of uterine enlargement, which may be mistaken for fibroids and need to be excluded include pregnancy, adenomyosis, benign ovarian tumor, etc.

MANAGEMENT

Women with asymptomatic uterine fibroids do not require any treatment. Treatment options for symptomatic fibroids are listed in **Figure 7.7**.

Surgical Treatment

Presently, the main modality of curative treatment in a patient with leiomyomas is surgery and acts as a definitive cure. If the woman has completed her family and does not wish to preserve her uterus, hysterectomy can be done. Myomectomy is an option for women, who desire future pregnancy or wish to preserve their uterus.

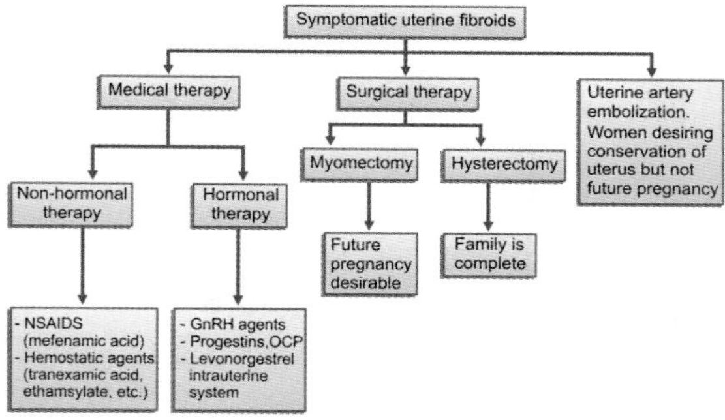

Figure 7.7: Treatment options for symptomatic fibroids

Hysterectomy: Hysterectomy can be performed in three ways: abdominally, vaginally and in some cases laparoscopically (Chapter 9).

Myomectomy: Surgical removal of myomas from the uterine cavity is termed as myomectomy. Myomectomy can be performed abdominally, laparoscopically or hysteroscopically.

- The advantages of hysteroscopic and laparoscopic myomectomy are that they can be performed as an outpatient procedure and allow faster recovery in comparison to conventional abdominal laparotomy. The steps for laparoscopic removal of a subserosal myoma are shown in **Figures 7.8A to H**
- Hysteroscopic myomectomy **(Figs 7.9A and B)** has been considered as an effective option for controlling menorrhagia in women with submucous fibroids.

COMPLICATIONS

- Severe pain, anemia
- Infertility
- Toxic shock syndrome
- *Torsion*: Torsion of the pedicle of a subserous pedunculated leiomyoma may interfere first with venous, then with the arterial supply
- *Ascites/Pseudomeigs syndrome*: Very mobile, pedunculated subserous tumors may produce ascites by causing mechanical irritation of the peritoneum. Sometimes, ascites may be accompanied by a right sided hydrothorax, resulting in pseudomeigs syndrome

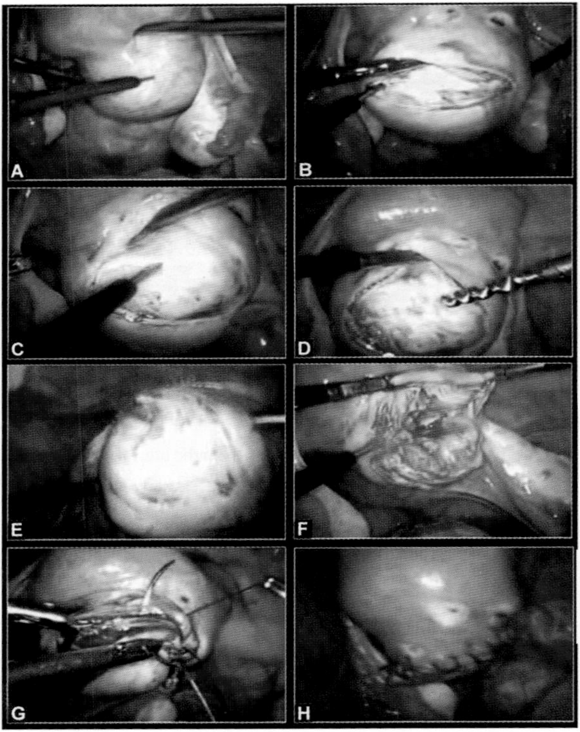

Figures 7.8A to H: Steps of laparoscopic myomectomy:(A) laparoscopic view showing the presence of a fibroid over the anterior surface of the uterus; (B) uterine incision is given over anterior wall of fibroid, which is progressively enlarged; (C) the myoma is gradually shelled out from the underlying myometrium with the help of blunt and sharp dissection; (D) inserting a myoma screw to facilitate the process of enucleation of myoma from the pseudocapsule; (E) the myoma has been shelled out completely; (F) the raw area left in the uterine myometrium following the removal of myoma; (G) the raw area left in the uterus after myoma removal is stitched together with vicryl sutures; (H) appearance of the myometrial suture line following the completion of surgery

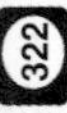

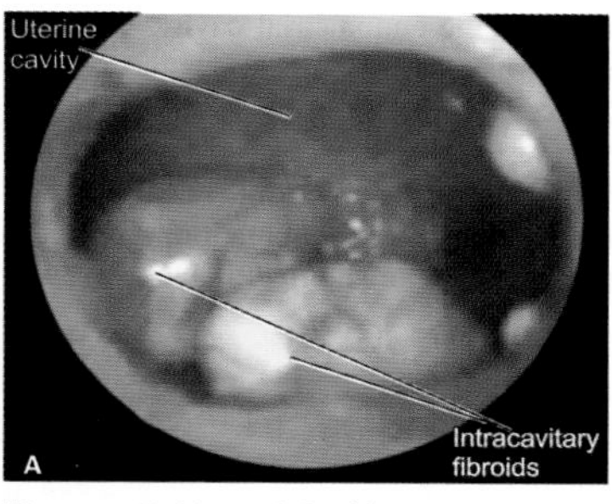

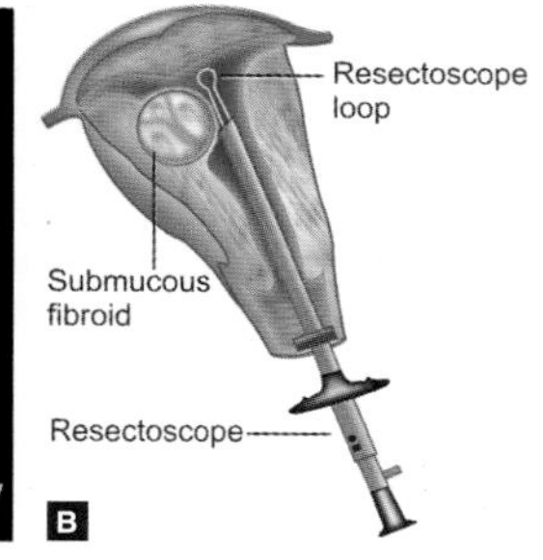

Figures 7.9A and B: Hysteroscopic myomectomy: (A) hysteroscopic view of the uterus showing submucous leiomyoma; (B) hysteroscopic resection of the leiomyoma

- *Infection*: A submucous leiomyoma may sometimes become infected and ulcerated at its lower pole
- *Secondary changes (degenerative changes)*
  - Atrophy: Shrinkage of the fibroid can occur as a result of reduced blood supply of the fibroid, usually following menopause
  - Hyaline degeneration: This is the commonest type of degeneration in which, a homogeneous substance that stains pink with eosin, replaces the fibrous tissue cells
  - Calcification: This is characterized by the deposition of phosphates and carbonates of calcium along the course of blood vessels, usually starting at the periphery
  - Myxomatous/cystic degeneration
  - Red/carneous degeneration: This type of degeneration of uterine fibroid usually develops during pregnancy and must be managed conservatively. It may be associated with constitutional symptoms like malaise, nausea, vomiting, fever and severe abdominal pain
  - Sarcomatous change: Occurrence of malignant changes in a leiomyoma is an extremely rare occurrence, occurring in only about 0.2% of tumors.

CLINICAL PEARLS

- Women suffering from leiomyomas, especially those in the perimenopausal group, who have continuous or irregular bleeding, should be subjected to a thorough endometrial evaluation in order to rule out the presence of endometrial cancer

- The nearer the leiomyomas are to the endometrial cavity, the more likely are they to produce menorrhagia
- Most fibroids remain uncomplicated during pregnancy. Some possible adverse effects related to the presence of fibroids during pregnancy include abortion, preterm labor, preterm prelabor rupture of membranes, placental abruption, IUGR, malpresentation, obstructed labor, cesarean section and cesarean hysterectomy, PPH, etc.

4. DYSMENORRHEA

INTRODUCTION

Dysmenorrhea has been defined by the ACOG as a gynecological medical condition characterized by presence of pain during the menstrual phase. The pain may be severe enough to interfere with normal activities of daily living. The pain could be sharp, throbbing, dull, nauseating, burning or shooting in nature. It may either precede menstruation by several days or may accompany it. However, it usually subsides as the menstrual bleeding ceases.

Dysmenorrhea can be of two types: primary (spasmodic or the 1st day pain) and secondary (congestive type). Dysmenorrhea is labeled as primary in the absence of underlying medical disease/pathology. Secondary dysmenorrhea on the other hand, is associated with an underlying medical disease/pathology. Some of the common causes of secondary dysmenorrhea include endometriosis, leiomyomas, adenomyosis, ovarian cysts, pelvic congestion, copper IUCDS, etc. Another type of dysmenorrhea is the membranous type, where the endometrium is shed in form of casts at the time of menstruation. The passage of casts is accompanied by painful uterine cramps.

ETIOLOGY

The pathophysiology of dysmenorrhea is not yet understood. Some of the probable factors include:

- Behavioral and psychological factors
- Muscular incoordination and uterine hyperactivity
- *Hormonal imbalance*: Stimulation of the uterus by progesterone could be another factor involved in its pathogenesis because dysmenorrhea usually occurs only with the ovulatory cycles
- *Prostaglandins*: Excessive amounts of prostaglandin PGF_2a could be responsible because they cause myometrial contraction and constriction

of small endometrial vessels to produce ischemia and breakdown of endometrium causing bleeding and pain
- *Other factors*: High levels of vasopressin may stimulate uterine activity.

DIAGNOSIS

Diagnosis is mainly based on the medical history of pain, menstrual history (relation to the 1st day of periods) and pelvic examination.

Symptoms

- *Relationship with the periods:* Pain is usually present a few hours before and after the onset of menstruation. It rarely lasts for more than 12 hours even in its severest form
- *Region*: Pain is usually present in the lower abdomen or umbilical or suprapubic regions
- *Character*: Pain is usually colicky in nature
- *Radiation of pain*: Radiation of the pain occurs towards the front and inner aspect of the thighs or lower back
- *Associated symptoms*: May be often associated with symptoms such as nausea/vomiting, diarrhea, constipation, headache, dizziness, disorientation, fainting, fatigue, etc.
- *Age of onset*: Pain reaches its maximum during the age of 18–24 years and then diminishes in severity
- *Relation with the ovulatory cycles*: Pain usually occurs in association with ovulation.

Pelvic Examination

Pelvic examination is within normal limits in cases of primary amenorrhea. On the other hand, in the cases of secondary dysmenorrhea, the underlying gynecological pathology can be detected on pelvic examination.

Investigations

In cases of secondary dysmenorrhea, the following investigations may be required to diagnose the underlying pathology:

- *Pap smear*
- *Imaging*: Gynecological ultrasound followed by CT scan and MRI, if required
- *Hysterosalpingography*: This helps in identification of intrauterine adhesions

- *Endocervical swabs and culture of peritoneal fluid*: This helps in diagnosing PID
- *Diagnostic laparoscopy/hysteroscopy*: This may be useful for diagnostic as well as curative purposes.

DIFFERENTIAL DIAGNOSIS

- *Corpus luteum hematoma*: This can be defined as hemorrhage into and from the corpus luteum. Patient experiences acute onset of sharp pain in the lower abdomen, moving from one side to the other, often accompanied by feeling of faintness and uterine bleeding. The main differentiating feature is that the pain occurs during the second half of a previously normal cycle
- *Ovulation pain (Mittelschmerz)*: This usually occurs during the 10th to 14th day of the menstrual cycle. The pain is usually localized to the hypogastrium or one of the two iliac fossae and may be at times accompanied by ovulation bleeding
- *Orthopedic conditions*: Orthopedic conditions such as disc lesions and arthritic changes in the spine may at times mimic dysmenorrheal pain.

MANAGEMENT

- The management of cases of dysmenorrhea is described in **Figure 7.10**
- NSAIDs are the most commonly used medicines and their use is restricted to the symptom days. They do not interfere with ovulation
- The following NSAIDS may be used: indomethacin 24 mg TDS or QID; ibuprofen 400 mg TDS; naproxen sodium 240 mg TDS; ketoprofen 40 mg TDS and mefenamic acid 240–400 mg BD or QID.

CLINICAL PEARLS

- Primary dysmenorrhea is widely prevalent, present in about 70% of teenagers and 30–40% of menstruating women
- Hormonal therapy is the treatment of choice for those women who desire contraception.

5. PREMENSTRUAL SYNDROME

INTRODUCTION

Premenstrual syndrome (PMS) or premenstrual tension includes a combination of physical, psychological and emotional symptoms, which the women experience for a few days (usually 7–10 days) preceding menstruation.

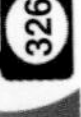

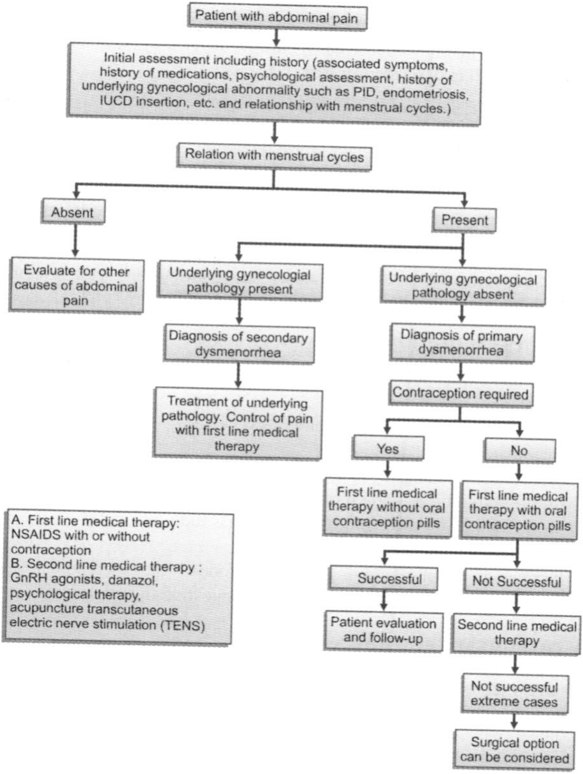

Patient with abdominal pain

↓

Initial assessment including history (associated symptoms, history of medications, psychological assessment, history of underlying gynecological abnormality such as PID, endometriosis, IUCD insertion, etc. and relationship with menstrual cycles.)

↓

Relation with menstrual cycles

- Absent → Evaluate for other causes of abdominal pain
- Present
  - Underlying gynecologial pathology present → Diagnosis of secondary dysmenorrhea → Treatment of underlying pathology. Control of pain with first line medical therapy
  - Underlying gynecological pathology absent → Diagnosis of primary dysmenorrhea → Contraception required
    - Yes → First line medical therapy without oral contraception pills
    - No → First line medical therapy with oral contraception pills
      - Successful → Patient evaluation and follow-up
      - Not Successful → Second line medical therapy → Not successful extreme cases → Surgical option can be considered

A. First line medical therapy: NSAIDS with or without contraception
B. Second line medical therapy : GnRH agonists, danazol, psychological therapy, acupuncture transcutaneous electric nerve stimulation (TENS)

Figure 7.10: Management of cases of dysmenorrhea

ETIOLOGY

- The cause of PMS is not completely understood and may be multifactorial
- It is commonly linked to the luteal phase of menstrual cycle
- Low levels of neurotransmitters such as β endorphins/serotonin, etc. may be responsible for producing irritability and behavioral changes

DIAGNOSIS

Diagnostic criteria for premenstrual syndrome devised by National Institute of Mental Health is described in **Box 7.3**.

Box 7.3: Diagnostic criteria for premenstrual syndrome

- A 30% increase in the intensity of symptoms of PMS (measured using a standardized instrument) from cycle days 4th to 10th as compared with the 6-day interval before the onset of menses
- Documentation of these changes in a daily symptom diary for at least two consecutive cycles.

Source: ACOG Practice Bulletin. Clinical management guidelines for obstetrician-gynecologists, Number 14, April 2000. Premenstrual syndrome. Obstet Gynecol. 2000;94:1-9.

Clinical Presentation

Some of the symptoms, which are commonly observed, include the following:

- Abdominal bloating, breast tenderness
- Headache
- Sleeplessness, fatigue
- Emotional liability and emotional outbursts
- Mood swings, depression, irritability, lassitude, insomnia
- Fluid retention
- Increase in appetite, craving for sweet foods
- Intestinal distension, colonic spasm, congestive dysmenorrhea.

DIFFERENTIAL DIAGNOSIS

PMS is a diagnosis of exclusion, usually established after excluding a variety of psychiatric and medical disorders described in **Box 7.4**.

Box 7.4: Differential diagnosis of PMS

Psychiatric disorders

- Anxiety and mood disorders (e.g. depression, anxiety, dysthymia, panic)
- Personality disorder
- Anorexia or bulimia.

Chronic medical disorders

- Diabetes mellitus
- Hypothyroidism
- Anemia.

Contd...

Contd...

Gynecological conditions
- Dysmenorrhea
- Perimenopause
- Use of oral contraceptive pills
- Substance abuse.

MANAGEMENT

Management of PMS is summarized in **Figure 7.11**.

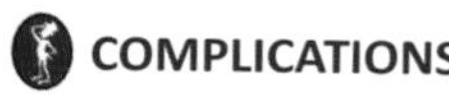

COMPLICATIONS

PMS may be a cause of individual misery, marital disharmony, absenteeism and even crimes such as murder and suicide.

CLINICAL PEARLS

- The key features, which point towards the diagnosis of PMS, are presence of symptoms consistent with PMS, occurrence of these symptoms only during the luteal phase of the cycle and negative impact of these symptoms on patient's functions and lifestyle
- Reassurance, counseling, psychotherapy and selective use of medicines is useful in most of the cases
- Symptoms of PMS usually regress rapidly with the onset of menses.

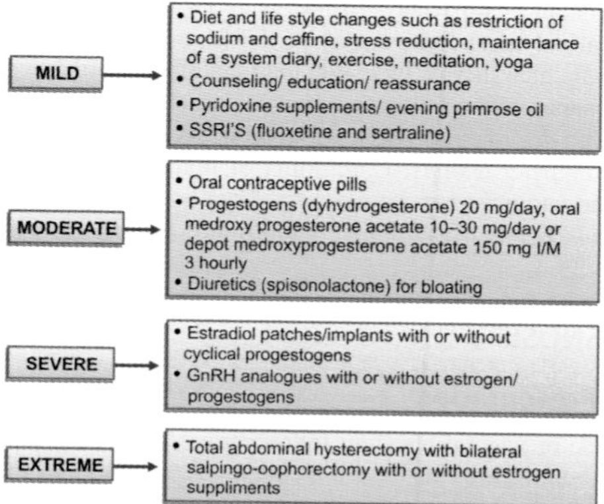

Figure 7.11: Management of PMS

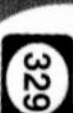

6. POSTMENOPAUSAL BLEEDING

INTRODUCTION

The menopause is defined by the WHO as the permanent cessation of menstruation resulting from the loss of ovarian follicular activity. Cessation of periods for at least 1 year after the age of 40 is considered as menopause. In fact, investigations must begin in case of vaginal bleeding any time after 6 months of cessation of periods. The most serious concern in postmenopausal and perimenopausal women with abnormal postmenopausal bleeding (PMB) is endometrial carcinoma.

ETIOLOGY

- Non-gynaecological causes including trauma, as bleeding disorders or a foreign body
- Prolonged use of HRT comprising of estrogens unopposed by progestogens or cyclical HRT
- *Vulvar lesions*: Vulvar trauma, vulvitis, tumors (benign and malignant)
- *Vaginal lesions*: Vaginal atrophy, senile vaginitis, vaginal tumors
- *Cervical lesions*: Cervical polyps, erosion, cervicitis, cervical malignancy, etc.
- *Endometrial lesions*: Endometrial cancer and/or hyperplasia (simple, complex and atypical), polyps, senile endometritis, tubercular endometritis
- Ovarian cancer, especially estrogen-secreting (theca cell) ovarian tumors
- Vaginal/vulvar malignancy
- Dysfunctional uterine bleeding, metropathia hemorrhagica
- Malignancy of the fallopian tube
- *Systemic disorders*: Hypertension, blood dyscrasias
- *Urinary tract lesions*: Carcinoma of bladder, bladder papilloma, urethral caruncle, etc.
- *Gastrointestinal tract lesions*: Hemorrhoids, anal fissure, rectal cancer, etc.

DIAGNOSIS

Clinical Presentation

- Episode of vaginal bleeding following cessation of periods (at least for 6 months) after the age of 40 years
- Abdominal pain

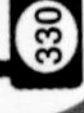

- Foul smelling discharge
- Presence of urinary and rectal symptoms may be associated with urinary or rectal causes of bleeding respectively, which may be at times mistaken for vaginal bleeding
- Triad of obesity, diabetes and hypertension serves as a risk factor for the development of endometrial cancer
- History of nulliparity is associated with an increased incidence of endometrial cancer
- Intake of drugs such as tamoxifen, tibolone and other combined HRT.

Abdominal Examination: There may be presence of an abdominal lump (suggestive of a tumor) on palpation.

Per Speculum and Per Vaginal Examination: This may help delineate the exact underlying pathology.

Investigations

- Cervical cytology (Pap smear or liquid based cytology) for suspected cervical pathology or detection of abnormal endometrial cells
- Assessment of endometrial thickness using transvaginal sonography **(Figs 7.12 and 7.13)**. Further evaluation of endometrial thickness by SIS or 3-D ultrasound may be done
- If endometrial thickness is greater than or equal to 4 mm, study of endometrial cytology using endometrial biopsy, aspiration, D&C or hysteroscopic guided D&C must be done
- Hysteroscopy may help in evaluation of focal lesions, polyps or uterine abnormalities
- Cystoscopy and proctoscopy in order to rule out urinary tract and rectal lesions respectively must be done.

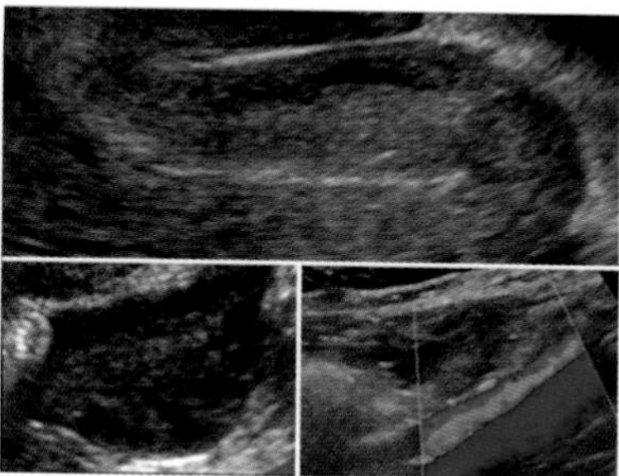

Figure 7.12: A patient presenting with post-menopausal bleeding in which TVS shows presence of thin hyperechogenic endometrium. Color Doppler demonstrates the presence of iliac vessels adjacent to the ovary with no growing follicle

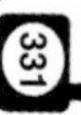

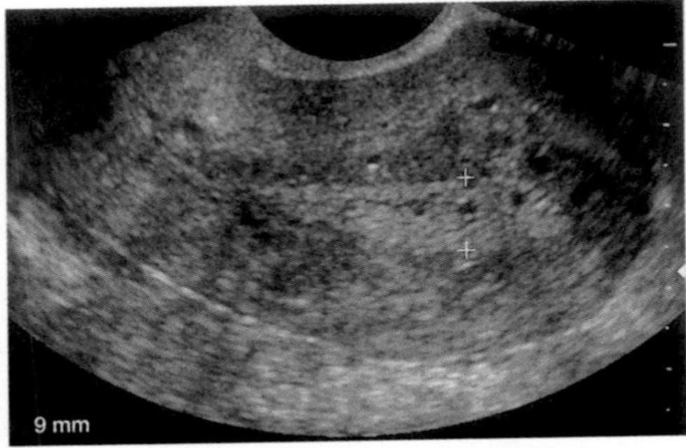

Figure 7.13: Transvaginal sonography in a patient with postmenopausal bleeding showing an endometrial thickness of 9 mm

DIFFERENTIAL DIAGNOSIS

Various causes of PMB which need to be differentiated have already been described under "etiology".

MANAGEMENT

- History and examination may help in delineating the exact underlying pathology
- The most important dictum regarding the management of PMB is that "this bleeding should be treated as malignant until proven otherwise"
- Treatment has to be tailored depending on the type of pathology discovered
- The patient should be kept under observation, if no obvious cause has been detected and there has been only one bout of bleeding
- Treatment of atrophic vaginitis comprises of application of local estrogens
- Endometrial polyps should be removed during hysteroscopic evaluation and sent for histopathology evaluation
- Endometrial hyperplasia without atypia responds well to hormone therapy
- Endometrial hyperplasia with atypia (simple or complex) responds well to surgical therapy.

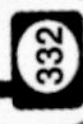

COMPLICATIONS

The most sinister complication associated with PMB is the presence of underlying malignancy. Other complications are same as those described with DUB.

CLINICAL PEARLS

- Most women with PMB will not have significant pathology; however, efforts must be made to rule out the presence of any underlying malignancy
- Normal age for menopause can be considered as 44–47 years
- In the women with PMB, the cut-off for endometrial thickness is considered as 4 mm. In women with PMB on hormone therapy or tamoxifen, the cut-off for endometrial thickness is considered as 8 mm.

CHAPTER 8

Gynecological Oncology

1. ENDOMETRIAL CANCER

INTRODUCTION

Endometrial cancer develops from the lining of the uterus known as the endometrium **(Fig. 8.1)**. It is the most common gynecologic cancer and the fourth most common cancers among women. Endometrial cancer usually affects women after menopause, commonly in the age groups of 50–65 years.

ETIOLOGY

The most important risk factor for endometrial cancer is hyperestrogenism or exposure to unopposed estrogen, both endogenous and exogenous. Other risk factors for endometrial cancer include:

- Woman of low parity or nulliparous women
- Early menarche and late menopause (associated with prolonged exposure to estrogen)
- Unopposed and unsupervised administration of HRT
- Chronic anovulation associated with DUB, infertility and PCOS
- Use of tamoxifen (for breast cancer) is associated with an increased risk of endometrial hyperplasia
- Triad of diabetes, obesity and hypertension increases the risk of cancer.

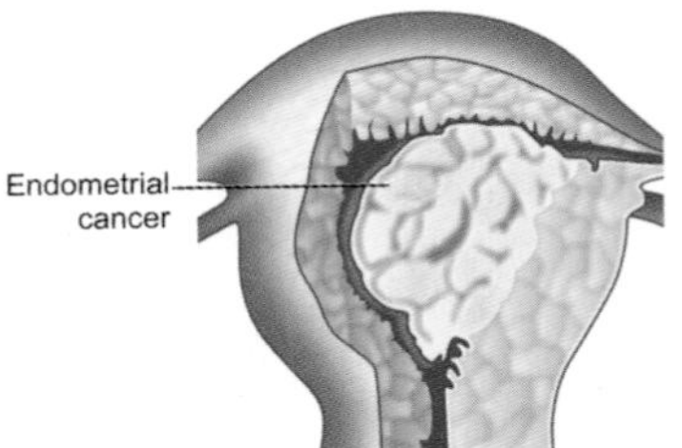

Figure 8.1: Endometrial cancer manifesting in form of an exophytic growth

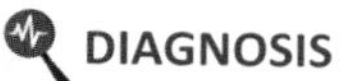

DIAGNOSIS

Symptoms

Bleeding abnormalities: Menorrhagia or irregular bleeding in perimenopausal women; postmenopausal bleeding.

Pelvic Examination

- Uterus may appear to be bulky due to associated fibroid or pyometra
- In advanced stages, the growth may be observed protruding through the os.

Per Speculum Examination

Sometimes metastatic vaginal growth may be visible.

Investigations

- *Cytological examination*: This includes investigations such as endometrial biopsy, endometrial aspiration, fractional curettage, etc.
- *Ultrasound*: Typically a TVS is required. Doppler ultrasound may reveal a low-resistance index **(Fig. 8.2)**
- *Hysteroscopy*: A hysteroscopic examination and guided biopsy may be performed to confirm the diagnosis.

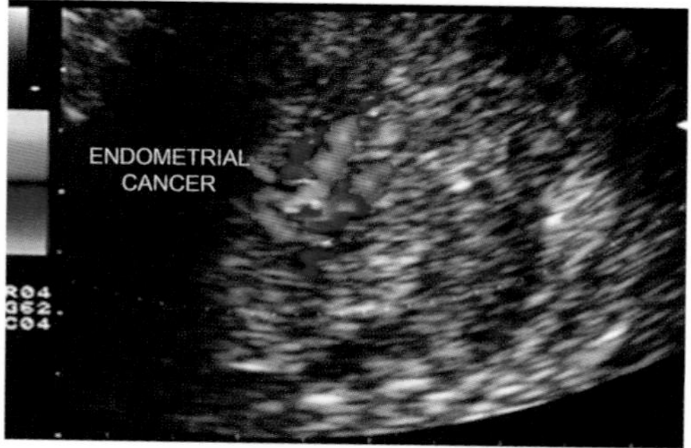

Figure 8.2: Thick heterogeneous endometrium with proliferation of blood vessels on color Doppler. This was found to be advanced stage of endometrial cancer

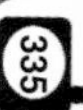

In case the diagnosis of endometrial cancer has been confirmed, the following investigations are performed to evaluate the spread of cancer:

- Blood tests (hematocrit)
- Kidney and liver function tests
- Chest X-ray
- CT
- MRI **(Fig. 8.3)**.

DIFFERENTIAL DIAGNOSIS

- Senile endometritis, tubercular endometritis
- Atypical hyperplasia, endometrial polyps
- Lesions such as cervical cancer may also cause postmenopausal bleeding.

MANAGEMENT

Cancer Staging

The detailed staging of endometrial cancer and stage-wise treatment is described in **Table 8.1.**

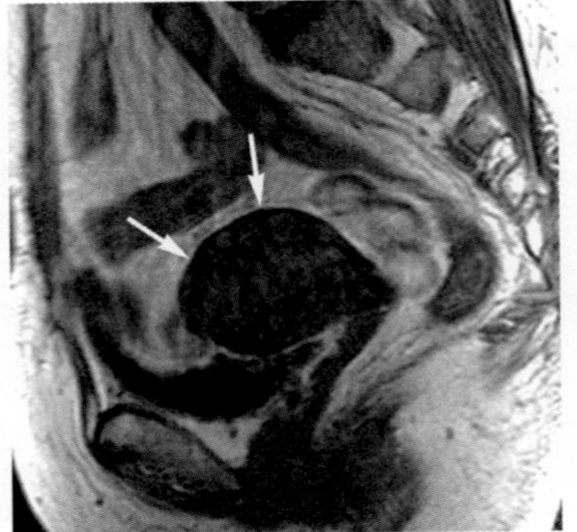

Figure 8.3: MRI scan showing endometrial adenocarcinoma

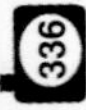

Table 8.1: FIGO staging of endometrial cancer and stage-wise treatment		
Stage	*Characteristics*	*Treatment*
Stage 0	*Cases of endometrial hyperplasia*	Total abdominal hysterectomy with salpingo-oophorectomy
Stage I (Grade 1, 2 or 3)	*Cancer confined to the corpus uteri* IA: Limited to the endometrium IB: Invasion of half or less than one half of myometrium IC: Invasion of one half or more than one half of myometrium	Extrafascial total abdominal hysterectomy and bilateral salpingo-oohorectomy with lymph node sampling. Removal of a vaginal cuff is usually not required in these cases. In the cases where lymph nodes are involved, postoperative radiotherapy may be required
Stage II (Grade 1, 2 or 3)	*Tumor involves the cervix, but does not extend beyond the uterus* IIA: Endocervical glandular involvement only IIB: Cervical stromal invasion	Radiation therapy (brachytherapy) is followed by surgery. External radiotherapy may be applied based on the histopathological findings. Alternatively, the surgeon may perform radical hysterectomy with bilateral salpingo-ophorectomy and pelvic lymphadenectomy
Stage III (Grade 1, 2 or 3)	*Local and/or regional spread* IIIA: Invasion of serosa and/or adnexa and/or positive peritoneal cytology IIIB: Vaginal metastases IIIC: Metastases to pelvic and/or para-aortic lymph nodes	For stage III tumors, the treatment involves TAH and bilateral salpingo-oophorectomy with selective lymphadenectomy, biopsies of suspicious areas, omental biopsy and debulking of tumor followed by radiotherapy. Chemotherapy with doxorubicin in the dosage of 60 mg/m^2 and other drugs including cisplatin and paclitaxel is also being tried
Stage IV (Grade 1, 2 or 3)	*Tumor becomes widespread* IVA: Invasion of bladder and/or bowel mucosa IVB: Distant metastases, including intra-abdominal metastases and/or inguinal lymph nodes	Treatment has to be individualized in those with stage IV tumors because cancer in this stage is usually nonoperable. Usually, palliative therapy comprising of a combination of surgery, radiotherapy, hormone therapy or chemotherapy is required

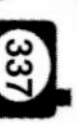

Indications for pelvic lymphadenectomy in cases of endometrial cancer are enlisted in **Table 8.2**. In the cases where lymph nodes are involved, postoperative radiotherapy may be required. Other indications for radiotherapy are listed in **Table 8.3**.

Table 8.2: Indications for pelvic lymphadenectomy

- The tumor histology is known to be clear cell type, serous, squamous or poorly differentiated grade III endometroid type
- Cut section shows that the myometrium has been invaded to more than half of its thickness
- The tumor has extended to the cervix or isthmus
- Size of the tumor is greater than 2 cm
- There is evidence of extrauterine disease

Table 8.3: Indications of radiotherapy

Postoperative vaginal irradiation
- Stage IA G3 tumors
- Stage IB G1 and G2 tumors
- Stage IB G3 and stage IIA (G1 and G2) tumors

External pelvic irradiation
- Tumors in stage IC (all grades), stage IIA (G3) and stage IIB (all grades), stage IIIA (all grades) or those with lymphovascular space invasion
- All patients with positive lymph nodes
- Patients with documented para-aortic and common iliac lymph node involvement
- Selected IVA patients

COMPLICATIONS

- Pyometra
- Uterine enlargement
- Menorrhagia, postmenopausal bleeding, intermenstrual bleeding, etc.
- Anemia due to blood loss and cancer cachexia
- Uterine perforation.

2. OVARIAN CANCER

INTRODUCTION

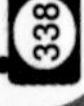

This type of cancer develops most often in women aged 50–70 years. In the United States, it is the second most common gynecologic cancer. Nearly 80% of the cancers are epithelial cell cancers, which originate from the surface epithelium of the ovaries. Other types of ovarian cancers include germ cell tumors, sex cord stromal cell tumors and metastatic cancers.

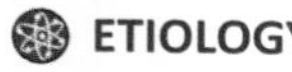

ETIOLOGY

Some of the risk factors for ovarian cancer are as follows:

- Old age, nulliparity, having the first child late in life
- Early menarche, late menopause
- Family history of cancer of the uterus, breast or large intestine. Mutations of the gene BRCA-1 (chromosome-17) and BRCA-2 (chromosome 13) are commonly implicated in its pathogenesis
- Risk increases with age (up to 70 years)
- Multiple ovulation in the IVF program.

DIAGNOSIS

Symptoms

Many women with ovarian cancer may not have any symptoms, until the cancer is in an advanced stage. Moreover, if the symptoms do appear they may be vague such as lower abdomen pain or discomfort, indigestion, bloating, loss of appetite, backache, cachexia, anemia, etc.

Abdominal Examination

A lump may be palpated on the abdominal examination. The malignant ovarian tumors are often bilateral, solid, fixed and may present with ascites.

Pelvic Examination

An adnexal mass, separate from the uterus, may be felt on pelvic examination. Fixed nodules may be palpated on the vaginal examination.

Investigations

- Ultrasonography: Presence of solid tumors with a thick capsule and papillary projections. There may be presence of low pulsatile index (< 1) and low resistance index (< 0.4) on Doppler ultrasound **(Figs 8.4A and B)**
- CT, MRI
- Biopsy of the tumor tissue
- Examination of the ascitic fluid
- Levels of CA 125: The levels of this antigen have been found to be raised in nearly 80% cases of epithelial cancers.

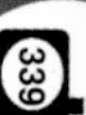

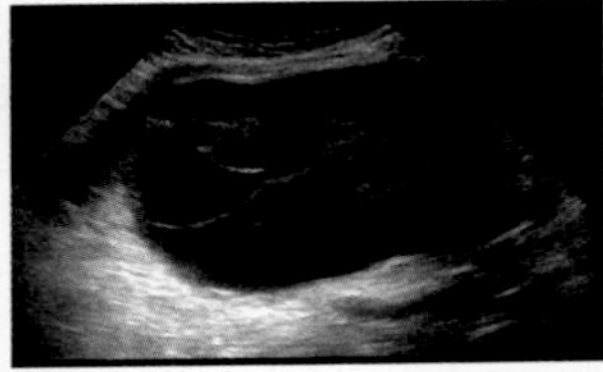

Figure 8.4A: Transvaginal scan showing multiseptated complex adnexal mass with heterogeneous solid areas

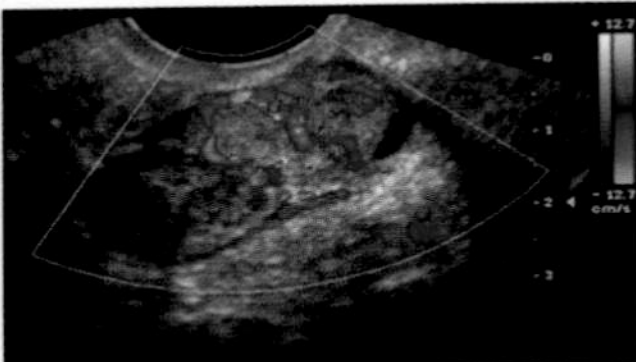

Figure 8.4B: TVS color Doppler in the same patient showing increased blood flow. Biopsy revealed ovarian cystadenocarcinoma

DIFFERENTIAL DIAGNOSIS

Peritoneal tuberculosis: Since this condition is also associated with raised CA 125 levels, it closely resembles ovarian cancer.

MANAGEMENT

The FIGO system, used for cancer staging, is summarized in **Table 8.4**.

Table 8.4: FIGO system for staging of ovarian cancer

Stage I: Limited to one or both ovaries

- IA: Involves one ovary; capsule intact; no tumor on ovarian surface; no malignant cells in ascitic fluid or peritoneal washings
- IB: Involves both ovaries; capsule intact; no tumor on ovarian surface; negative washings
- IC: Tumor limited to ovaries with any of the following: capsule ruptured, tumor on ovarian surface or positive peritoneal washings

Stage II: Pelvic extension or implants

- IIA: Extension or implants onto uterus or fallopian tube; negative washings
- IIB: Extension or implants onto other pelvic structures; negative washings
- IIC: Pelvic extension or implants with positive peritoneal washings

Stage III: Microscopic peritoneal implants outside of the pelvis or limited to the pelvis with extension to the small bowel or omentum

- IIIA: Microscopic peritoneal metastases beyond pelvis
- IIIB: Macroscopic peritoneal metastases beyond pelvis, less than 2 cm in size
- IIIC: Peritoneal metastases beyond pelvis > 2 cm or lymph node metastases

Stage IV: Distant metastases to the liver, lungs and pleura or outside the peritoneal cavity

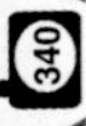

The gold standard treatment of ovarian cancer comprises of laparotomy followed by maximal reduction of the tumor mass. The surgical staging is followed by definite surgery or debulking, which is usually followed by chemotherapy or radiotherapy.

Stage IA (Grade I Disease): Primary treatment for stage 1 epithelial ovarian cancer is surgical, i.e. a total abdominal hysterectomy and a bilateral salpingo-oophorectomy and surgical staging.

Stage IA and IB (Grade 2 and 3) and Stage IC: Treatment options in these cases include additional chemotherapy or radiotherapy besides surgery as described above. Radiotherapy could be administered either in the form of intraperitoneal radiocolloids (P32) or whole abdominal radiation. Chemotherapy could be in form of either cisplatin or carboplatin or combination therapy of either of these drugs with paclitaxel for 3-4 cycles. For patients with no clinical evidence of disease and negative tumor markers at the completion of chemotherapy, a reassessment laparotomy or "second-look" surgery may be performed.

Stage II, III and IV: Debulking surgery or cytoreductive surgery is performed in these cases. This involves an initial exploratory procedure with the removal of as much disease as possible (both tumor and the associated metastatic disease).

COMPLICATIONS

- *Poor prognosis*: Cancer of the ovaries has the worst prognosis in comparison to any other type of gynecologic cancer. As a result, it is the fifth most common cause of cancer deaths in women
- *Metastasis*: The ovarian cancer is one of the most aggressive types of cancers, which can spread directly to the surrounding tissues; through the lymphatic system to other parts of the pelvis and abdomen and through the bloodstream to the distant body organs, mainly the liver and lungs
- Ascites and/or pleural effusion and/or peritonitis
- *Side-effects related to chemotherapy*: These include anorexia, bone marrow damage, constipation, diarrhea, hair loss, increased risk of infection, etc.

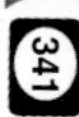

CLINICAL PEARLS

- Protective factors for ovarian cancer include multiparity, breast feeding, use of OCPs and anovulation
- Ovarian cancer rarely causes vaginal bleeding.

3. CANCER OF THE CERVIX

3.1. CERVICAL INTRAEPITHELIAL NEOPLASIA

INTRODUCTION

Cervical intraepithelial neoplasia (CIN) can be described as the preinvasive stage of cancer cervix. It denotes a continuum of disorders ranging from mild through moderate to severe dysplasia and carcinoma in situ (CIS) **(Fig. 8.5)**. Cancer of cervix usually is the end stage of the spectrum of these disorders. CIN can be considered as a precancerous lesion in which a part or the full thickness of the stratified squamous cervical epithelium is replaced by cells showing varying degrees of dysplasia. This is different from the invasive cancer as in this case the basement membrane remains intact. According to the WHO, cervical dysplasia has been categorized into mild (CIN1), moderate (CIN2) or severe dysplasia (CIN 3) and a separate category called CIS (carcinoma in situ). However according to the classification of the Bethesda System, all cervical epithelial precursor lesions have been divided into 2 groups: low grade squamous intraepithelial lesion (LSIL) including CIN1, and high grade squamous intraepithelial lesion (HSIL) including CIN2, CIN3 and CIS.

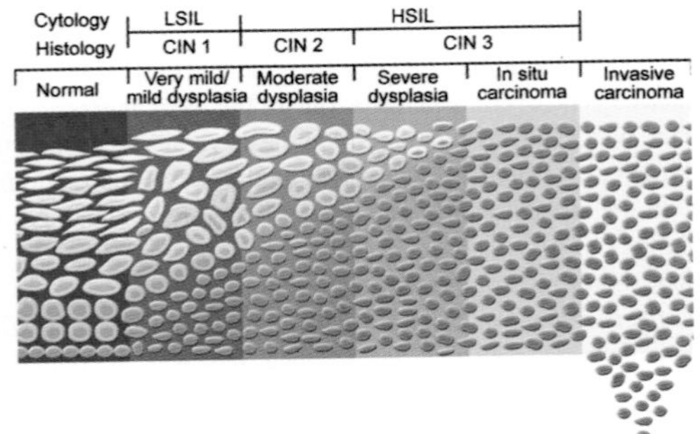

Figure 8.5: Progression of cervical dysplasia

DIAGNOSIS

Symptoms

Presence of dysplasia may be associated with minimal findings on clinical examination.

Per Speculum Examination

On inspection, the cervix often appears normal, or there may be cervicitis or erosion which bleeds on touch.

Investigations

- *Pap smear*: A Pap smear must be done at the time, when the patient is not actively bleeding. Pap smear involves cytological analysis of the cells from the squamocolumnar junction, which is an area of squamous metaplasia and the site of oncogenic transformation. **Figure 8.6** shows the Pap smear kit, while **Figure 8.7** demonstrate the procedure for taking a Pap smear
- *Cervical punch biopsy*: If any locally visible lesion on the cervix is seen, a cervical punch biopsy must be immediately performed **(Fig. 8.8)**. If the Pap smear shows severe dysplasia (HSIL) the next step is to perform a colposcopic directed biopsy and endocervical curettage
- *Visual inspection of cervix*: In areas where facilities for Pap smear screening do not exist, visual inspection with 5% acetic acid (VIA) or visual inspection with Lugols iodine (VILI) can be done. Application of 5% acetic acid causes areas of abnormality to turn acetowhite in appearance. With Schiller's iodine the abnormal area remains unstained, while the normal cervical cells take up iodine and turns mahogany brown
- *Colposcopy*: Colposcopy is an office-based procedure during which the cervix is examined under illumination and magnification before and after application of dilute acetic acid and Lugol's iodine. The characteristic features of malignancy and premalignancy on colposcopy include changes such as acetowhite areas, abnormal vascular patterns, mosaic pattern, punctuation and failure to uptake iodine stain
- *Cervicography*: This procedure involves taking the photograph of the entire cervical os with a 35 mm camera after application of 5% acetic acid. The photographs are then sent to the colposcopist for evaluation in order to select areas for biopsy.

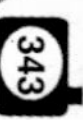

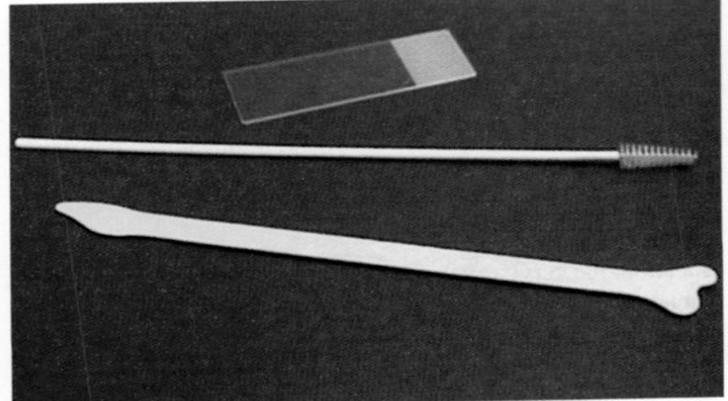

Figure 8.6: Pap smear kit

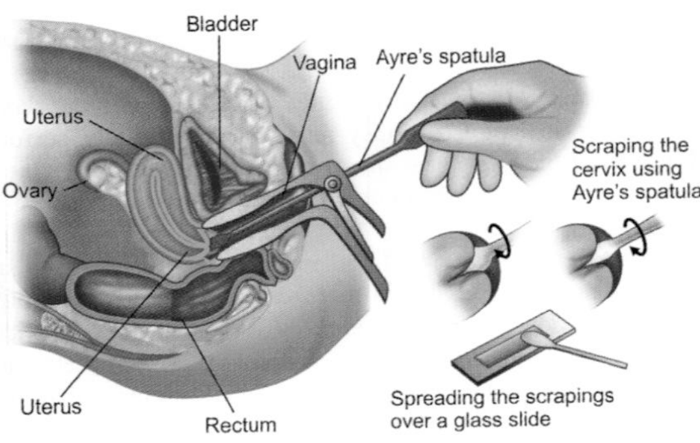

Figure 8.7: Procedure of taking a pap smear

DIFFERENTIAL DIAGNOSIS

- Cervicitis
- Infection of the cervix (*Human papilloma virus, Herpes simplex virus, Treponema pallidum*, etc.)
- Tubercular lesions of cervix
- Hyperkeratosis and parakeratosis

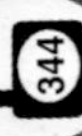

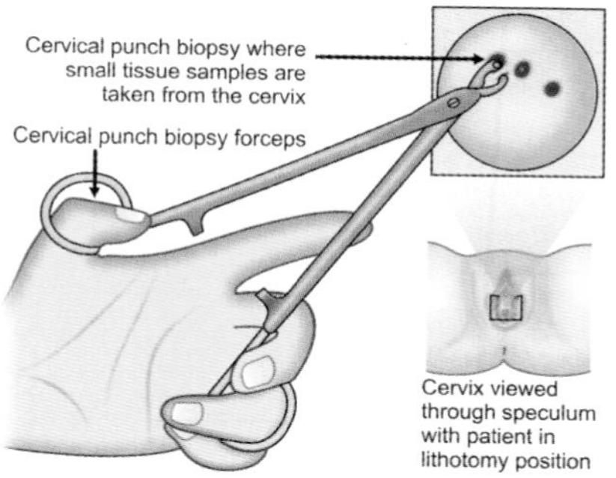

Figure 8.8: Cervical punch biopsy

- Endocervical polyps
- Squamous papillomas
- Cervical endometriosis.

MANAGEMENT

Management of patients with preinvasive lesions has been described in **Figure 8.9**. In case a preinvasive cervical lesion is detected on colposcopy, the various treatment options, which are available, are as follows:

- Local destructive methods such as cryosurgery, fulguration/ electrocoagulation and laser ablation
- Excision of the abnormal tissue with cold knife conization, laser conization, large loop excision of transformation zone (LLETZ), loop electrosurgical excision procedure (LEEP) and needle excision of transformation zone (NETZ). Surgical options such as therapeutic cone biopsy can be both diagnostic and therapeutic.

COMPLICATIONS

- Progression to invasive cancer
- Complications related to therapy: excessive bleeding and cervicovaginal infections.

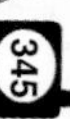

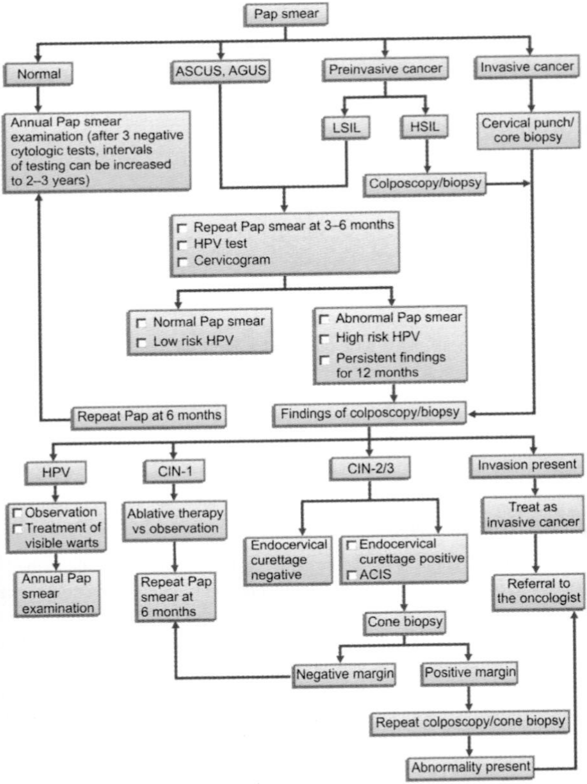

Pap smear

Normal

ASCUS, AGUS

Preinvasive cancer

Invasive cancer

Annual Pap smear examination (after 3 negative cytologic tests, intervals of testing can be increased to 2–3 years)

LSIL

HSIL

Cervical punch/ core biopsy

Colposcopy/biopsy

- Repeat Pap smear at 3–6 months
- HPV test
- Cervicogram

- Normal Pap smear
- Low risk HPV

- Abnormal Pap smear
- High risk HPV
- Persistent findings for 12 months

Repeat Pap at 6 months

Findings of colposcopy/biopsy

HPV

CIN-1

CIN-2/3

Invasion present

- Observation
- Treatment of visible warts

Ablative therapy vs observation

Treat as invasive cancer

Endocervical curettage negative

- Endocervical curettage positive
- ACIS

Annual Pap smear examination

Repeat Pap smear at 6 months

Referral to the oncologist

Cone biopsy

Negative margin

Positive margin

Repeat colposcopy/cone biopsy

Abnormality present

Figure 8.9: Management of patients with preinvasive lesions

CLINICAL PEARLS

- The severer varieties of dysplasias may progress to invasive cancer in about 10–30% of cases in 5–10 years time
- The peak incidence of occurrence of dysplasias appears to be 10 years earlier than that of frank invasive cancer

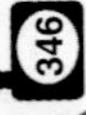

- The ACOG, (2003) recommends that all women must receive screening Pap smears by approximately 3 years after onset of vaginal sexual intercourse, but no later than age of 21. Screening should be done at least once every 2 or 3 years
- Satisfactory colposcopy requires visualization of the entire squamocolumnar junction and transformation zone for presence of any visible lesions
- HSIL changes have the greatest risk of turning cancerous in the future, thus these need to be definitively treated. Other types of changes also may require further testing, but may not need treatment.

3.2. INVASIVE CANCER OF THE CERVIX

INTRODUCTION

Cervical cancer usually affects women aged 35–55, but it can also affect women as young as 20. Regular testing with Pap smears and HPV vaccination can help prevent cervical cancer.

ETIOLOGY

Some risk factors for cervical cancer are as follows:

- History of having sexually transmitted diseases such as *Herpes simplex, Human papilloma virus* (16, 18, 31, 33) or condylomata
- Young age at the time of first sexual intercourse (coitus before the age of 18 years)
- Delivery of the first child before the age of 20 years
- Having multiple sexual partners
- Multiparity with poor birth spacing between pregnancies
- Poor personal hygiene and poor socioeconomic status
- History of smoking cigarettes or drug abuse
- History of disorders of immune system (e.g. AIDS)
- History of having preinvasive lesions.

DIAGNOSIS

Symptoms

- *Abnormal bleeding*: This may manifest as irregular vaginal bleeding, postcoital bleeding, bleeding in between periods, etc.
- *Discharge*: There may be offensive vaginal discharge or leucorrhea.

Pelvic Examination

- *Cervical growth*: A growth may be present on the cervix, which bleeds upon touching. The growth may be cauliflower-like-proliferative growth or an ulcerative lesion
- *Uterus*: Uterus may be bulky due to pyometra
- *Induration*: Involvement of uterosacral ligaments may present as an area of thickened induration on pelvic and rectal examination.

Investigations

- *PAP smear*: Pap smear is able to accurately detect cervical cancers in up to 90% of the cases in the early stages, even before the symptoms have developed
- *Colposcopic examination and biopsy*: In case an abnormality is detected on pap smear, a colposcopic examination and biopsy may be performed to further confirm the diagnosis
- *Tissue biopsy*: Histopathological examination helps in establishing the accurate diagnosis. Different types of biopsies, which can be performed are punch biopsy, endocervical curettage, cone biopsy, etc.
- *Imaging studies*: These include ultrasound (transabdominal, transvaginal and color Doppler) and CT examination **(Figs 8.10 to 8.14)**
- *Investigations for staging*: Various investigations, which help in the staging include cystoscopy, chest X-ray, sigmoidoscopy, CT, MRI, barium enema, bone and liver scans and positron emission tomography.

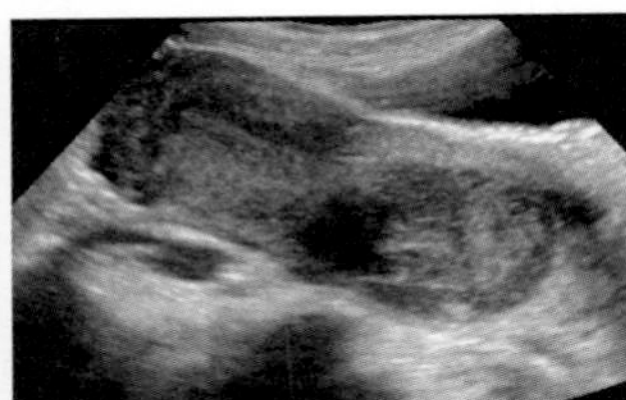

Figure 8.10: Transabdominal sonography showing solid heterogeneous cervical mass

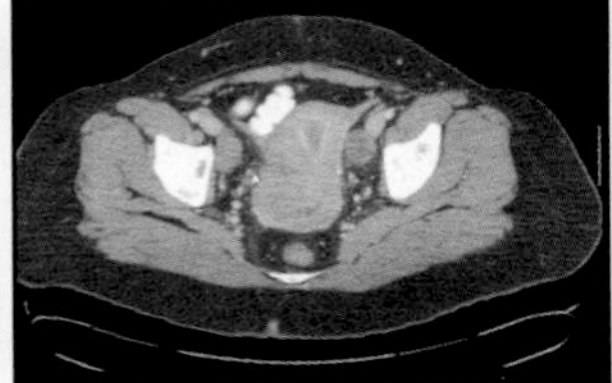

Figure 8.11: CT scan of the same patient showing a large lobulated cervical mass with central hypoattenuation

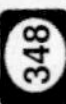

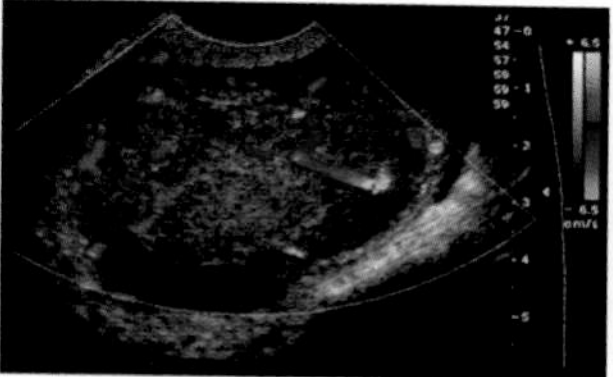

Figure 8.12: Color Doppler of the same patient showing randomly distributed irregular vessels in the mass arising from the posterior aspect of the cervix

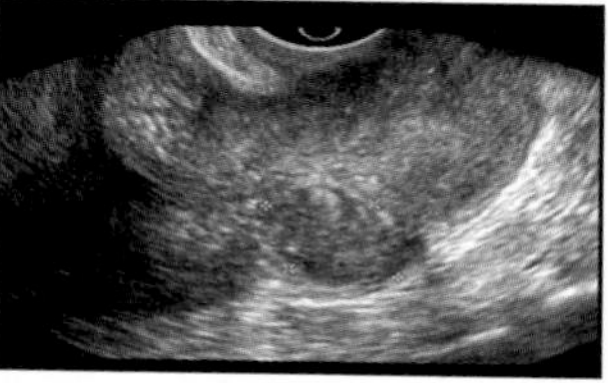

Figure 8.13: TVS of cervix of a 47 year old patient with severe suprapubic pain. Transvaginal sonography shows presence of a solid cervical mass measuring 3 × 2 × 2.5 cm

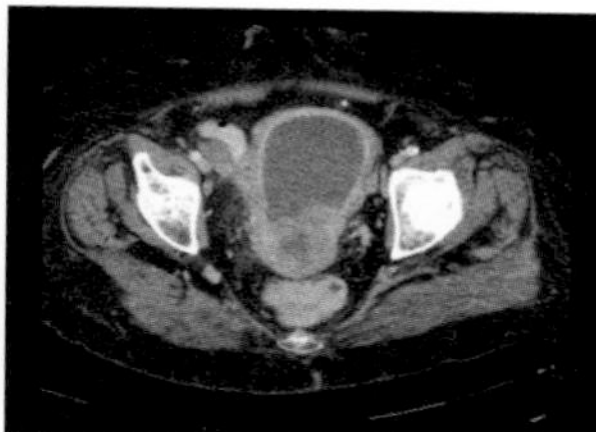

Figure 8.14: CT scan of the same patient showing spread of the cancer

DIFFERENTIAL DIAGNOSIS

- Ulcerative growths such as tubercular and syphilitic ulcers
- Fibroid polypus
- Sarcoma of the cervix (rarely).

Biopsy of the cervical lesion helps in establishing the diagnosis in most of the cases.

MANAGEMENT

Staging system for cervical cancer as devised by FIGO is described in **Table 8.5**, while the TNM staging of cervical cancer is described in **Table 8.6**.

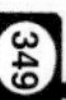

Table 8.5: FIGO staging system for cervical cancer

Stage	*Characteristics*
0	CIS, intraepithelial neoplasia
I	Carcinoma strictly confined to the cervix
	IA Invasive cancer identified only microscopically. All gross lesions, even with superficial invasion are stage IB cancers. Invasion is limited to measured invasion of stroma $\leq$ 5 mm in depth and $\leq$ 7 mm in width
	IA1 Measured invasion of stroma > 3 mm in depth and $\leq$ 7 mm in width
	IA2 Measured invasion of stroma > 3 mm and $\leq$ 5 mm in depth and $\leq$ 7 mm in width
	IB Clinical lesions confined to the cervix or preclinical lesions greater than IA
	IB1 Clinical lesions $\leq$ 4 cm in size
	IB2 Clinical lesions > 4 cm in size
II	Carcinoma extends beyond the cervix, but not to the pelvic wall; carcinoma involves the vagina but not as far as the lower one third.
	IIA No obvious parametrial involvement
	IIB Obvious parametrial involvement
III	Carcinoma has extended to the lateral pelvic wall; on rectal examination no cancer-free space is found between the tumor and the pelvic wall; tumor involves the lower one-third of the vagina; and /or including all cases with a hydronephrosis or nonfunctioning kidney, unless they are known to be related to another cause
	IIIA No extension to the pelvic wall, but involvement of the lower one-third of the vagina
	IIIB Extension to the pelvic wall and hydronephrosis or nonfunctioning kidney or both
IV	Carcinoma has extended beyond the true pelvis or has clinically involved the mucosa of the bladder or rectum
	IVA Spread to adjacent organs

Lymph nodes

Regional lymph nodes (N) include paracervical, parametrial, hypogastric (obturator), common, internal and external iliac, presacral and sacral group of lymph nodes

NX: Regional lymph nodes cannot be assessed

N0: No regional lymph nodes metastasis

N1: Regional lymph nodes metastasis

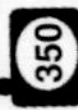

The treatment of cervical cancer varies with the stage of the disease (**Table 8.6**). For early invasive cancer, surgery is the treatment of choice. In more advanced cases, radiation combined with chemotherapy is the current standard of care. In patients with disseminated disease, chemotherapy or radiation provides symptom palliation.

Table 8.6: Stage-wise treatment of cervical cancer

TNM stage	*FIGO stage*	*Treatment*
Tis	0 CIS	LEEP, laser therapy, conization and cryotherapy
T1a1	IA1	Simple hysterectomy with or without pelvic lymph node dissection. Lymph node dissection is not required, if the depth of invasion is less than 3 mm and no lymphovascular invasion is noted on microscopic examination. Patients with lymphatic or the vascular channel infiltration require treatment as in stage IB
T1a2	IA2	Extended hysterectomy and lymph node sampling may be recommended in cases with stage IA2 disease Postoperative radiotherapy may be administered in cases where the nodes are positive
T1b	IB	The treatment options for stage IB is surgical treatment or radiotherapy or both combined surgery and radiotherapy. Radiotherapy can be either in the form of external beam or intracavitary radiotherapy. Surgery includes a radical hysterectomy (Wertheims hysterectomy). Oophorectomy is usually not necessary in premenopausal women
T2a	IIA	Treatment for stage IIA is similar to that described for I B
T2b	IIB	In stage IIB, III and IV cancer, radiation therapy has become the mainstay of treatment. However, in some cases combination chemotherapy and radiotherapy is employed
T3	III	Same as that described for IIB
—	IV	Same as that described for IIB
M1	IVB	Patients with distant metastases (stage IVB) also require chemotherapy with or without radiotherapy, to control systemic disease. In advanced cases of cervical cancer, the most extreme surgery called pelvic exenteration may be employed

COMPLICATIONS

- Infertility
- Therapy related complications: Complications related to treatment modalities such as surgery, chemotherapy and radiotherapy
- Cancer recurrence
- High rate of mortality and morbidity.

CLINICAL PEARLS

- Wertheims hysterectomy involves removal of the entire uterus, both adnexa, medial one-third of parametrium, uterosacral ligaments, upper 2–3 cm cuff of the vagina and dissection of pelvic lymph nodes
- Pelvic exenteration involves removal of all of the organs of the pelvis including the bladder and rectum.

4. VAGINAL CANCER

INTRODUCTION

Vaginal cancer is a disease in which malignant cells mainly involve the vagina. Vaginal cancer is not common. When found in early stages, it can often be cured. There are two main types of vaginal cancer: squamous cell carcinoma (which is more common) and adenocarcinoma. Vaginal cancer is found most often in women aged 60 or older, typically following the cessation of sexual activity.

ETIOLOGY

Risk factors for vaginal cancer are as follows:

- Exposure to diethylstilbestrol in utero (clear cell adenocarcinoma)
- 60 years or more in age
- Trophic ulcers in women with procedentia
- Prolonged and neglected use of ring pessary in cases of prolapse
- Infection with human papilloma virus
- History of cervical dysplasia or cervical cancer
- Exposure to radiation for the treatment of cancer cervix.

DIAGNOSIS

Symptoms

- Abnormal vaginal bleeding/discharge, which is not related to the menstrual periods

- Pain during sexual intercourse
- Pain in the pelvic area
- A lump in the vagina
- Bladder/bowel symptoms (in case of involvement of these structures).

Per Speculum Examination

Areas of involvement may be visible as diffuse, velvety, raised lesions or whitish ulcerative patches. They may bleed on touch.

Pelvic Examination

Pelvic examination along with the rectal examination helps in determining the extent of spread.

Investigations

- *Pap smear*: Cytological examination
- Staining with Schiller's iodine
- Colposcopic examination
- *Biopsy*: If a Pap smear shows abnormal cells a biopsy may be done during colposcopy
- *Other investigations*: Investigations such as a chest X-ray, cystoscopy, proctoscopy, barium enema, CT scan, MRI, etc. may be done to evaluate the spread of cancer.

DIFFERENTIAL DIAGNOSIS

- Vaginal condyloma or vaginal endometriosis
- Vaginitis or vaginal inflammation
- Metastatic lesions in vagina as a result of primary growth in cervix, endometrium, etc.

MANAGEMENT

Staging and treatment of vaginal cancer is described in **Table 8.7**.

Table 8.7: Staging and treatment of vaginal cancer

Cancer stage	*Description*	*Treatment*
Stage 0 (CIS) [Vaginal intraepithelial neoplasia	Squamous cell cancer is found in tissue lining the inside of the vagina	○ Wide local excision, with or without a skin graft ○ Partial or total vaginectomy, with or without a skin graft

Contd...

Contd...

Cancer stage	*Description*	*Treatment*
(VAIN)]		○ Topical chemotherapy (fluorouracil cream) ○ CO_2 Laser surgery ○ Internal radiation therapy
Stage I	Cancer limited to the vaginal walls	○ Internal radiation therapy, with or without external radiation therapy to lymph nodes or large tumors ○ Wide local excision or vaginectomy with vaginal reconstruction. Radiation therapy may be given after surgery ○ Vaginectomy and lymphadenectomy, with or without vaginal reconstruction. Radiation therapy may be given after the surgery
Stage 2	Cancer has spread from the vaginal walls to the tissues around the vagina, but not up to the pelvic side walls	○ Both internal and external radiation therapy to the vagina, with or without external radiation therapy to lymph nodes ○ Vaginectomy or pelvic exenteration, with or without radiation therapy
Stage 3	Cancer has spread from the vagina to the lymph nodes in the pelvis or groin, or to the pelvic walls, or both	Both internal and external radiation therapy, with or without surgery
Stage IV A	Extension beyond the true pelvis with or without the involvement of the pelvic lymph nodes, bladder and/or the rectum	Both internal and external radiation therapy, with or without surgery
Stage IV B	Distant metastasis such as the lungs. Cancer may also have spread to the distant lymph nodes	○ Radiation therapy as palliative therapy to relieve symptoms and improve the quality of life. Chemotherapy may also be given

COMPLICATIONS

- *Metastasis*: Metastasis of vaginal cancer can occur to distant organs, such as lung, liver, etc.
- *Therapy related complications*: Complications related to treatment modalities such as radiation, surgery and chemotherapy.

CLINICAL PEARLS

- The prognosis in these cases depends upon the cancer stage, grade and the tumor size
- New types of treatment are being tested in clinical trials. These include radiosensitizers, which make tumor cells more sensitive to radiation therapy
- Treatment of recurrent vaginal cancer may include pelvic exenteration and radiation therapy.

5. VULVAR CANCER

INTRODUCTION

Vulvar cancer, which affects the vulva, (region of female external genitalia including various anatomical structures such as labia majora, mons pubis, labia minora, clitoris, vestibule and the vaginal introitus) is the fourth most common gynecologic cancer, accounting for 3–4% of these cancers in the United States **(Fig. 8.15)**. Vulvar cancer usually occurs after menopause. The average age at diagnosis is 70 years.

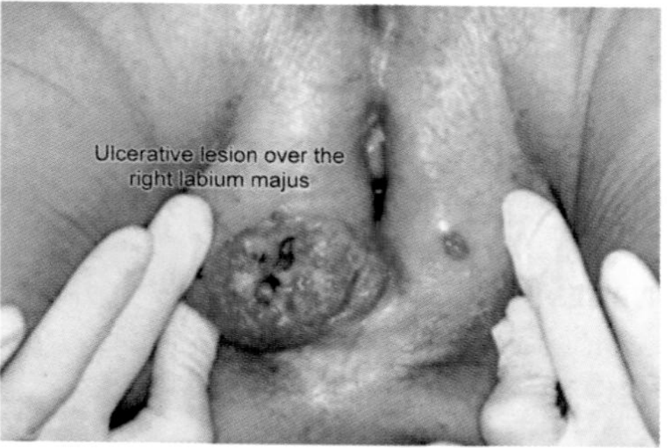

Figure 8.15: Vulvar cancer

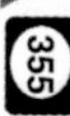

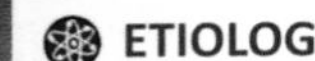

ETIOLOGY

The risk factors for developing vulvar cancer are presence of precancerous/ dysplastic changes, lichen sclerosus, etc. in the vulvar tissues.

DIAGNOSIS

Clinical Presentation

Symptoms: In 50% of cases, presentation is in the form of a lump or a mass along with a long standing history of pruritis, which may be related to vulvar dystrophy.

Per speculum examination: There may be a lesion in labia majora, labia minora, clitoris, perineum, vagina, urethra, anus, etc.

Pelvic Examination: This may help detect abnormalities in the cervix, uterus and adnexa.

Investigations

- Biopsy of the abnormal skin over the vulva
- Pap smear to be obtained from the cervix
- Colposcopic examination of the cervix and vagina
- Wedge biopsy of the lesions is commonly performed. In case the lesion is less than 1 cm in diameter, an excisional biopsy may be performed.

DIFFERENTIAL DIAGNOSIS

- Paget disease of the vulva
- Vulvar intraepithelial neoplasia
- Non-neoplastic vulvar lesions such as lichen sclerosis, squamous cell hyperplasia and vulvar vestibulitis
- Infectious lesions (e.g. herpes simplex virus, human papilloma virus, syphilis, etc.)

MANAGEMENT

The revised FIGO staging and treatment for vulvar cancer is described in **Table 8.8**.

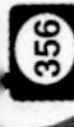

Table 8.8: Revised FIGO staging and treatment for vulvar cancer

FIGO stage	*Clinical/Pathological*	*Treatment*
Stage 0	CIS, intraepithelial cancer	Laser ablation, surgical excision
Stage I	Tumor confined to the vulva or perineum, < 2 cm in greatest dimension and nodes are negative Ia Stromal invasion < 1 mm Ib Stromal invasion > 1 mm	The management of patients with T1 cancer of the vulva is individualized. Radical local excision, rather than a radical vulvectomy is advocated for the primary lesions for patients with T1 tumors. Some type of vulvar reconstruction is usually required after radical local excision. Groin dissection is usually required for the cases of vulvar cancer having more than 1 mm of stromal invasion. In case of two or more positive groin nodes, postoperative groin and pelvic radiation must be administered
Stage II	Tumor confined to vulva and/or perineum, > 2 cm in greatest dimension and nodes are negative	Management of patients with T2 and early T3 tumors comprises of radical vulvectomy with bilateral inguinal-femoral lymphadenectomy. Pelvic and groin irradiation may be administered in cases where there are two or more positive groin nodes
Stage III	Tumor of any size with: • adjacent spread to the lower urethra or anus • unilateral regional lymph node metastasis	Pelvic exenteration in combination with radical vulvectomy and bilateral groin dissection may be required. Bornow's combination therapy, comprising of combined radiosurgical approach (involving the use of intracavitary radium with or without external irradiation), has been suggested in patients with advanced vulvar cancer, as an alternative to pelvic exenteration
Stage IV	Tumor invades the distant organs IVa Invasion of upper urethra, bladder mucosa, rectal mucosa, pelvic bone or bilateral lymph-node metastasis IVb Any distant metastasis including the pelvic lymph nodes	Same as that for stage III

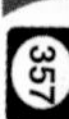

COMPLICATIONS

- Metastasis to distant organs such as lungs, liver, pelvic bones, etc.
- Complications related to surgery such as wound infection, sexual dysfunction, venous thromboembolism, etc.

6. CANCER OF THE FALLOPIAN TUBES

INTRODUCTION

Fallopian tube cancer, also known as tubal cancer, develops in the fallopian tubes that connect the ovaries and the uterus. It is very rare and accounts for only 1–2% of all cases of gynecologic cancers. The most common type of tumor is an adenocarcinoma and typically affects women between the ages of 50 and 60 years. It is bilateral in nearly one-third cases.

ETIOLOGY

- Women who have inherited the BRCA1 gene (linked with the development of ovarian and breast cancer) are also at an increased risk of developing fallopian tube cancer
- It is more common in nulliparous menopausal women.

DIAGNOSIS

Symptoms

- Abnormal vaginal bleeding/amber colored discharge, especially after menopause
- Abdominal pain or a feeling of pressure in the abdomen.

Pelvic Examination

A pelvic mass at the time of diagnosis may be present in up to two-thirds of patients.

Investigations

- *Pap smear*: Unreliable test for the diagnosis of fallopian tube cancer
- *Uterine biopsy*: Negative findings on the biopsy of the uterine curettings and a negative hysteroscopic examination in a patient with postmenopausal bleeding should raise the suspicion of fallopian tube cancer

- *Imaging*: Transvaginal ultrasound may show presence of an adnexal mass **(Fig. 8.16)**. Doppler flow velocimetry may show low resistance blood flow in the mass **(Fig. 8.17)**
- *CA 125 Test*: An estimated 85% of women with gynecological disease have increased levels of CA 125.

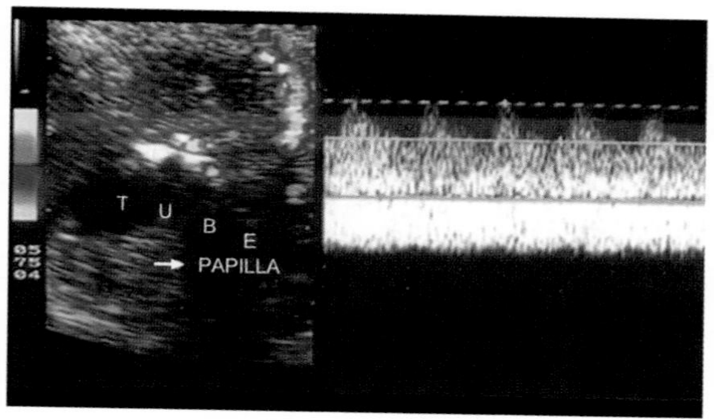

Figure 8.16: Patient with fallopian tube cancer having sausage shaped adnexal mass with presence of papillomatous protrusions and solid parts

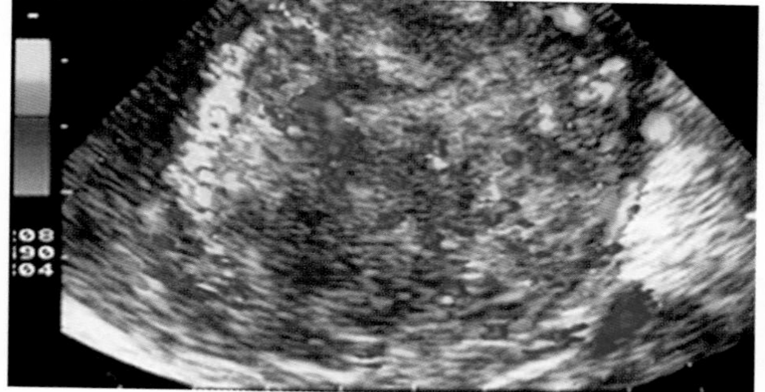

Figure 8.17: Color Doppler shows increased venous blood flow signals

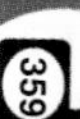

DIFFERENTIAL DIAGNOSIS

- Pyosalpinx
- Tubercular lesion of the tube
- Other malignancies of genital tract such as endometrial, cervical, vaginal, etc.

MANAGEMENT

Staging for fallopian tube cancer is described in **Table 8.9.** Treatment for fallopian tube cancer usually involves surgery and comprises of total abdominal hysterectomy with bilateral salpingo-ophorectomy, pelvic lymph node sampling and omentectomy. Postoperative radiotherapy, chemotherapy and hormonal therapy with progestogens may be required depending upon the spread of cancer.

Table 8.9: Staging of the cancer of fallopian tubes

Stage	*Description*
I	Tumor is confined to the tubal muscle and the mucosa
II	The tumor has invaded tubal serosa II A: Tumor has not spread to the pelvic organs IIB: Tumor has spread to the adjacent pelvic organs
III	Tumor has spread outside the pelvic cavity into the abdominal cavity, but not outside the abdominal cavity
IV	Spread to extra-abdominal organs is present

COMPLICATIONS

- *Metastasis*: This is a highly malignant tumor, which spreads rapidly to the surrounding as well as distant tissues
- *High mortality rate*: Prognosis is poor with the 5-year cure rate of approximately 25%.

CLINICAL PEARLS

- Surgical staging is an important aspect of treatment in these cases
- Since fallopian tube cancer is so rare, and its symptoms are non-specific and can resemble other problems, it can be difficult to diagnose
- It is more common for fallopian tube cancer to arise as a result of metastasis from cancer in other parts of the body, such as the ovaries or endometrium, rather than for cancer to actually originate in the fallopian tubes as a primary growth.

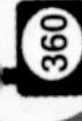

CHAPTER 9

Gynecological Surgery

1. PRINCIPLES OF GYNECOLOGICAL SURGERY

These are described in **Box 9.1**.

Box 9.1: Principles of gynecological surgery

Ethics in Surgery

Some of the ethical principles which must be incorporated into medical and surgical practice include the following:

- *Beneficence*: the principle of "avoiding any harm"
- *Justice*: The doctor should be fair in the process of treating the patients
- *Respect for patients*: The doctors must show respect for their patients by treating them as autonomous individuals and obtaining informed consent before undertaking a surgical procedure
- Clinicians are responsible for maintaining their own medical and surgical competence
- Respecting the patient's confidentiality at each stage.

Preoperative Care

The main aim of preoperative assessment before anesthesia and surgery is to help improve outcome by identifying potential anesthetic difficulties; identifying existing medical conditions; improving safety by assessing and quantifying risk; planning of perioperative care; providing the opportunity for explanation and discussion and by allaying the patient's fear and anxiety. Good preoperative preparation comprises of adequate patient assessment through appropriate clinical history and examination, and preanesthetic evaluation. The clinical examination must include a complete gynecological history and examination as well as complete evaluation of the pulmonary, cardiovascular, gastrointestinal, urinary, musculoskeletal and neurological systems.

Preoperative Management One Day Prior to Surgery

- *Diet and nutrition*: For all practical purposes, the patient may be allowed to have a light and easily digestible diet, the night before the morning of surgery. After midnight, the patient must be NPO

Contd...

Contd...

- *Sedation*: Mild sedative drugs may be administered on the night before the surgery to help allay the patient's anxiety
- *Bowel preparation*: Women undergoing abdominal surgery in which entry into the bowel is anticipated, complete bowel preparation must be performed by use of laxatives or preoperative enema, either the evening before or on the morning of surgery
- *Preoperative antibiotics*: A single dose of prophylactic broad-spectrum antibiotics immediately prior to the surgery is sufficient for most of the cases. A repeat dose may be required if the surgery is likely to last for longer than 8 hours
- *Thromboprophylaxis*: This may be required because gynecological surgery may be associated with a high incidence of deep vein thrombosis and pulmonary embolism.

Anesthesia

Preanesthetic check-up: During the preanesthetic check-up performed prior to surgery, anesthetist gets the opportunity to discuss with the patient, the advantages and complications of each type of anesthetic procedure. During this time, the anesthetist must also gain the patient's consent for anesthetic procedure.

Types of Anesthesia: The types of anesthesia used most commonly for the obstetric and gynecological surgeries include general anesthesia and regional anesthesia (spinal, epidural or combined spinal and epidural). Local anesthesia blocks such as pudendal nerve block **(Fig. 9.1)** and paracervical blocks **(Fig. 9.2)** are also commonly used for minor surgeries.

Intraoperative Principles

- Surgery must be done along the lines of tissue planes
- Tissues must be handled gently
- Adequate access to the operation field and good source of light are important prerequisites before undertaking any surgery
- Use of appropriate retractors and bowel packing helps in obtaining adequate access
- Asepsis: An important principle which is required for achieving asepsis is reduction of three things: time duration for performance of surgery; trauma to the tissues and trash (contamination of tissues by bacteria or foreign bodies). Hand washing for 3–5 min prior to any surgical procedure is important for the maintenance of asepsis.

Types of Surgical Incisions

Characteristics of various types of abdominal incisions are described in **Table 9.1**. Nowadays, transverse incisions are more commonly employed and are associated with the best cosmetic results. These incisions are

Contd...

Contd...

much stronger in comparison to the midline incisions. They are less painful and associated with reduced postoperative discomfort, rate of wound evisceration and hernia formation

Sutures

A suture is any strand of material used to approximate tissue or ligate vessels. Though, the ideal suture has yet not been created, broadly, the various types of suture materials can be of two types: absorbable and nonabsorbable **(Box 9.2)**.

Surgical Needles

The surgical needles have three components: eye, body and the point **(Fig. 9.3)**.

Surgical Knots

The surgical knots can be of two basic types: flat knots and the sliding knots. Flat knots can be of three types: square **(Fig. 9.4)**, surgeon's and Granny's **(Fig. 9.5)**.

Postoperative Care

Postoperative care can be divided into three phases:

Immediate postoperative care: This involves the period immediately following surgery when the patient is still in the operation theater. The parameters, such as airway, breathing and circulation (ABC), must be monitored soon after the surgery. The patient must be eventually shifted to the recovery area when the patients' vitals have stabilized.

Early postoperative care: The care in the ward during the early postoperative period can be summarized by acronym SOAP, which can be described as follows:

- S: Subjective: how does the patient feel?
- O: Objective: assessment of objective parameters such as pules, blood pressure, temperature and fluid balance
- A: Assessment: physical examination
- P: Plan: plan of care for the next 24 hrs (bleeding, signs of infection, etc.)

Various parameters which need to be taken into consideration during this period are as follows:

- Medications: Adequate analgesia must be prescribed. These may include oral medicines such as paracetamol and NSAIDS, patient controlled analgesia (PCA), opioids, epidural analgesia, etc. In case, the patient complains about nausea, she should be administered antiemetic medications. The other medications which must be prescribed include antibiotics and prophylactic therapy for DVT

Contd...

Contd...

- Fluid and electrolyte balance: Maintenance of fluid balance is important during this phase. The nursing care professionals must be instructed to inform the surgeon in case the urinary output becomes less than 30 ml per hr
- Nutrition and dietary requirements: Patient who had uncomplicated surgery may be given a regular diet on the first postoperative day if the bowel sounds are present; abdominal examination reveals no distension and the patient is no longer nauseated from anesthesia

Late postoperative care: This involves the period after which the patient is discharged home and comprises of the following components:

- *Wound care*: The surgeon must individualize care of each wound, but the sterile dressing placed in the operating room is generally left intact for 24 hours unless signs of infection (e.g. increasing pain, erythema and drainage) develop
- *Requirement for hormone replacement therapy*: Estrogen deficiency may occur in patients who have undergone bilateral oophorectomy at the time of surgery
- *Physical activity*: The patient should be encouraged to ambulate as early as possible in the postoperative period in order to reduce the risk of development of venous thromboembolism.

Postoperative Complications

- *Hemorrhage:* In patients with severe anemia prior to the surgery or severe intraoperative bleeding, blood must be transfused
- *Postoperative febrile morbidity*: Common cause of fever is a high metabolic rate that occurs due to stress of the surgical procedure. Other causes of fever may include pneumonia, UTIs and wound infections
- *Pulmonary complications*: Most important pulmonary complications after pelvic or abdominal surgery include atelectasis, pneumonia and pulmonary thromboembolic diseases
- *Urinary infection and/or retention*
- *GIT complications*: Slight postoperative nausea and vomiting due to the use of anesthetic agents is common problem amongst postoperative patients. Two other common gastrointestinal complications include postoperative ileus and postoperative intestinal obstruction
- *Venous thrombotic events (VTEs)*: These include complications such as DVT and PE. These can be considered as important causes of postoperative mortality. The major sites of thrombus formation are soleal venous sinuses of the calf and venous arcade, which join the posterior tibial and peroneal veins draining the soleal muscle.

Some of the preventive measures which can be taken to reduce the risk of embolism include preoperative and postoperative prophylaxis with unfractionated heparin or low molecular weight heparin and concomitant

Contd...

Contd...

use of embolic stockings or intermittent pneumatic compression stockings. Early mobilization in the postoperative period encourages the muscle pumping function of the legs, thereby reducing the venous stasis.

- *Postoperative infections*: Common postoperative infections include pelvic infections such as pelvic cellulitis, vaginal cuff hematoma and/or abscess, pelvic vein thrombosis, postoperative adnexal abscess, cellulitis, osteomyelitis pubis, incisional wound infection and cystitis. Nonpelvic infections may include infections such as pneumonia, bacteremia, pyelonephritis, etc. Steps which can be taken to reduce the incidence of postoperative infection include administration of prophylactic antibiotics 30 mins prior to the incision or at the time of induction of anesthesia; use of meticulous surgical techniques at the time of surgery; ensuring adequate hemostasis at the time of surgery; judicious use of cautery; gentle handling of the tissues, etc.
- *Wound dehiscence*: Dehiscence can be defined as the separation of the sutured layers of the abdominal wall and may be classified as partial or complete
- *Wound infection*: Wound infection has been reported to occur in 2–4% of all clean abdominal incisions and up to 35% of all grossly contaminated incisions. Copious irrigation of wound with nonirritating physiologic solutions also helps in significantly reducing the chances of wound contamination

Table 9.1: Characteristics of lower abdominal incisions

Incisions	*Pfannenstiel*	*Vertical*	*Cherney*	*Maylard*
Extent of the incision	Transverse skin incision made approximately 4 cm above the superior border of pubis **(Fig. 9.6)**	The incision is made from just above the pubis to below the **(Fig. 9.7)** umblicus	Rectus muscles are detached from their insertion over the pubic bone **(Fig. 9.8)**	Involves the transverse incision of rectus muscle, along with skin, fascia and rectus sheath **(Fig. 9.9)**
Pelvic exposure	Least extensive	Extensive	Extensive	Most extensive
Upper abdomen	None	Most extensive	Least extensive	Extensive
Hemorrhage	Moderate	Minimal	Moderate	Maximal

Contd...

Contd...

Incisions	*Pfannenstiel*	*Vertical*	*Cherney*	*Maylard*
Hernia formation	Minimal	Maximum	Minimal	Moderate
Risk of evisceration	Minimal	Maximum	Minimal	Moderate
Speed	Minimal	Maximum	Moderate	Minimal

Box 9.2: Different types of sutures

Absorbable Sutures

Natural

- Catgut
  - Plain
  - Chromic

Synthetic

- Polyglactin 910 (Vicryl)
  - Uncoated
  - Coated
  - Polyglycolic acid (Dexon)
  - Poliglecaprone (Monocryl)
  - Polydioxanone (PDS) (Quill)
  - Polyglyconate (Maxon)

Nonabsorbable Sutures

- *Natural nonabsorbable sutures*: Silk, cotton and stainless-steel wire (Flexon)
- *Synthetic nonabsorbable sutures*: Nylon (Dermalon, Surgilon); polypropylene (Prolene, Novafil) and braided synthetics (Dacron®, Tevdek).

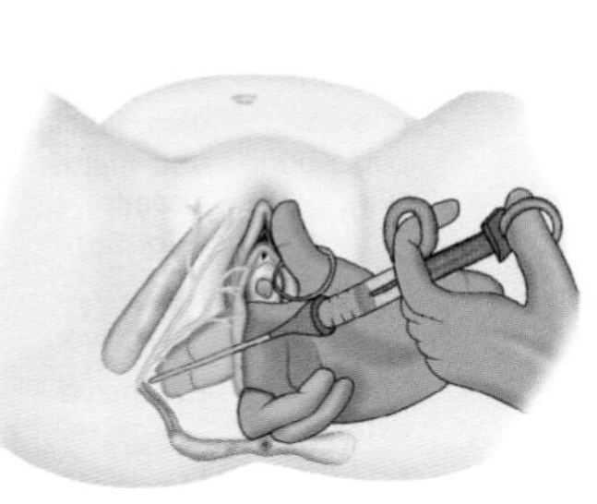

Figure 9.1: Pudendal nerve block

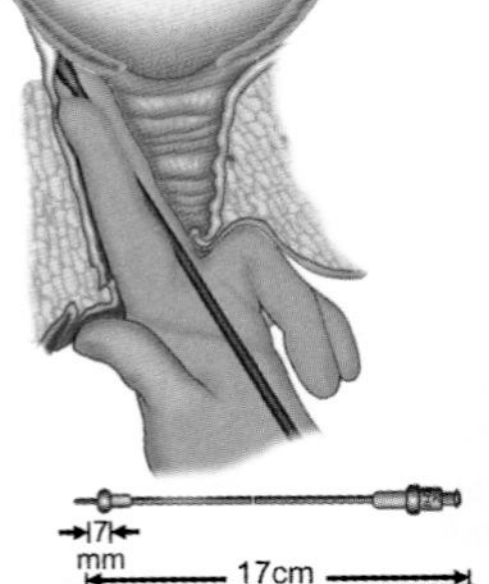

Figure 9.2: Paracervical nerve block

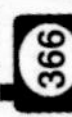

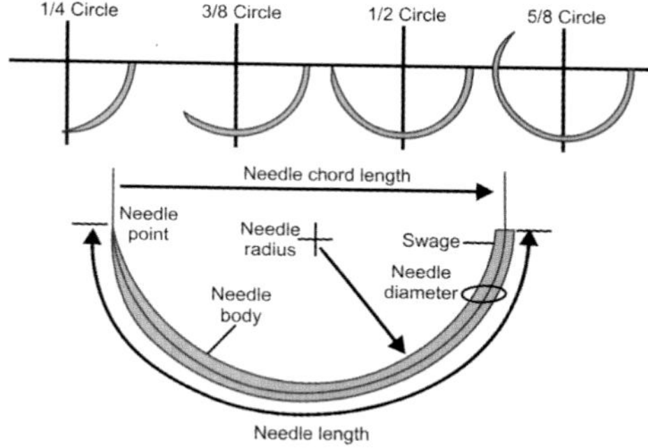

Figure 9.3: Various needle configurations and characteristics of a curved surgical needle

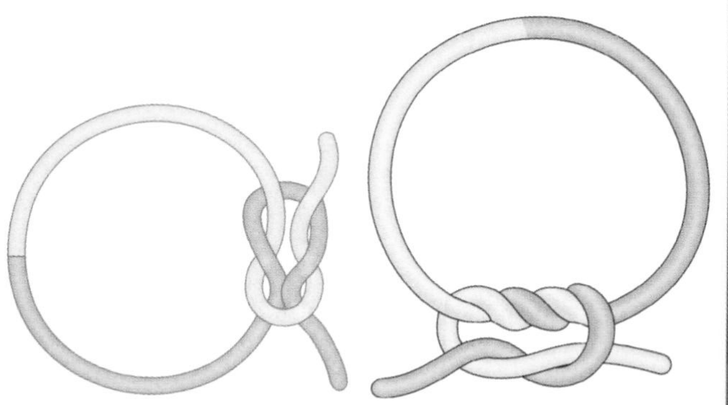

Figure 9.4: Square knot

Figure 9.5: Granny's knot

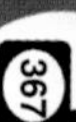

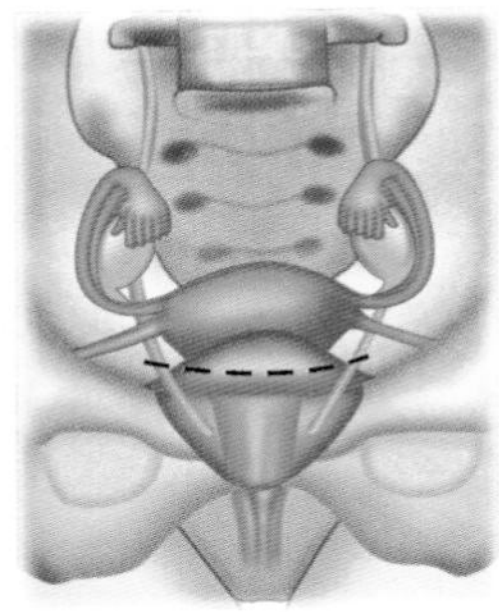

Figure 9.6: Pfannenstiel incision

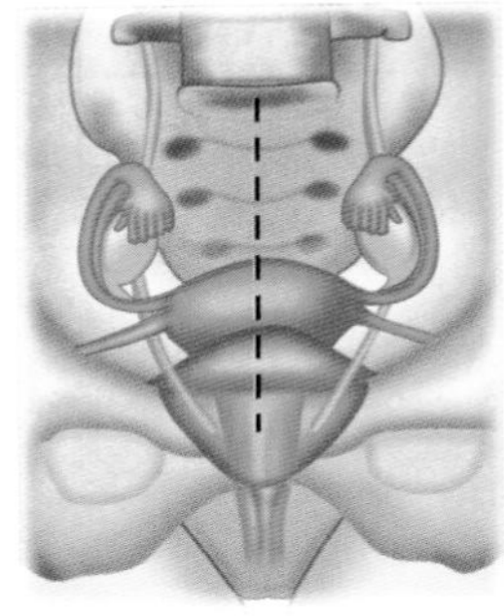

Figure 9.7: Vertical incision

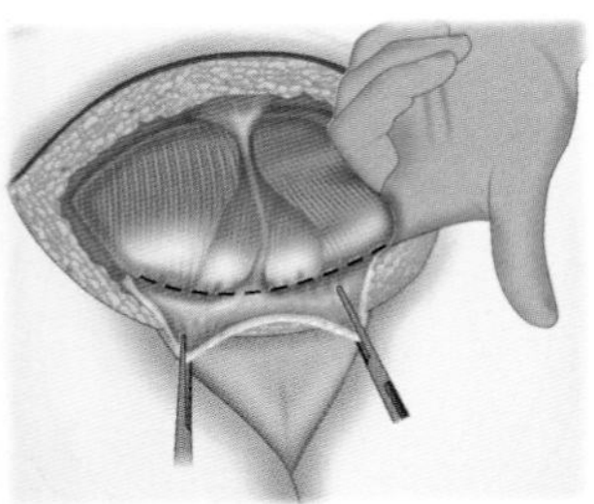

Figure 9.8: Cherney's incision: transection of the tendons of the rectus muscle

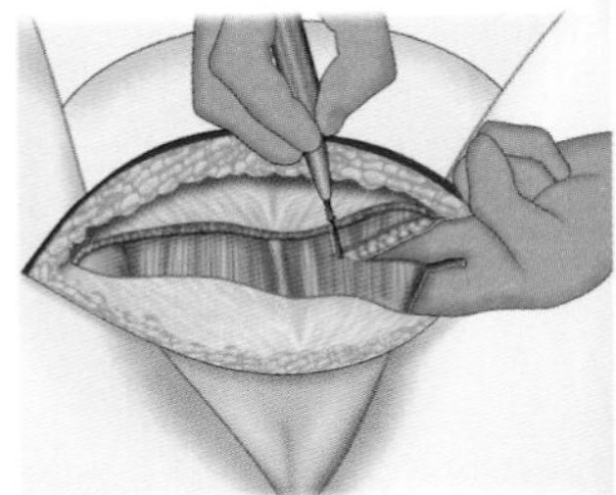

Figure 9.9: Maylard incision: transection of the rectus muscle

CLINICAL PEARLS

- Importance must be given towards maintenance of patient-physician relationship. It is important for a male gynecologist to take history and perform vaginal examination in presence of a third party or a chaperone (a female nurse or the patient's female relative or friend)
- Among the various steps taken to maintain asepsis, use of preoperative shaving has not been observed to alter the rate of wound infection

- Oral NSAIDs form the first line of management for mild-to-moderate pain. For patients who cannot tolerate NSAIDs or who require stronger dosage of analgesics, combinations of paracetamol and opioids are the next best choice.

2. ABDOMINAL HYSTERECTOMY

INTRODUCTION

Abdominal hysterectomy is a commonly performed gynecological procedure utilized for removal of the uterus (with or without removal of ovaries) in cases of benign and malignant gynecological diseases. Depending on the route through which the hysterectomy is performed, it can be classified as abdominal hysterectomy (performed through an abdominal incision), vaginal hysterectomy (performed through vaginal incision) or as a laparoscopic procedure [laparoscopic hysterectomy(LH)] or laparoscopic assisted vaginal hysterectomy (LAVH).

INDICATIONS

Hysterectomy is commonly performed for the following indications:

- *Fibroid uterus*: Especially in cases of symptomatic fibroids
- *Malignancies of the genital tract*: These may include endometrial cancer; cancer of the cervix or severe cervical dysplasia (CIN grade III) and cancer of the ovary
- *Endometriosis*: A hysterectomy may be recommended when medication and minimal invasive surgery fails to cure endometriosis
- Persistent vaginal bleeding
- *Uterine prolapse*: Moderate or severe prolapse of the uterus
- *Complications during childbirth*: Hysterectomy may be performed as an emergency procedure to control atonic primary PPH.

SURGICAL MANAGEMENT

Preoperative Preparation

- A complete history and physical examination
- *Routine preoperative investigations*: Investigations such as complete blood count with platelet count, fasting blood glucose, kidney function test and liver function test must be performed. Other preoperative investigations include tests such as endometrial biopsy or aspiration, Pap smear and ultrasound examination

- *Informed consent*: Written informed consent must be obtained from the patient prior to the surgery
- *Nil per orally*: The patient should not take either food or water by mouth for at least 6 hours prior to the time of scheduled surgery
- *Analgesics and antibiotics*: Painkillers, mild sedatives and antibiotics may be prescribed before the procedure
- *Part preparation*: The abdomen and genital area may be shaved and prepared for the surgery
- *Bowel preparation*: An enema may be administered to the patient 6–10 hours prior to the surgery
- *Anesthesia*: Abdominal hysterectomy can be performed under spinal or general anesthesia
- *Patient position*: The patient is put in approximately 15° Trendelenburg position for the surgery
- *Cleaning and draping*: Under all aseptic precautions the lower abdominal area, the genital area and upper parts of the thighs are cleaned and draped using sterile aseptic technique
- *Foley catheter*: The bladder is catheterized with the help of Foley's catheter.

Steps of Surgery

The procedure of abdominal hysterectomy is illustrated in **Figures 9.10 to 9.21**.

Abdominal closure is the final concluding step of abdominal hysterectomy. Prior to closing the abdomen, all the stumps must be inspected for hemostasis.

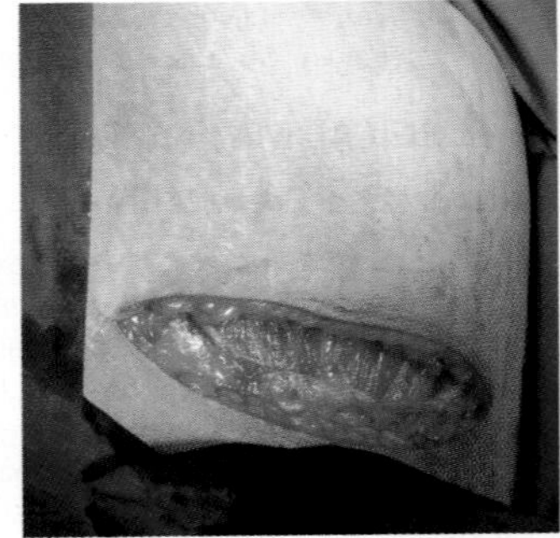

Figure 9.10: Opening the abdomen using a Pfannenstiel transverse abdominal incision

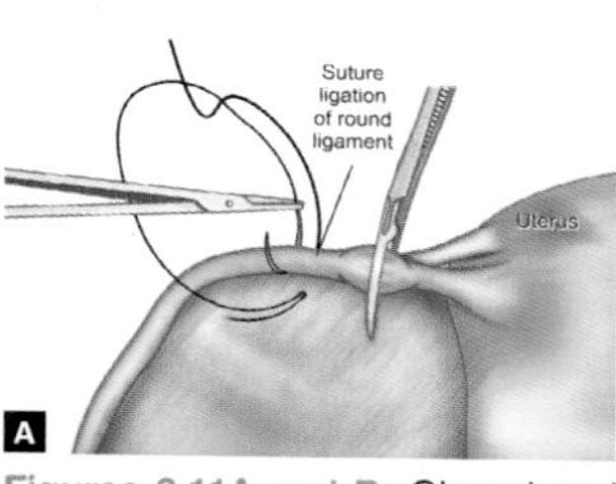

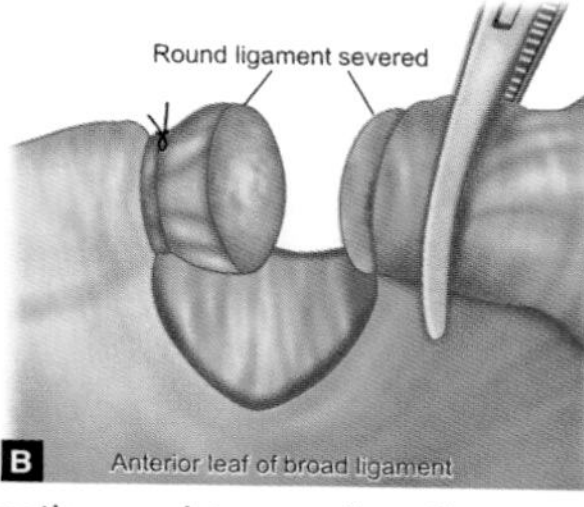

Figures 9.11A and B: Clamping, ligating and transecting the round ligaments, and incising the anterior leaf of broad ligament

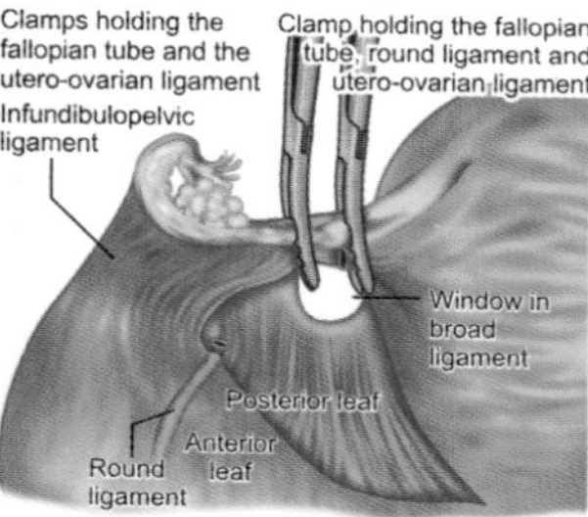

Figure 9.12: Clamping, cutting and ligation of the fallopian tubes and utero-ovarian ligaments in case the tubes and ovaries are to be preserved

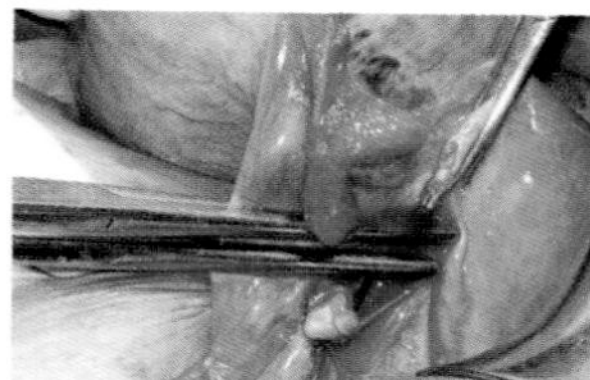

Figure 9.13: Clamping, cutting and ligating the infundibulopelvic ligaments, in case the tubes and ovaries have to be removed

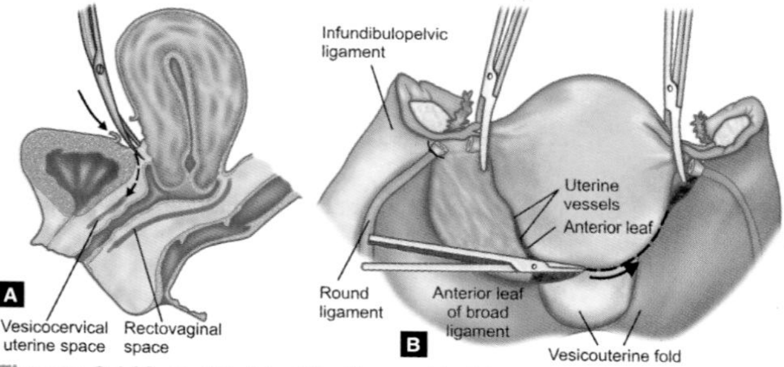

Figures 9.14A and B: Identification and incision of the vesicouterine fold of peritoneum, which is extended over the anterior leaf of broad ligament

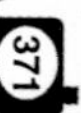

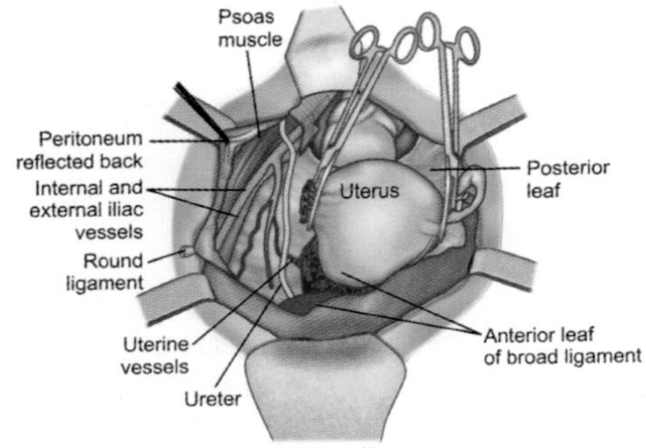

Figure 9.15: Identification of the ureter as it crosses the common iliac vessels by following the external iliac artery cephalad to the bifurcation

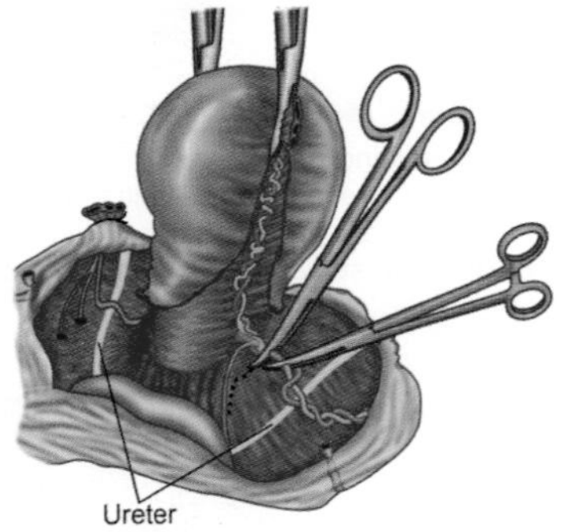

Figure 9.16: Clamping, cutting and ligating the uterine vessels after skeletonizing the vessels

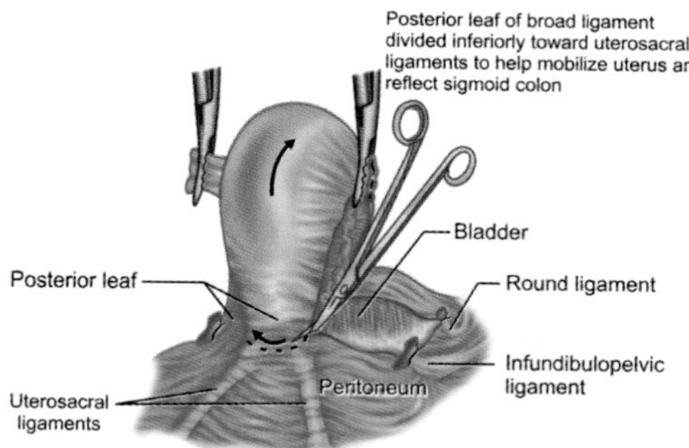

Figure 9.17: The posterior leaf of broad ligament is then incised to the point where the uterosacral ligaments join the cervix and the rectum is mobilized from the posterior cervix

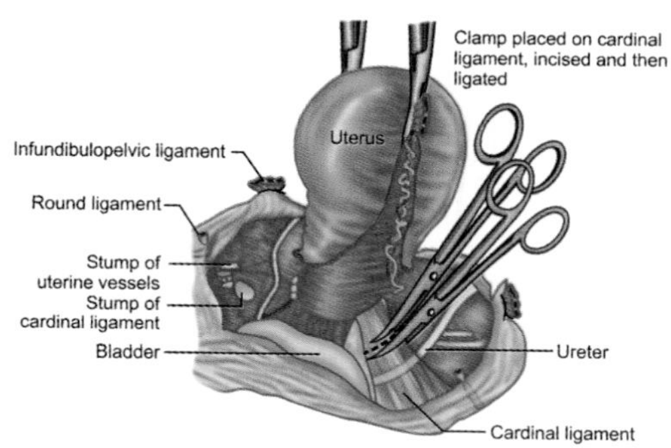

Figure 9.18: Diagrammatic representation of clamping, cutting and ligating the Mackendrot's and uterosacral ligaments

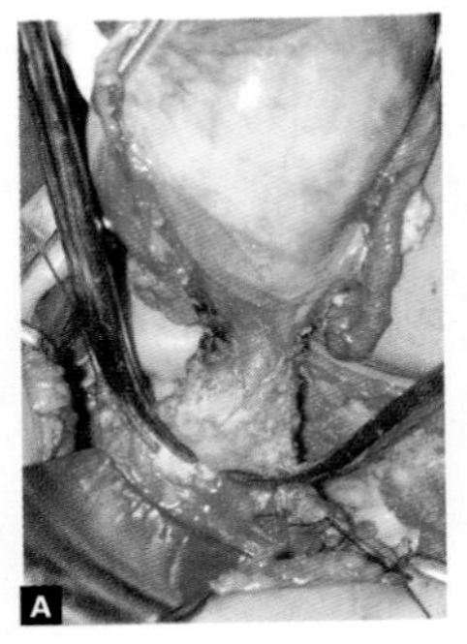

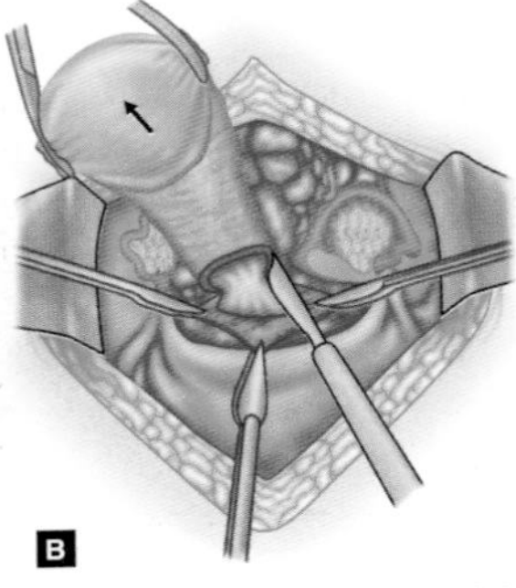

Figures 9.19A and B: Identification, clamping and cutting of the vaginal angles

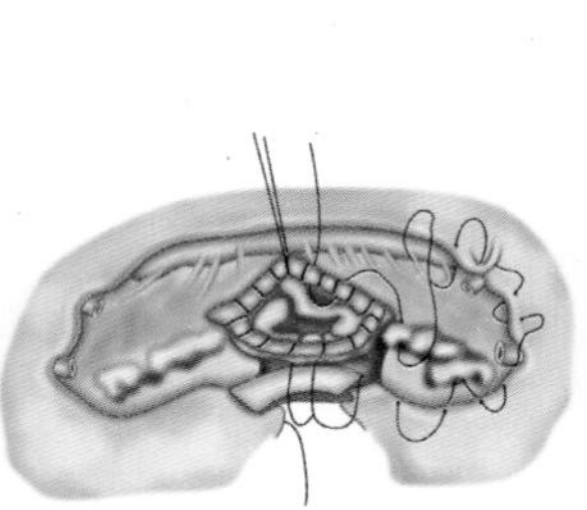

Figure 9.20: Vaginal cuff is left open with running locking stitch sutures placed along the cut edge of vaginal mucosa

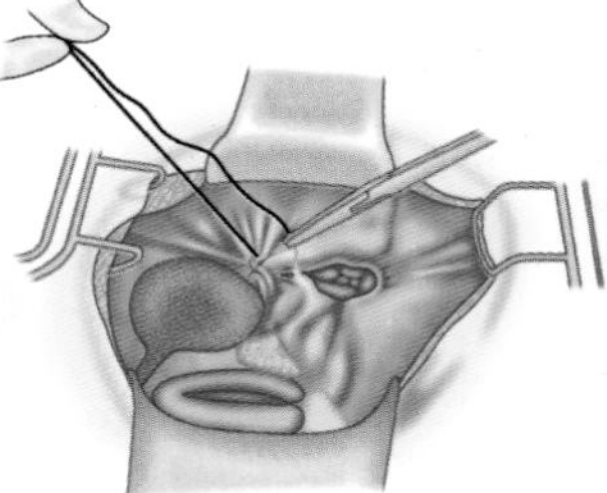

Figure 9.21: Reperitonization of the pelvis

Postoperative Care

- The patient must be closely observed for the signs of hemorrhage for the first few hours following the surgery
- Intravenous and oral pain-killer medications can provide relief from postoperative pain. PCA can be utilized for adequate control of pain
- Foley's catheter may be removed in the morning following surgery or the patient may remain catheterized for 1–2 days to help her pass urine

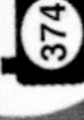

- Intravenous fluids are administered for the first 24 hours following surgery
- Lifting of heavy weights or vaginal sexual intercourse must be discouraged for at least 4–6 weeks until the vaginal cuff heals completely
- Skin sutures are removed on 7th to 10th postoperative day.

COMPLICATIONS

Immediate Postoperative Period

- *Hemorrhage*: Primary and reactionary, immediately following surgery or secondary hemorrhage after 24 hours of surgery
- Injury to adjacent structures such as bladder, intestines and ureter
- Anesthetic complications
- *Shock*: Hypovolemic shock
- *Urinary complications*: These may include complications such as retention, cystitis, anuria and incontinence such as overflow, stress or true incontinence
- *Pyrexia*: Pyrexia more than 100.8°F, commonly due to infection
- *Hematoma*: Cuff or rectus sheath hematoma
- Wound dehiscence
- Paralytic ileus and intestinal obstruction
- *Venous complications:* Phlebitis, DVT and PE.

Remote

- Vault granulation, vault prolapse
- Prolapse of fallopian tubes
- Incisional hernia
- Postoperative adhesion formation
- High mortality rate
- Early surgical menopause in case of salpingo-oophorectomy.

CLINICAL PEARLS

- Abdominal hysterectomy must be reserved only for cases where the vaginal route is contraindicated and LAVH is either difficult or risky
- In order to avoid clamping the ureters, at the time of hysterectomy, the lowest clamp must be placed first, at the level of internal os and at right angles to the lower uterine segment

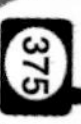

- The ovaries are usually removed at the time of abdominal hysterectomy in the women above the age of 40 years in order to prevent the occurrence of ovarian carcinoma at a later date.

3. VAGINAL HYSTERECTOMY

INTRODUCTION

Vaginal hysterectomy is based on the same principle as that of abdominal hysterectomy, it is just that the uterus is removed through the vaginal route rather than the abdominal route and the various steps as described previously with abdominal route are now performed vaginally.

INDICATIONS

When the hysterectomy is performed for utero-vaginal prolapse, the vaginal route is more commonly used. However, the absence of prolapse is not a contraindication for vaginal route. Only in cases where the vaginal route is not possible, should a surgeon consider LAVH or abdominal route.

SURGICAL MANAGEMENT

Preoperative Preparation

Preoperative preparation is same as that with abdominal hysterectomy described previously.

Steps of Surgery

The steps of surgery are described in **Figures 9.22 to 9.33**.

Postoperative Care

Postoperative care is same as that for abdominal hysterectomy described previously.

COMPLICATIONS

Postoperative complications are same as that with abdominal hysterectomy, described previously.

CLINICAL PEARLS

- The main advantages of the vaginal hysterectomy are that there is no visible scar, healing is faster in comparison to abdominal hysterectomy and there is an overall reduced rate of morbidity and mortality

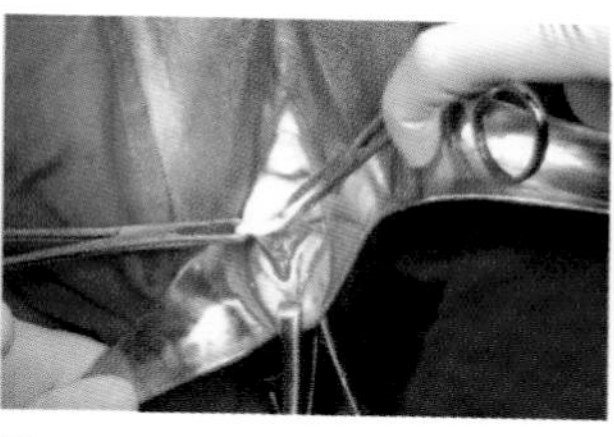

Figure 9.22: The anterior and posterior lips of the cervix are grasped with a single or double-toothed tenaculum and traction is applied in the downwards direction

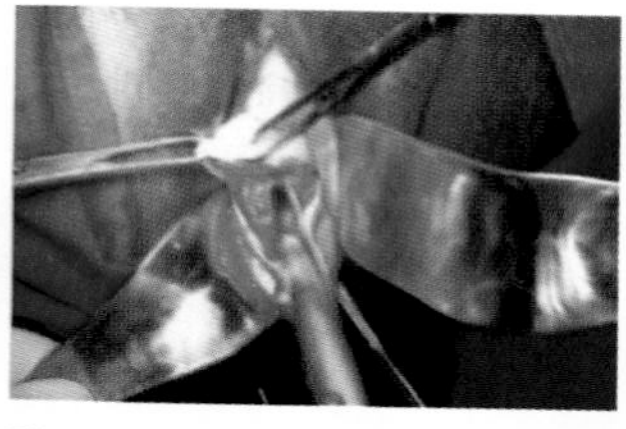

Figure 9.23: A circumferential incision is made in the vaginal epithelium at the junction of the cervix just below the bladder sulcus

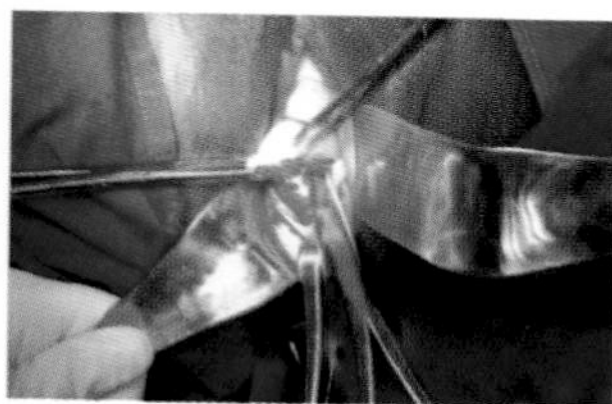

Figure 9.24: The vaginal epithelium may be dissected sharply from the underlying tissues or pushed bluntly with an open sponge

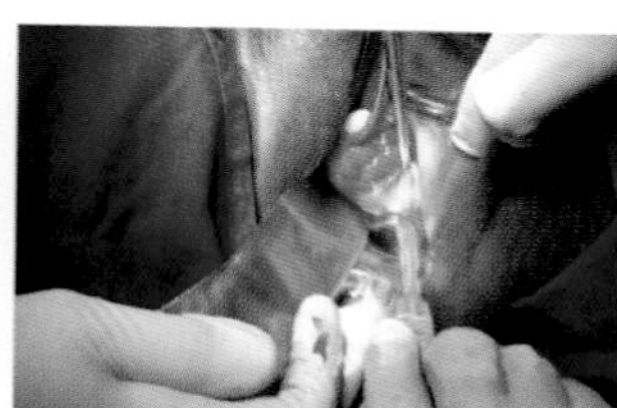

Figure 9.25: The circular vaginal incision is extended posteriorly and laterally

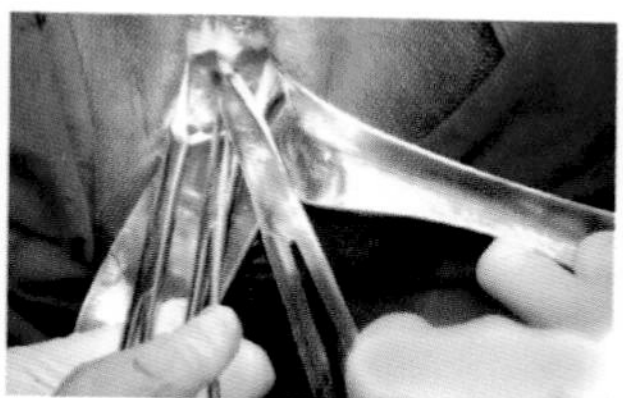

Figure 9.26: Identifying and incising the Pouch of Douglas

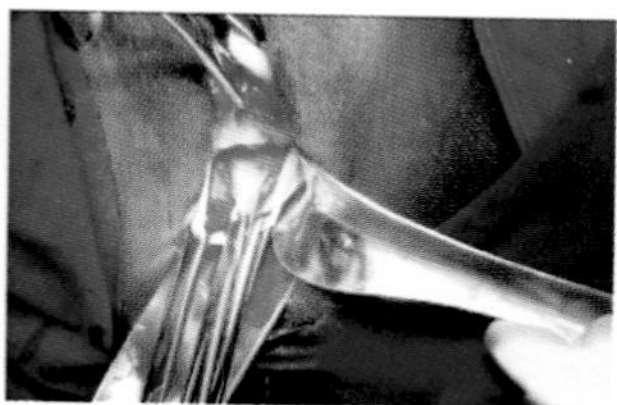

Figure 9.27: Separating the posterior vaginal wall from Pouch of Douglas

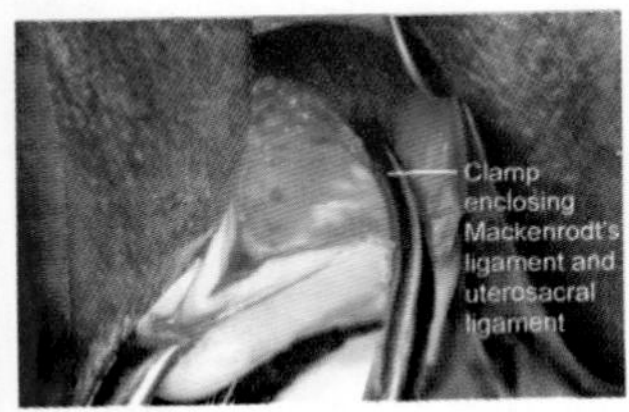

Figure 9.28: With the retraction of lateral vaginal wall and counter traction on the cervix, first the uterosacral ligaments and then the cardinal ligaments are identified, clamped, cut and suture ligated

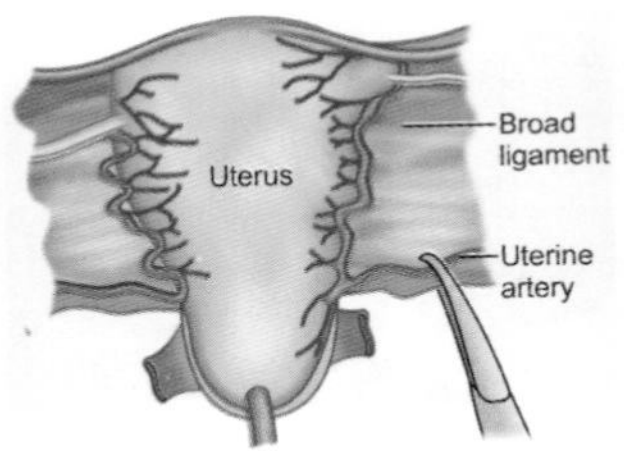

Figure 9.29: The uterine vessels are identified, clamped, cut and suture ligated

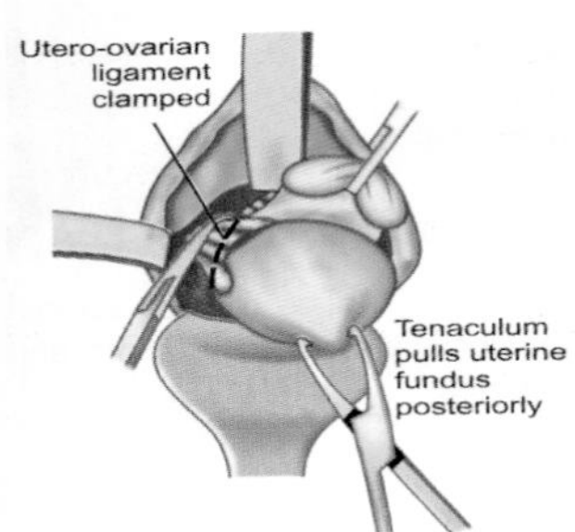

Figure 9.30: A tenaculum is placed onto the uterine fundus in a successive fashion in order to deliver the fundus posteriorly

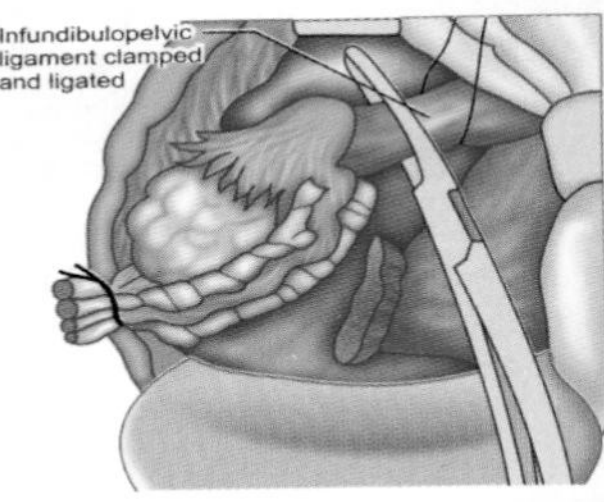

Figure 9.31: If the ovaries have to be removed, a Heaney's clamp is placed across the infundibulopelvic ligaments and the ovaries and tubes are excised

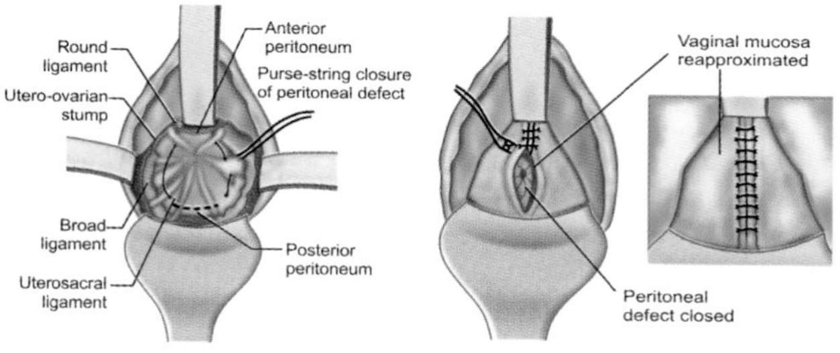

Figure 9.32: If the peritoneal closure is performed, the peritoneum is reapproximated in a purse-string fashion using continuous absorbable sutures

Figure 9.33: The vaginal mucosa can be reapproximated in a vertical or horizontal manner using either interrupted or continuous sutures

- The main disadvantages associated with vaginal hysterectomy are that there is less room for the surgeon to visualize and operate, the procedure can only be used for smaller sized uterus and there is a higher chance for causing injury to the adjoining organs
- Vaginal hysterectomy, however, cannot be performed in presence of certain complications, such as uterus greater than 12 weeks in size; invasive cancer of the cervix or inaccessible cervix; vesicovaginal fistula or rectovaginal fistula and uterine pathology such as endometriosis with severe adhesions or presence of large uterine myomas, adenomyosis, etc.

4. LAPAROSCOPIC ASSISTED VAGINAL HYSTERECTOMY

INTRODUCTION

Numerous approaches can be taken by the surgeons towards use of minimally invasive surgery at the time of hysterectomy. These include LAVH, LH and laparoscopic supracervical hysterectomy (LSH).

The procedure of LAVH is quite similar to the procedure of vaginal hysterectomy described above, but in this case laparoscopy is used for better dissection of the abdominal tissues.

SURGICAL MANAGEMENT

Preoperative Preparation

- *Anesthesia*: The procedure is performed under general anesthesia
- *Patient position*: Patients are placed in a dorsal lithotomy position with pneumoboots.

Rest of the steps for preoperative preparation is same as that described with abdominal hysterectomy previously.

Steps of Surgery

The steps of surgery are described in **Figures 9.34 to 9.39**.

The anterior and posterior leaves of the broad ligament are separated with the help of a Harmonic scalpel. The vesicouterine peritoneal fold is identified and the bladder is mobilized off the lower uterine segment. Rest of the procedure of hysterectomy is carried out vaginally.

Following the closure of vaginal cuff, the pelvis can then be irrigated and hemostasis at all sites assured. The port sites are then closed.

Postoperative Care

The postoperative care is same as that described for abdominal hysterectomy previously.

CLINICAL PEARLS

- The LAVH can be considered as an alternative to abdominal hysterectomy because it is associated with reduced rate of complications such as blood loss, bowel complications, shorter duration of hospital stay, speedier return to normal activities and fewer abdominal wall infections
- LAVH is associated with a higher rate of complications (such as injuries to the urinary tract) and increased operative time in comparison to the vaginal hysterectomy. However, these problems are likely to get alleviated as the surgeons gain more and more experience in the use of this procedure
- If the hysterectomy is possible by all the three routes in the best interests of the patient, the order of preference would be vaginal, LAVH followed by the abdominal route.

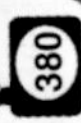

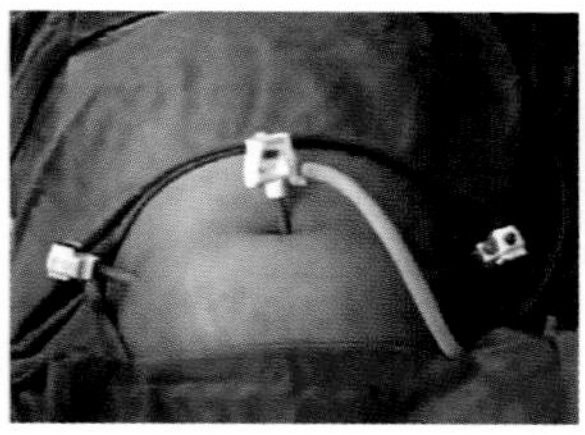

Figure 9.34: Insertion of laparoscope and others surgical tools

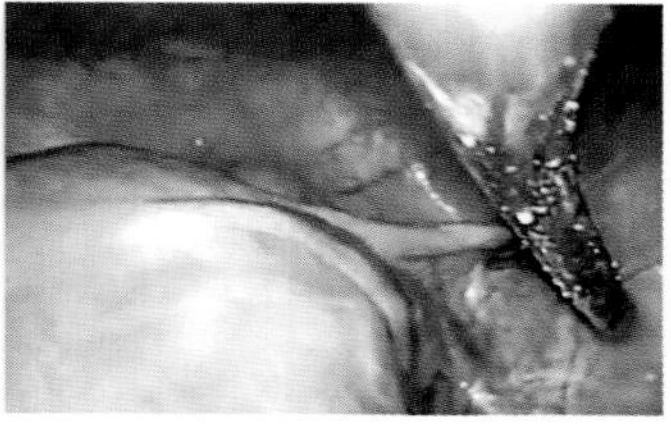

Figure 9.35: Laparoscopic clamping of round ligament

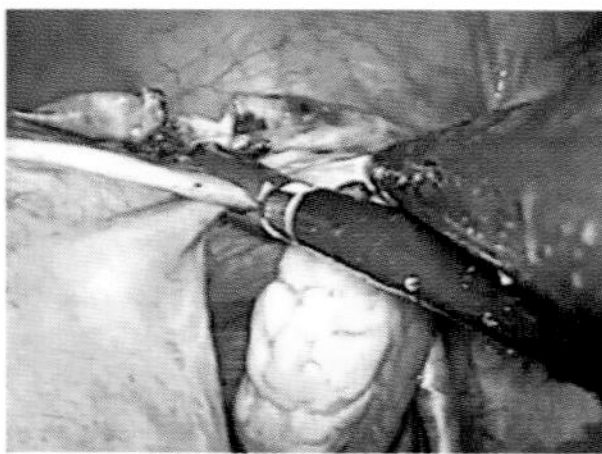

Figure 9.36: Laparoscopic clamping of fallopian tube and utero-ovarian ligament

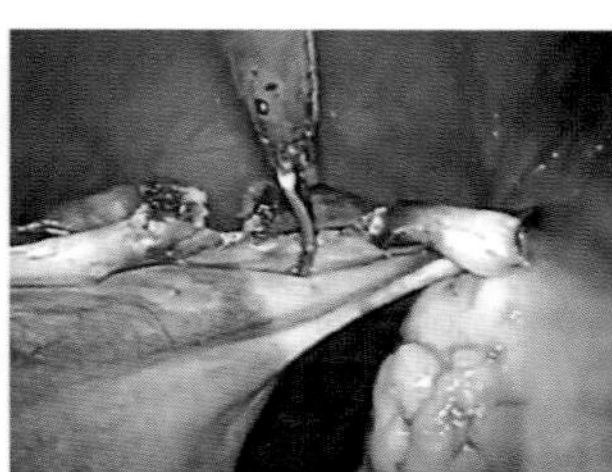

Figure 9.37: Laparoscopic cutting of fallopian tube and utero-ovarian ligaments

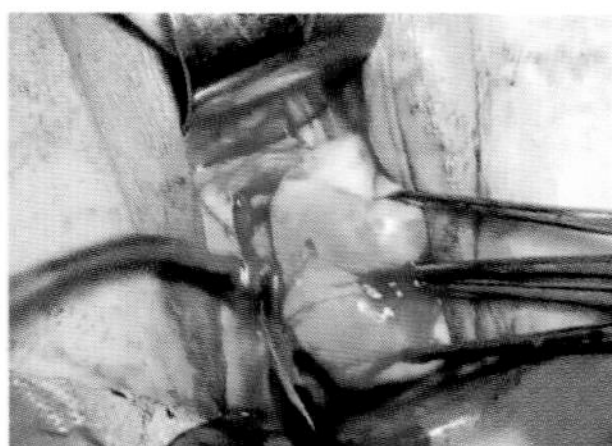

Figure 9.38: Vaginal delivery of the uterus

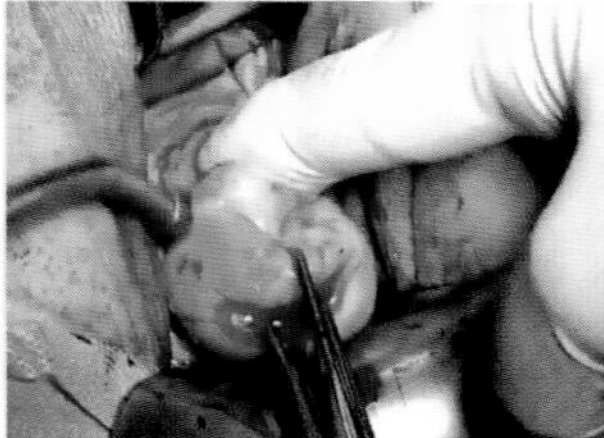

Figure 9.39: Separation of cervix from the vaginal apex

5. DIAGNOSTIC AND OPERATIVE LAPAROSCOPY

INTRODUCTION

Laparoscopy is a type of endoscopy, which helps in visualization of peritoneal cavity. Compared with laparotomy, laparoscopy is a form of minimal invasive surgery which is associated with a low complication rate, reduced pain, better cosmetic results, reduced rate of adhesion formation, shorter recovery time and reduced duration of hospital stay. Laparoscopic equipment is illustrated in **Figures 9.40 to 9.44**.

INDICATIONS

Diagnostic Laparoscopy

- Assessment of the pelvis in cases of acute or chronic pelvic pain, adnexal masses, ectopic pregnancy, endometriosis, adnexal torsion or other pelvic pathology
- Determination of tubal patency through transcervical dye instillation (chromopertubation)
- *Laparoscopic biopsy*: To aid in diagnosis of endometriosis or malignancy.

Therapeutic Laparoscopy

- Tubal sterilization
- Lysis of adhesions
- Treatment of endometriosis and ectopic pregnancy
- Ovarian cystectomy
- Oophorectomy
- Myomectomy
- Hysterectomy
- Oncologic procedures
- Ovarian drilling.

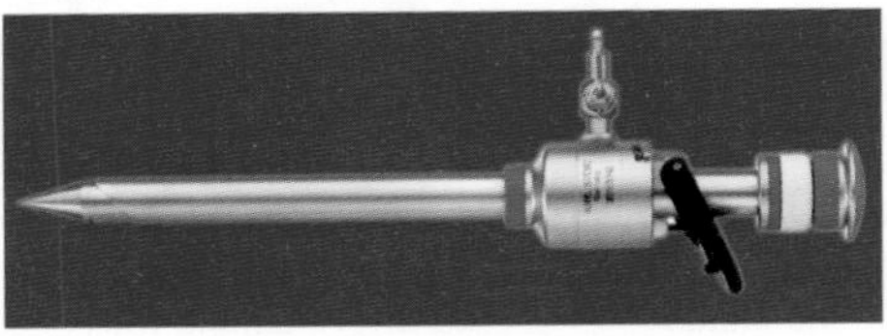

Figure 9.40: Primary trocar and cannula

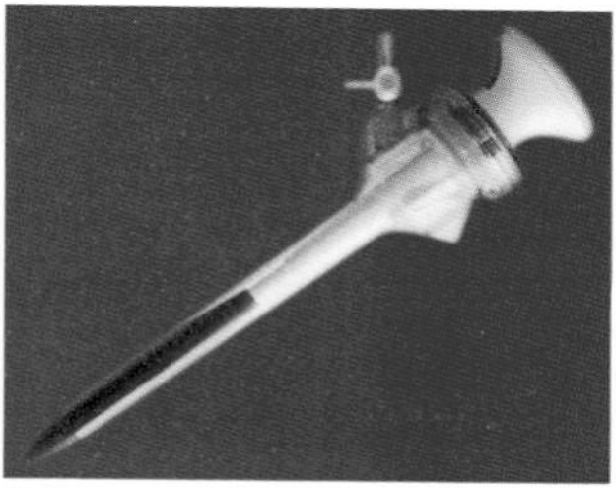

Figure 9.41: Disposable trocar

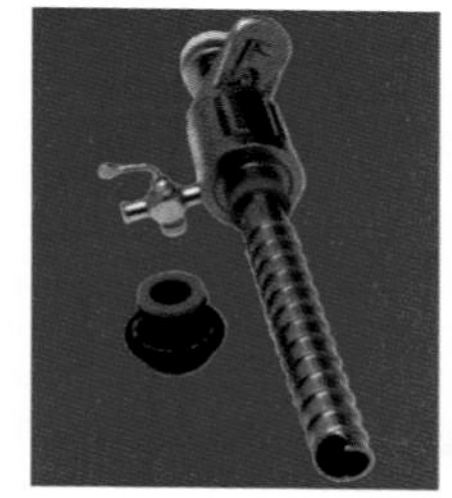

Figure 9.42: EndoTIP® reusable visual access cannula

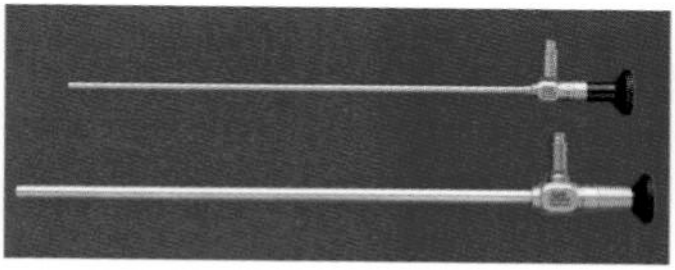

Figure 9.43: Laparoscopic telescope

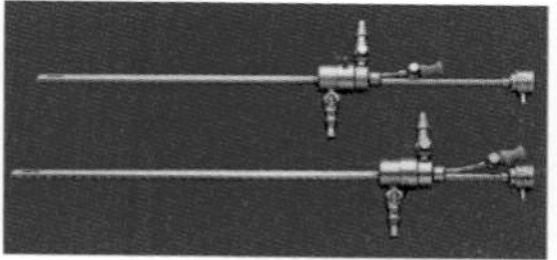

Figure 9.44: Operative telescope

SURGICAL MANAGEMENT

Preoperative Preparation

- *Laboratory studies*: These include complete blood cell count; pregnancy test (to rule out pregnancy) and urine analysis (to rule out any urinary infection)
- *Informed consent*: Informed consent must be taken from the patient after explaining the nature of the procedure, risks, complications and alternatives
- *Preoperative medications*: Use of GnRH agonists prior to surgery may help a few patients
- *Prophylactic antibiotics*: These help in reducing the risk of postoperative infections after gynecological surgery
- *Preoperative gastrointestinal preparation*: The patient must be instructed to remain NPO after midnight to avoid risk of aspiration
- *Other preoperative considerations*: In case the surgeon is suspecting a major blood loss during laparoscopy, establishment of intravenous access may be required prior to starting the case

- *Bladder catheterization*: Ideally, prior to the placement of Veress cannula or the primary trocar, the bladder must be catheterized to minimize the risk of bladder injury
- *Deep vein thrombosis prophylaxis*: DVT prophylaxis helps in preventing the risk of thromboembolism
- *Patient positioning*: Gynecologic laparoscopy procedures are usually performed with the patient in the low dorsal lithotomy position with the buttocks extended over end of the table. Once the primary trocar is placed, the patient is usually placed in no more than 25° Trendelenburg position to help keep the bowel out of the pelvis so as to obtain a clear view of the abdominal and pelvic organs **(Fig. 9.45)**
- *Skin preparation*: Clipping the pubic hair above the symphysis may be required. The site of surgery is prepared by cleaning and draping the abdominal skin by antiseptic solutions. Following this, specially designed fenestrated laparoscopy drapes are placed over the site of surgery
- *Anesthesia*: General anesthesia with endotracheal intubation is most commonly used for laparoscopy.

Steps of Surgery

- *Veress needle insertion*: Veress needle is commonly placed through a small subumbilical incision about 3–4 mm in size
- *Carbon dioxide insufflation*: After confirming the position of Veress needle, CO_2 insufflation can begin at the rate of 3 L/min
- *Insertion of primary trocar and cannula*: After adequate amount of intra-abdominal pressure has been created, trocar and cannula

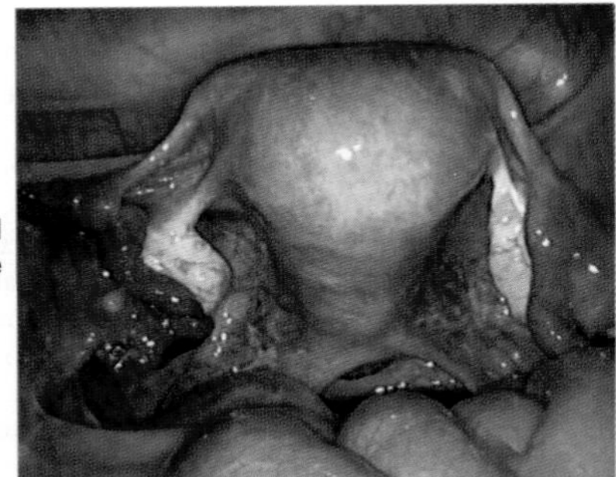

Figure 9.45: Normal laparoscopic view of the pelvis

(most commonly 5 mm or 10 mm in diameter) are placed at an angle similar to that of the Veress needle, aiming at the hollow of the sacrum

- *Placement of secondary trocars*: Secondary trocars are required for most operative gynecologic laparoscopy procedures and are placed lateral to the inferior epigastric vessels on both the sides
- *Introduction of the laparoscopic telescope*: The trocar is removed from its sleeve (cannula) and the laparoscopic telescope then inserted inside through the cannula
- *Performance of laparoscopic procedures*: Depending on the indication of laparoscopic surgery, diagnostic or operative procedures are performed next.

Postoperative Care

- The patient must be prescribed a light/liquid diet because the bowel function may take several days to normalize
- Mild-moderate painkillers (NSAIDS) may be prescribed for pain relief
- In most of the cases, the patient is able to return to full activity within 72 hours after most gynecologic laparoscopic procedures
- At the time of discharge, the patients should be instructed to contact their physician if she experiences extensive pain or bleeding at any point.

COMPLICATIONS

- Complications related to surgery such as infection and generalized bleeding, etc.
- *Gas embolism*: Embolization is usually caused by inadvertent placement of the Veress needle into a major vessel during attempts to insufflate the abdominal cavity with carbon dioxide
- *Retroperitoneal vessel injury*: This is one of most life-threatening complications in laparoscopy and may occur during insertion of Veress needle or primary trocar
- *Abdominal wall vessel injury*: Injury to the epigastric vessels (inferior and superficial) and the superficial circumflex iliac vessel may occur during the placement of secondary ports
- *Intestinal injury*: Both the small and large intestine can be injured during laparoscopy
- *Urologic injuries*: Injury to the bladder or ureters can occur during trocar placement or during the use of power instruments, stapling or suturing devices

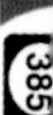

- *Incisional hernia*: With the use of larger ports (> 5 mm), the incidence of incisional hernias has increased
- *Nerve injuries*: Patient positioning during laparoscopic surgery is associated with a low risk of potentially serious nerve injury to either the lower or upper extremities (e.g. brachial plexus injury)
- *Anesthetic complications*: Complications related to anesthetic medications can also occur.

CLINICAL PEARLS

- In the past, many of the procedures, which would have been performed only through laparotomy, can now be performed using laparoscopic techniques
- Some of the innovations, which have been introduced in the field of laparoscopy, include: robotic surgery; natural orifice transluminal surgery (NOTES) and single incision laparoscopic surgery (SILS). Of these three developing technologies, robotic surgery presently has the largest impact on clinical care.

6. DIAGNOSTIC AND OPERATIVE HYSTEROSCOPY

INTRODUCTION

Hysteroscopy is a minimally invasive procedure, involving the direct inspection of the cervical canal and endometrial cavity through a rigid, flexible or contact hysteroscope **(Fig. 9.46)**. The procedure allows for the diagnosis intrauterine pathology (submucous fibroids, endometrial cancer, etc.) and serves as a method for surgical intervention (operative hysteroscopy). **Figures 9.47 to 9.50** show the hysteroscopic equipment.

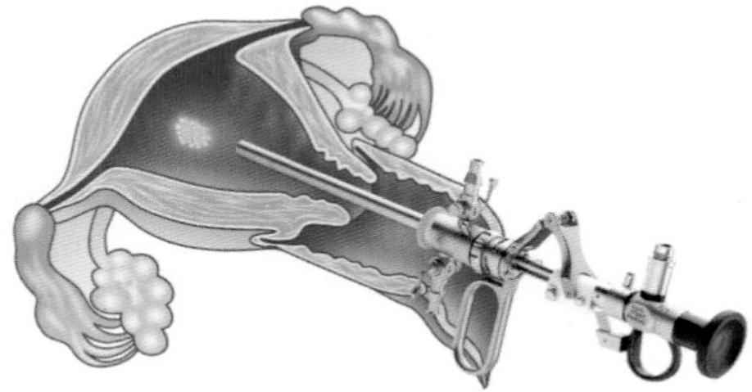

Figure 9.46: Diagrammatic view of a hysteroscope inside the uterine cavity

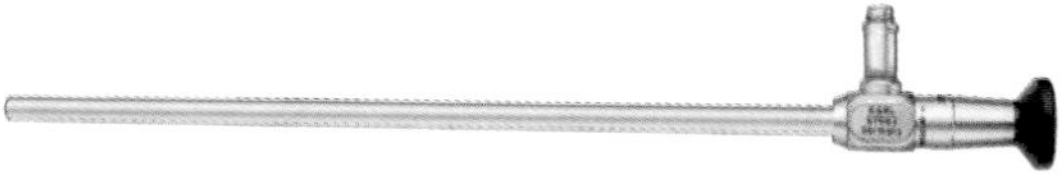

Figure 9.47: Telescope

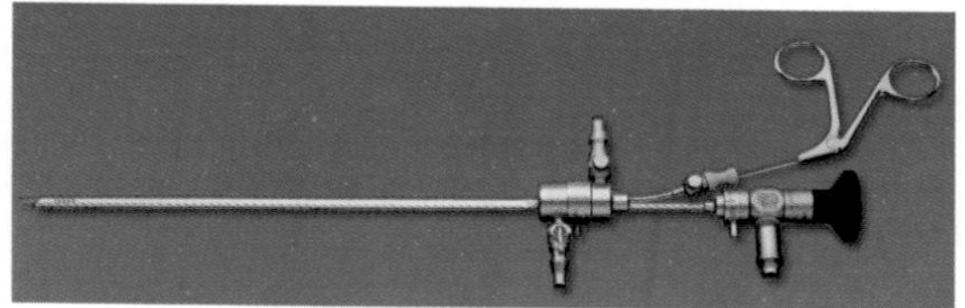

Figure 9.48: Operative hysteroscope with instruments through the operative channel

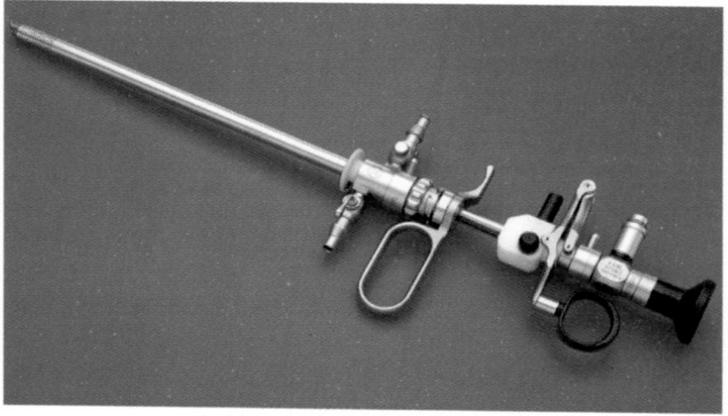

Figure 9.49: Resectoscope (Karl Storz)

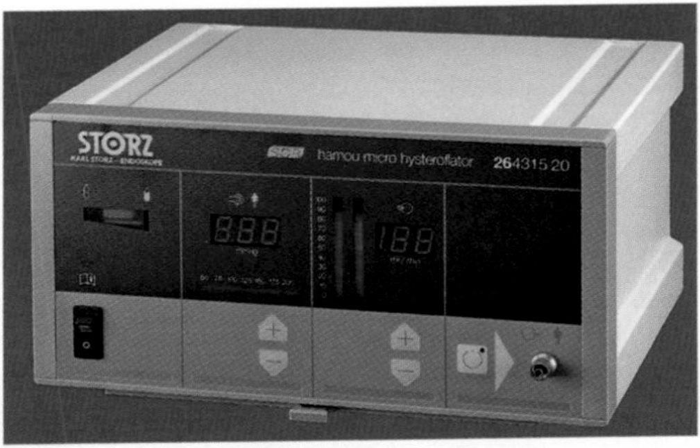

Figure 9.50: Hysteromat of hamou helps in providing a constant flow of low-viscosity fluid, which helps in maintaining sufficient pressure to keep the uterine walls distended

INDICATIONS

Diagnostic Indications

- Diagnosis of causes of infertility and/or abnormal bleeding
- Diagnosis of congenital uterine abnormalities
- Diagnosis of lost or misplaced intrauterine devices.

Operative Indications

- Treatment of abnormal uterine bleeding
- Polypectomy: Removal of endometrial polyps
- Adhesiolysis
- Myomectomy for submucosal fibroids
- Treatment of congenital uterine malformations or Müllerian abnormalities
- Removal of misplaced/embedded intrauterine contraceptive devices
- Sterilization
- Targeted endometrial biopsy
- Management of cornual and interstitial tubal blockage.

SURGICAL MANAGEMENT

Preoperative Preparation

- *Timing of the procedure*: Hysteroscopy is best done in the immediate postmenstrual phase
- *Anesthesia*: Paracervical block using 1% lidocaine is usually sufficient for diagnostic hysteroscopy procedures. Operative hysteroscopic interventions on the other hand, are usually performed under general endotracheal anesthesia
- Informed consent
- History and physical examination
- Pain prophylaxis
- *Patient position*: The patient is placed in a standard lithotomy position with legs apart in order to maximize the vaginal access. The perineum and vagina are gently swabbed with a suitable antiseptic solution.

Steps of Surgery

- The posterior vaginal wall is retracted using Sim's speculum. The anterior edge of cervix is grasped with the help of a single-toothed tenaculum
- Cervix must carefully be dilated with a Hegar's dilator until the operative sheath of hysteroscope negotiates through the cervix
- The telescope is inserted into the operative or resectoscope sheath
- The sheath is flushed with a distending medium and a light cable is attached
- With the distension medium flowing, the hysteroscope can be inserted inside the uterine cavity under direct vision or coupled to the TV camera
- The uterine cavity is thoroughly scanned
- After a clear view has been obtained, the operating device (electrode or scissors) is inserted inside the uterine cavity and slowly advanced in order to make contact with the endometrium
- In some cases, it may be advantageous to perform a laparoscopy simultaneously.

Postoperative Care

- Following the procedure, especially operative hysteroscopy, the patient must be observed for at least 6–12 hours for the signs of any potential complications such as tachycardia, hypotension, diminished urinary output, fever and abdominal distention, pain, nausea, vomiting, etc.

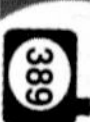

COMPLICATIONS

- *Traumatic injury*: This includes traumatic injury to the cervix and rarely uterus, injury to the bowel and bladder, etc.
- Uterine perforation
- Intraoperative and postoperative bleeding
- *Infection:* Infection rarely occurs if the procedure is performed using strict aseptic precautions
- *Electrical and laser injuries*: In cases of suspected thermal injury, laparoscopy or laparotomy must be done to determine the exact extent of injury
- *Complications caused by the distention media*: This can result in fatal complications due to gas embolism or fluid overload with electrolyte imbalances
- *Endometrial cancer*: Abnormal bleeding in the patients who have undergone hysteroscopic resection of the endometrium must be duly investigated to rule out the risk of endometrial cancer
- Hematometra
- *Uterine rupture*: Uterine rupture during pregnancy has been reported in cases where women have become pregnant following endoscopic procedures such as myoma or septum resection.

CLINICAL PEARLS

- Hysteroscopic myomectomy has currently become the standard minimally invasive surgical procedure for treating patients with submucous fibroids
- Contraindications for the performance of hysteroscopy include presence of recent or active PID; acute cervicovaginal infection; active uterine bleeding, which might obscure the operative field; and presence of intrauterine pregnancy.

CHAPTER 10

Disorders of the Uterus

1. PELVIC PROLAPSE

INTRODUCTION

Uterine prolapse can be described as a descent or herniation of the uterus into or beyond the vagina. Weakness of the anterior compartment results in cystocele and urethrocele **(Fig. 10.1)**, whereas that of the middle compartment in the descent of uterine vault or uterine prolapse **(Fig. 10.2)** and enterocele **(Fig. 10.3)**. The weakness of the posterior compartment results in rectocele **(Fig. 10.4)**. Baden-Walker Halfway system for evaluation of pelvic organ prolapse is described in **Table 10.1** and **Figures 10.5A to D**.

Table 10.1: Baden-Walker Halfway system for evaluation of pelvic organ prolapse

Stage	*Definition*
0	Normal position for each respective site
I	Descent of the cervix to any point in the vagina above the introitus
II	Descent of the cervix uptil the introitus
III	Descent of the cervix halfway past the hymen
IV	Total eversion or procidentia

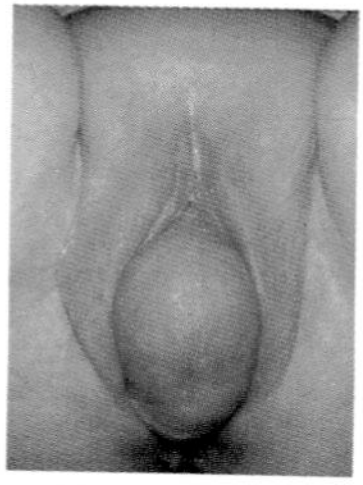

Figure 10.1: Urethrocele and cystocele

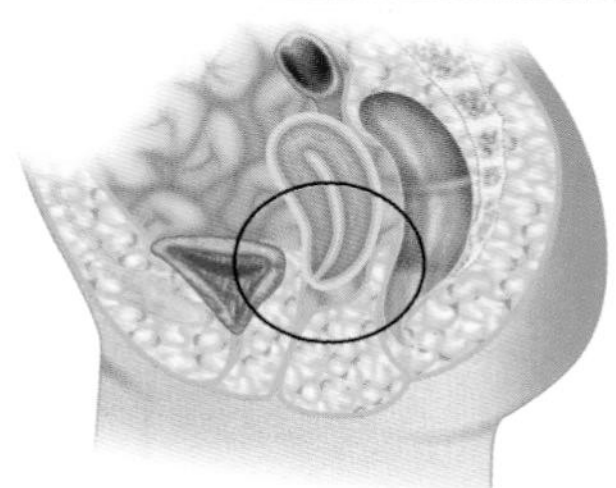

Figure 10.2: Descent of uterine vault

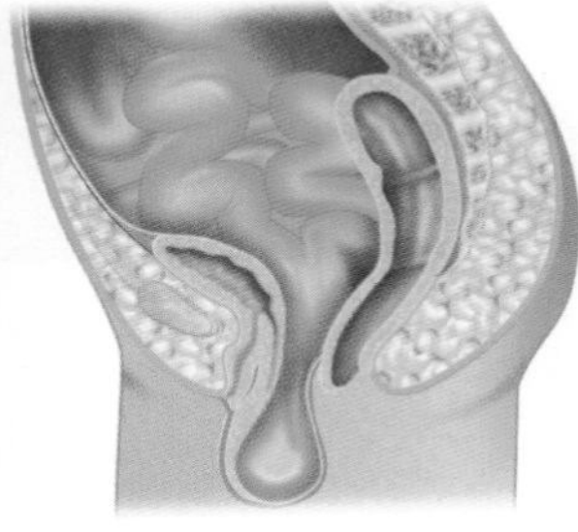

Figure 10.3: Enterocele

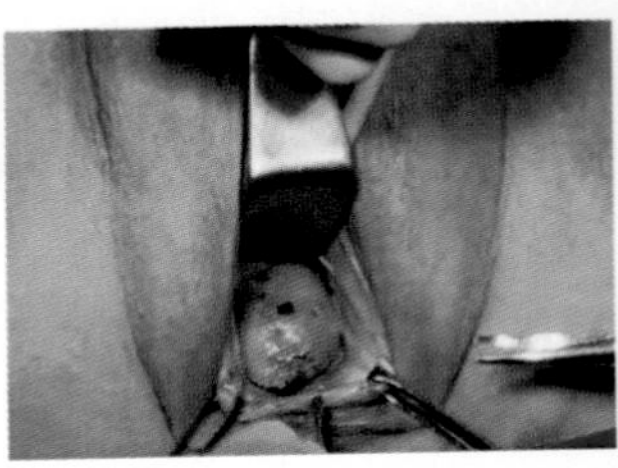

Figure 10.4: Rectocele

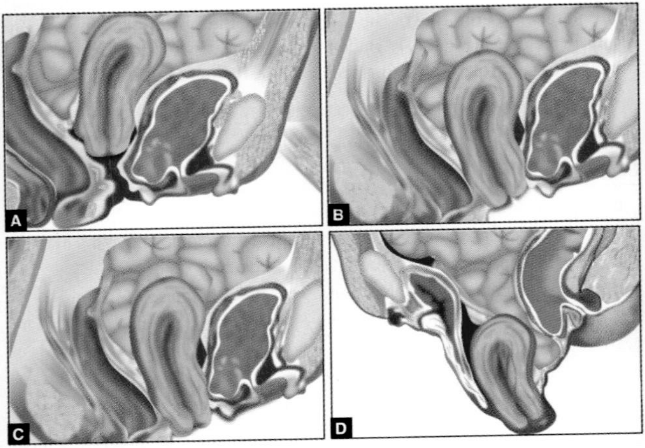

Figures 10.5A to D: Stages of uterine prolapse: (A) stage I uterine prolapse; (B) stage II uterine prolapse; (C) stage III uterine prolapse; (D) uterine procidentia

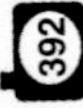

ETIOLOGY

Various causes of prolapse are as follows:

- Weakness and atonicity of the pelvic floor muscles and ligaments that support the female genital tract
- Injury to the pelvic floor muscles during repeated childbirths, causing their excessive stretching
- Reduced estrogen level following menopause is another important cause for atonicity and reduced elasticity of the muscles of pelvic floor
- It can occur in nulliparous women due to conditions such as spina occulta and split pelvis.

Indications of various surgeries performed for prolapse are listed in **Table 10.2**.

Table 10.2: Indications for various surgeries performed for uterine prolapse

Hysterectomy

- Removal of a nonfunctioning organ in postmenopausal women
- Concomitant uterine or cervical pathology (e.g. large fibroid uterus, endometrial carcinoma, etc.)
- Patient desires removal of the uterus

Anterior Colporrhaphy

- Presence of cystocele, urethrocele or a cystourethrocele
- Repair of anterior defects

Posterior Colpoperineorrhaphy

- Presence of a rectocele
- Repair of posterior defects

Manchester Operation

- Childbearing function is not required
- Malignancy of the endometrium has been ruled out
- Absence of UTI
- Presence of a small cystocele with only a first- or second-degree prolapse
- Absence of an enterocele
- Symptoms of prolapse are largely due to cervical elongation
- Patient requires preservation of menstrual function

Le Fort Colpocleisis

- No sexual activity at present or no plans for sexual activity in future
- Patient is medically fragile

DIAGNOSIS

Clinical Presentation

- Minor prolapse can be asymptomatic
- The main complaint in cases of uterovaginal prolapse is a feeling of something coming down the vagina, sensation of lump in the vagina, a feeling of pelvic insecurity and low backache. The symptoms are relieved by lying flat
- Blood stained vaginal discharge may be present in the cases of procidentia and decubitus ulcerations
- Urinary symptoms, such as difficulty in passing urine and recurrent UTIs, may be associated with cystocele and cystourethrocele
- Presence of rectocele may be associated with symptoms such as difficulty with defecation or incomplete defecation.

Investigations

The diagnosis of pelvic prolapse is established on the basis of history and clinical examination. Routine investigations which must be ordered prior to surgery include: CBC with hematocrit; urine routine and microscopy; kidney function tests; chest X-ray and ultrasound examination.

MANAGEMENT

The only definitive cure for prolapse is surgery. Various surgical options, which can be used in cases of prolapse, are enumerated in **Box 10.1**.

Box 10.1: Surgical options which can be used in cases of prolapse

- Vaginal hysterectomy, posterior culdoplasty, colporrhaphy
- Vaginal hysterectomy, closure of enterocele sac, total colpectomy, colporrhaphy, colpocleisis
- Combined vaginal colporrhaphy and abdominal hysterectomy
- Moschcowitz culdoplasty, sacral colpopexy and suprapubic urethrocolpopexy
- Manchester operation

Principles of Surgery

- The aim of surgery is to restore the pelvic anatomy and human physiologic functions such as micturition, defecation and sexual functioning

- In patient with advanced degree of prolpase, additional procedures like sacrospinous ligament fixation, sacral colpopexy, etc. may be required to provide adequate support to the vaginal vault
- The vagina should be suspended in its normal posterior direction over the levator plate and rectum, pointing into the hollow of the sacrum, towards S3 and S4
- Normal vaginal length should be maintained because a shortened vagina is likely to prolapse again
- The primary site of damage should be identified first and over-repaired in order to reduce the chances of recurrence
- The gynecologist must repair all relaxations, even if they are minor in order to prevent recurrence in future
- The cul-de-sac should be closed and rectocele repaired in all cases. A posterior colpoperineorrhaphy should be preferably performed in all cases, where possible
- Colpocleisis can be considered for patients, in whom preservation of the sexual functioning is not important.

Preoperative Preparation

- Medical treatment for chronic cough or constipation must be administered
- If decubitus ulceration is present over the prolapsed tissue, it first needs to be treated by the application of glycerine acriflavine pack or ring pessaries
- Surgery must be undertaken only when the associated infections (UTI, PID, etc.) have been aggressively treated
- Preoperative estrogen therapy must be given, especially to the elderly postmenopausal patients, in whom vaginal epithelium is thin and inflamed
- Full dose of antibiotics (80 mg of gentamycin, 1 gram of ampicillin and 500 mg of metronidazole) must be administered 2 hours before surgery to prevent postoperative pelvic infections.

Steps of Surgery

Anterior Repair

Surgical steps for anterior colporrhaphy are described in **Figures 10.6 to 10.11**.

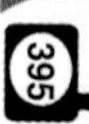

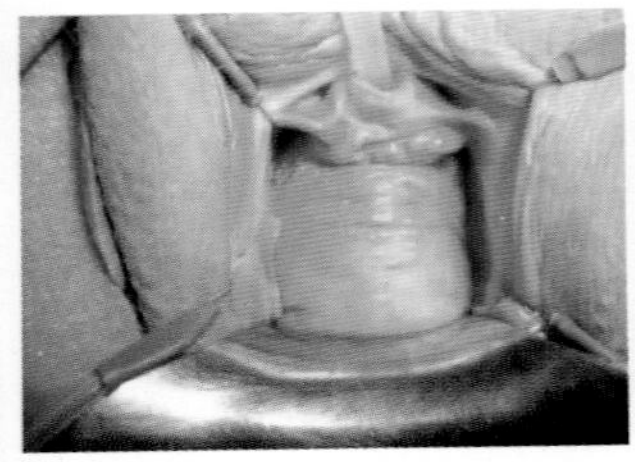

Figure 10.6: Appearance of cystocele just before giving the incision

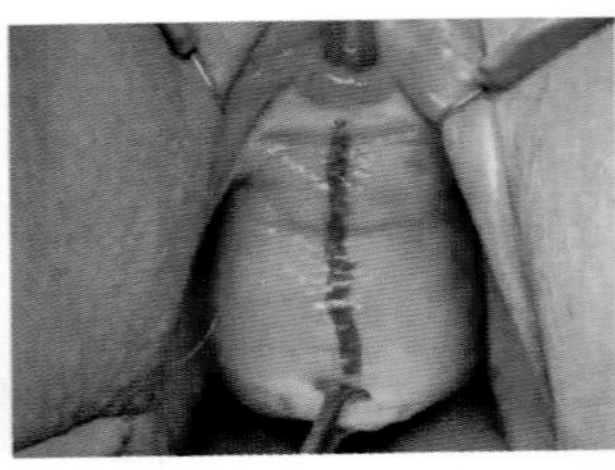

Figure 10.7: An inverted T-shaped skin incision is given over the skin overlying the cystocele

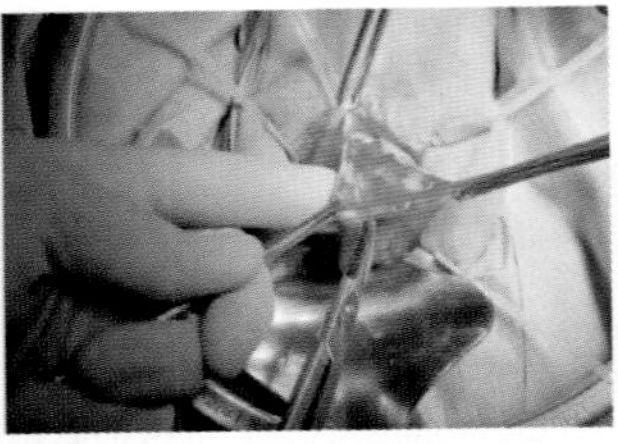

Figure 10.8: Dissection of the underlying fascia to separate the vaginal skin from the underlying fascia

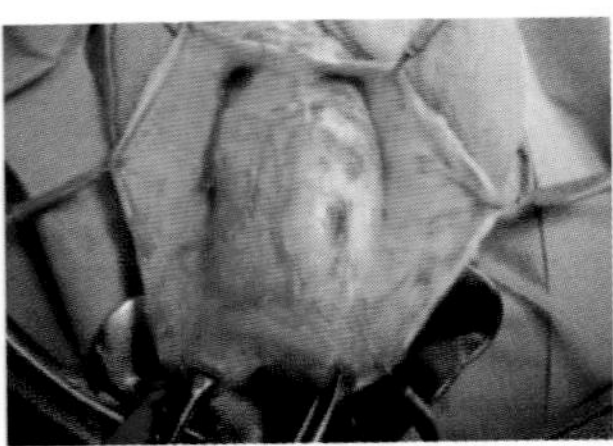

Figure 10.9: Dissection as described previously is continued until the midline defect in pubocervical fascia is visualized

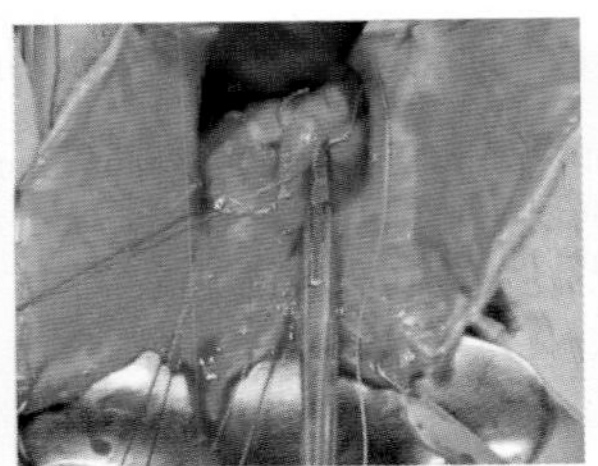

Figure 10.10: The tissue under the bladder is plicated and pulled together in the midline, thus reducing the bulge

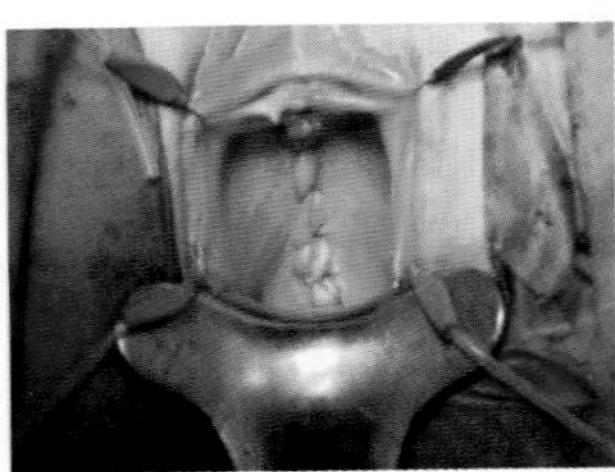

Figure 10.11: Excessive vaginal skin is cut following which the vaginal epithelium closed

Posterior Colporrhaphy and Colpoperineorrhaphy

This process involves nonspecific midline plication of the rectovaginal fascia, after reducing the rectocele, the steps of which are illustrated in **Figures 10.12 to 10.17**.

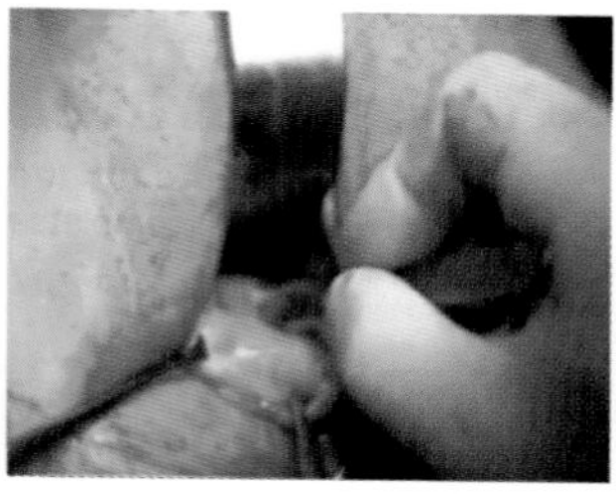

Figure 10.12: Rectocele identified and skin incised: the dotted line represents the skin incision, performed in this posterior repair procedure

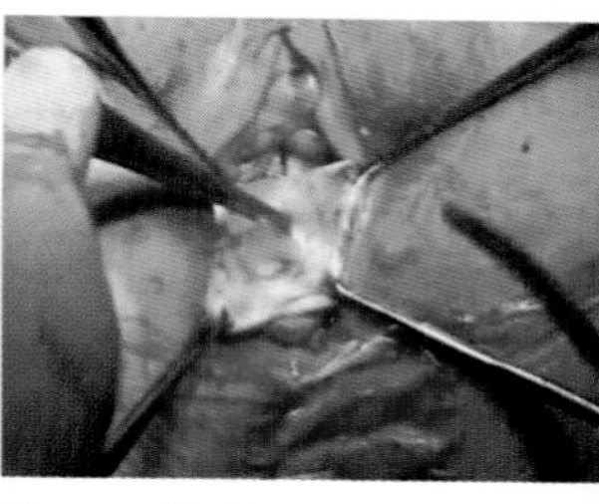

Figure 10.13: The defect in rectovaginal fascia is readily identified and the rectal wall is found protruding through this break

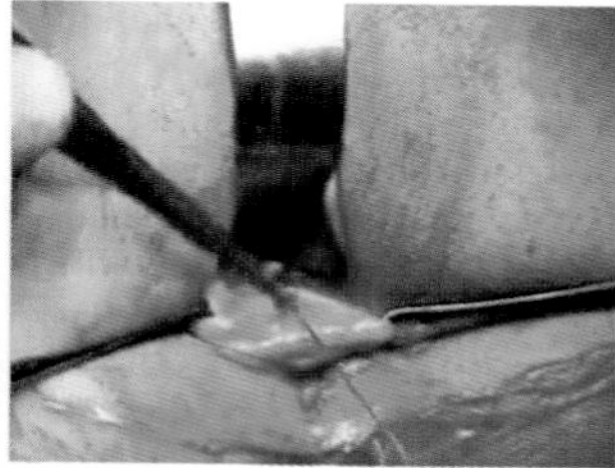

Figure 10.14: The rectovaginal fascia is reattached to the perineal body, where the distal defect was located

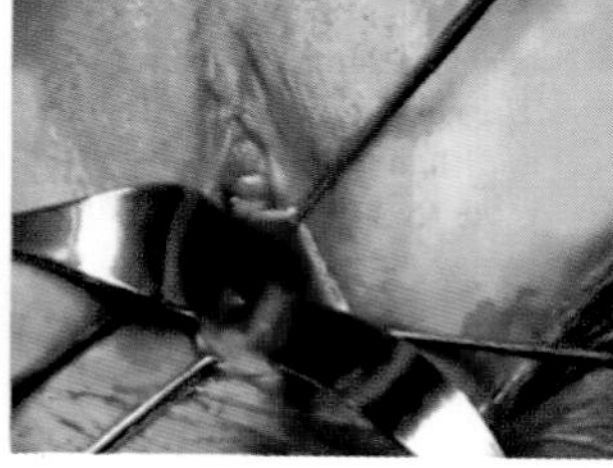

Figure 10.15: The rectovaginal fascial defect has been repaired

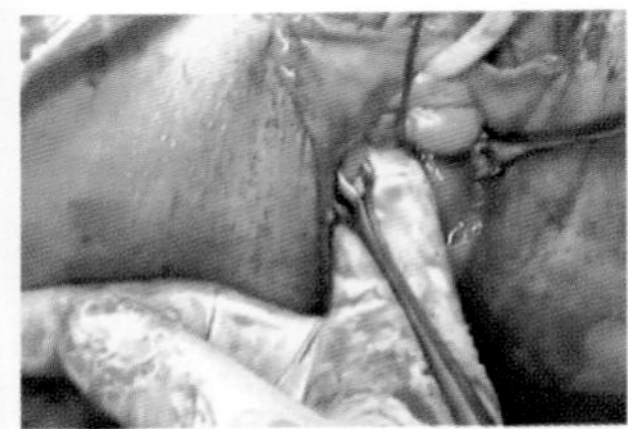

Figure 10.16: The rectovaginal fascia is reattached to the iliococcygeal muscles bilaterally with permanent sutures

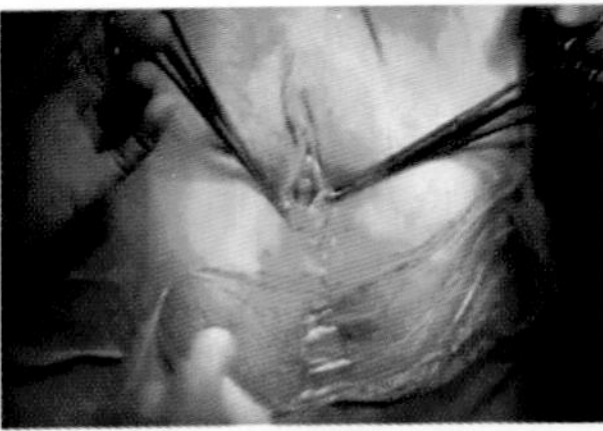

Figure 10.17: Closure of the vaginal epithelium (skin) completes the operation

Manchester Repair

Manchester repair is performed in those cases where removal of the uterus is not required. The procedure for Manchester repair (also called Fothergill operation) is described in **Figures 10.18 to 10.21**.

Postoperative Care

- Vaginal and pelvic discomfort in the 1st week following surgery can be largely avoided by sitting in sitz baths once or twice daily
- The patient should be asked to avoid sexual intercourse and lifting heavy weights for the first 6 weeks following surgery
- The patient must be instructed to come for a follow-up visit at 15 days and then again after 6 weeks to assess, if the surgical wound has properly healed and whether the patient can resume her normal day-to-day activities.

COMPLICATIONS

Uterine prolapse, if not corrected, can interfere with bowel, bladder and sexual functions and result in the development of the following complications:

- Ulceration, infection/sepsis (including that due to pessary use)
- Urinary incontinence, constipation
- Fistula formation, postrenal failure
- Decubitus ulceration.

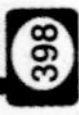

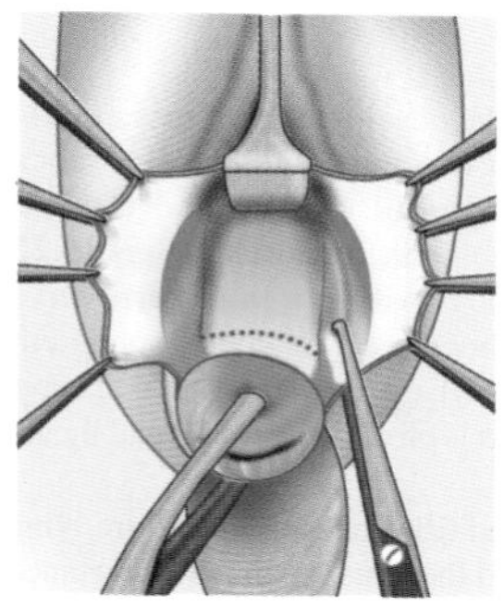

Figure 10.18: The bladder is dissected from the cervix. A circular incision is given over the cervix. The base of cardinal ligament is exposed, clamped and cut

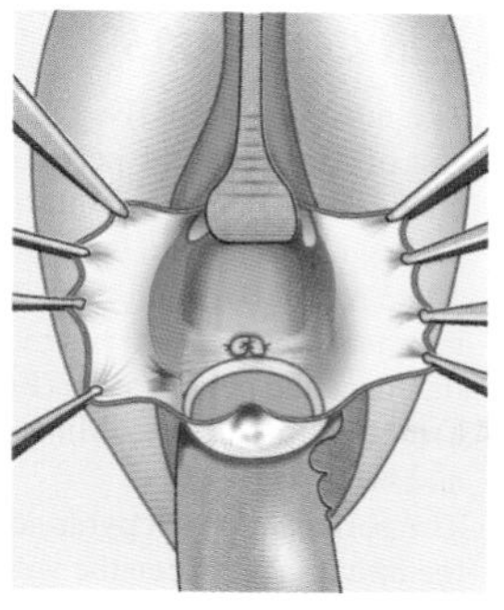

Figure 10.19: The cervix is amputed and posterior lip of cervix is covered with a flap of mucosa. The base of cardinal ligament is sutured over the anterior surface of cervix

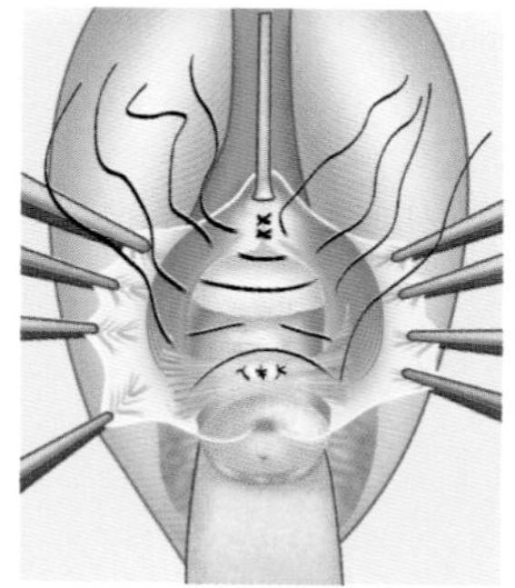

Figure 10.20: Approximation of pubovesicocervical fascia in the midline

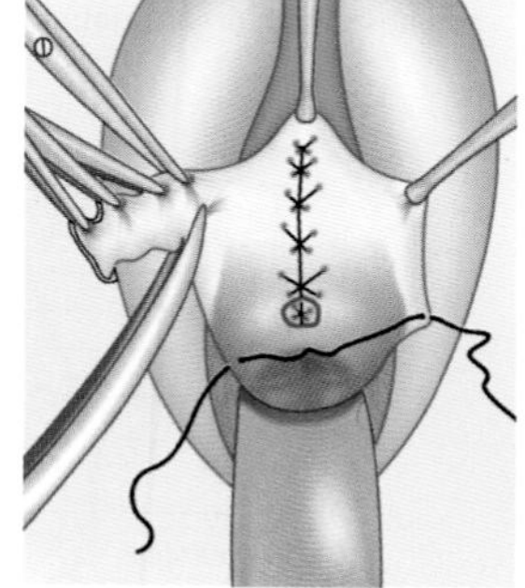

Figure 10.21: The fascial approximation has been completed and excessive vaginal mucosa has been excised

CLINICAL PEARLS

- The most important risk factor for the development of prolapse is the loss of strength of the pelvic support structures. Muscles [Levator ani, coccygeus, obturator internus, piriformis, superficial transverse perineal muscles and deep transverse perineal muscles **(Figs 10.22 to 10.23 A and B)**] and ligaments of the pelvic floor [transverse cervical ligaments, uterosacral ligament, pubocervical ligament, pubourethral ligament and pelvic fascia **(Fig. 10.24)**] are the main source of support to the pelvic structures. Minor support is provided by the broad ligament and round ligaments
- The perineal body, a pyramid-shaped fibromuscular structure lying at the midpoint between the vagina and the anus, assumes importance in providing support to the pelvic organs as it provides attachment to the following eight muscles of the pelvic floor: superficial and deep transverse perineal muscles; levator ani muscles of both the sides; bulbocavernosus anteriorly and the external anal sphincter posteriorly **(Fig. 10.25)**
- Expectant management, including the pelvic floor exercises (Kegel exercises) and vaginal pessaries are currently the mainstay of nonsurgical management amongst patients with mild degree uterine prolapse, with no or minimal symptoms.

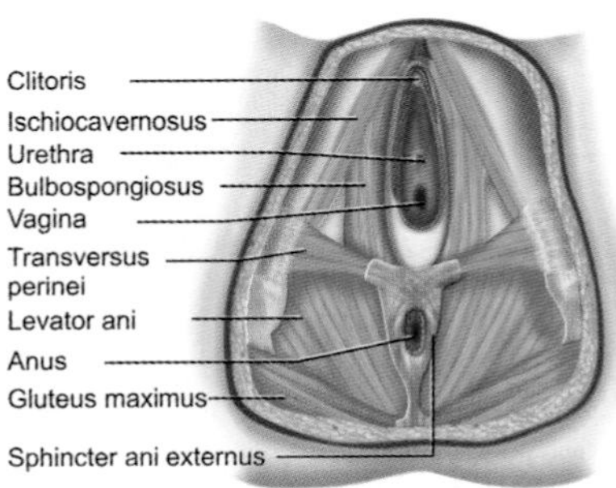

Figure 10.22: Muscles of the pelvic floor including muscles of the pelvic diaphragm (levator ani muscle); muscles of the urogenital diaphragm (deep transverse perineal muscle); superficial muscles of the pelvic floor (superficial transverse perineal muscle, external anal sphincter and bulbospongiosus)

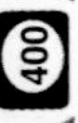

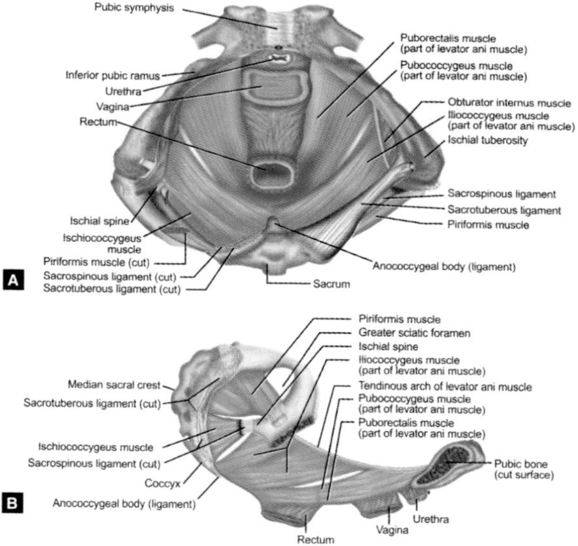

Pubic symphysis
Inferior pubic ramus
Urethra
Vagina
Rectum
Puborectalis muscle (part of levator ani muscle)
Pubococcygeus muscle (part of levator ani muscle)
Obturator internus muscle
Iliococcygeus muscle (part of levator ani muscle)
Ischial tuberosity
Sacrospinous ligament
Sacrotuberous ligament
Piriformis muscle
Ischial spine
Ischiococcygeus muscle
Piriformis muscle (cut)
Sacrospinous ligament (cut)
Sacrotuberous ligament (cut)
Anococcygeal body (ligament)
Sacrum
A
Piriformis muscle
Greater sciatic foramen
Ischial spine
Iliococcygeus muscle (part of levator ani muscle)
Tendinous arch of levator ani muscle
Pubococcygeus muscle (part of levator ani muscle)
Puborectalis muscle (part of levator ani muscle)
Median sacral crest
Sacrotuberous ligament (cut)
Ischiococcygeus muscle
Sacrospinous ligament (cut)
Coccyx
Anococcygeal body (ligament)
Pubic bone (cut surface)
Urethra
Vagina
Rectum
B

Figures 10.23A and B: Levator ani muscle: (A) inferior view and (B) lateral view

Anterior
Pubic symphysis
Retropubic space (opened)
Pubovesical ligament
Urinary bladder
Vesical fascia
Tendinous arch of levator ani
Cervix
Transverse cervical ligament
Rectouterine pouch
Uterosacral (rectouterine ligament)
Rectum
Rectal fascia
Presacral space (opened)
Sacrum
Posterior

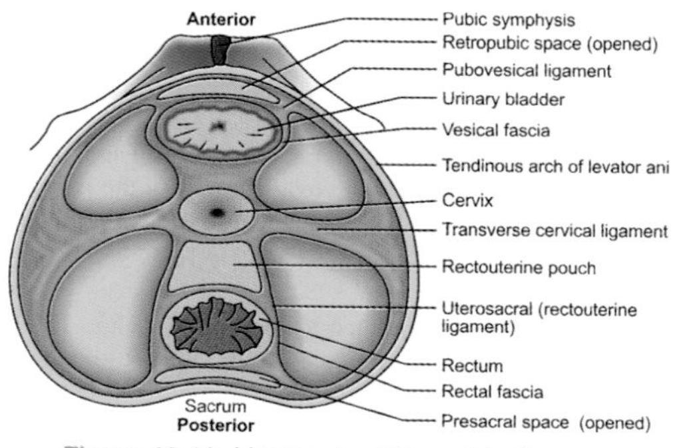

Figure 10.24: Ligaments of the pelvic floor

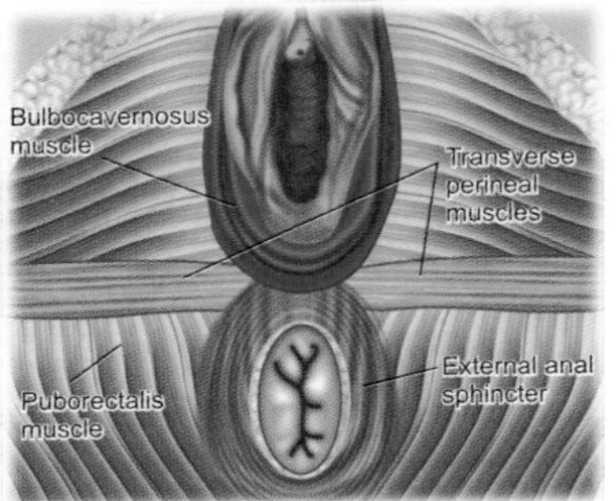

Figure 10.25: Attachments of perineal body

2. UTERINE RETROVERSION

INTRODUCTION

Normal uterine position is that of anteversion and anteflexion, i.e. the uterine body is bent forwards at the uterocervical junction over the bladder **(Fig. 10.26A)**. Retroversion is a type of uterine displacement in which the uterine body is displaced backwards at the uterocervical junction **(Fig. 10.26B)**. Retroversion could be either fixed or mobile.

ETIOLOGY

Mobile Retroversion

- *Congenital*: Some women may be simply born with a retroverted uterus, which is otherwise normal
- *Conditions, which push the uterus backwards*: These include uterine prolapse, anterior myomas and ovarian cysts of the pelvis
- *Physiological causes*: Such as menopause and early pregnancy.

Fixed Retroversion

Fixed retroversion could be related to conditions such as PID (salpingo-oophoritis), pelvic tumors, chocolate cysts of the ovary and pelvic endometriosis.

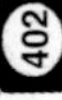

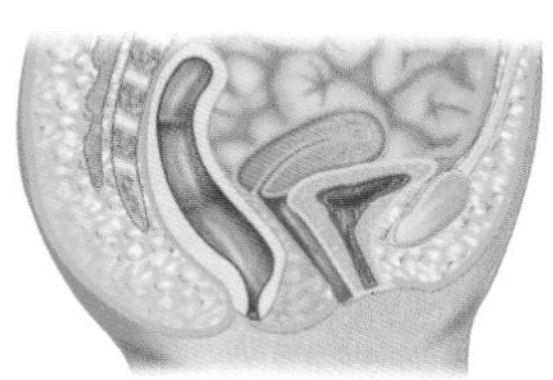

Figure 10.26A: Uterus in the position of anteversion and anteflexion

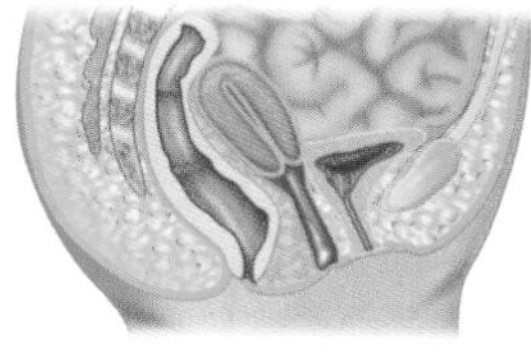

Figure 10.26B: Retroverted uterus: long axis of the uterus is directed backward

DIAGNOSIS

Clinical Presentation

The two main symptoms are dyspareunia and dysmenorrhea. Other symptoms may include:

- *Menorrhagia*: This could be related to myohyperplasia, DUB or pelvic congestion
- *Pressure symptoms*: This could be related to pressure over the rectum or bladder neck. There may be as associated backache
- *Infertility*: This could be due to the fact that the cervical canal may not be accessible to the mobile sperms. Moreover, fixed retroversion due to salpingo-oophoritis may cause tubal blockage.

Investigations

- Diagnosis is mainly established on the basis of findings of pelvic examination. On bimanual examination, a mass is felt in the pouch of Douglas. Since this mass moves with the cervix, it can be considered to be a part of the uterus. Uterus may be tender to touch
- *Hodge pessary test*: If application of Hodge pessary **(Fig. 10.27A)** helps in providing relief against the symptoms related to retroversion **(Fig. 10.27B)**, the clinician can assume that surgery undertaken to correct the uterine position would be useful.

DIFFERENTIAL DIAGNOSIS

- Pelvic prolapse
- Endometriosis
- Pelvic inflammatory diseases

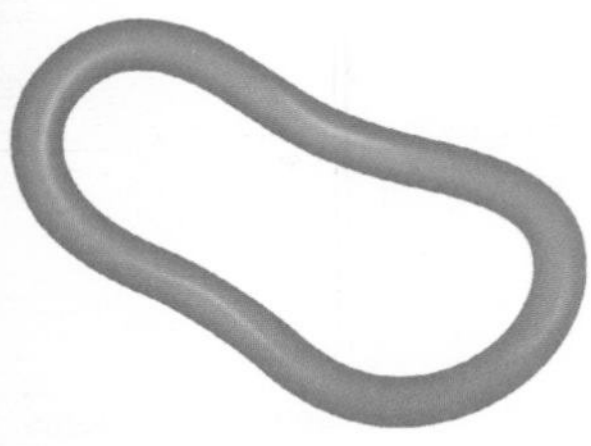

Figure 10.27A: Hodge pessary

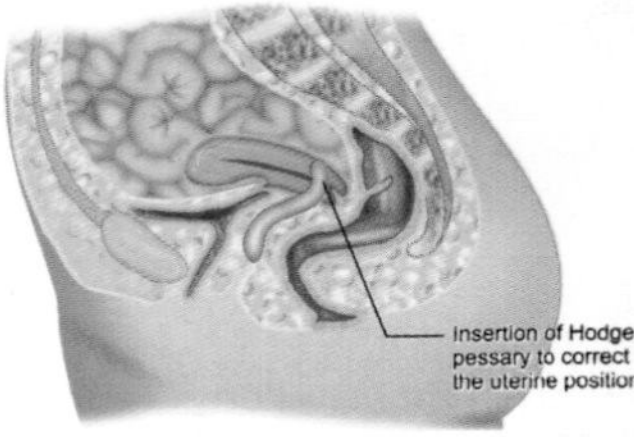

Figure 10.27B: Hodge pessary used for correction of uterine retroversion

The various conditions can be differentiated from one another with help of pelvic examination.

MANAGEMENT

In asymptomatic cases of mobile retroversion, no treatment is required. Insertion of a pessary may be required in symptomatic cases, where the uterus is bimanually replaced and a Hodge pessary is inserted inside to keep the uterus in an anteverted position. It is usually retained for 3 months in position and then removed.

Surgical Treatment

Surgical treatment may be required in the cases of fixed retroversion and comprises of the following options:

- *Modified Gillam's Ventrosuspension*: This is the most commonly used surgical option in which the round ligaments are anchored to the anterior rectus sheath
- Plication of the round ligaments
- *Balby-Webster's operation*: Round ligaments are anchored to the posterior surface of the uterus by passing them through the anterior and posterior leaves of the broad ligament.

COMPLICATIONS

- DUB or menorrhagia resulting in anemia or other related complications
- Infertility
- Dyspareunia, leading to difficulty at the time of sexual intercourse and resultant marital dysharmony
- Urinary incontinence
- UTI.

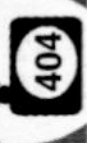

CLINICAL PEARLS

- In majority of women, there are no problems due to retroverted uterus
- If, during pregnancy, the uterus becomes impacted into the pelvis, the woman must be advised to lie on her abdomen for a day or two.

3. CHRONIC PELVIC PAIN

INTRODUCTION

ACOG has defined chronic pelvic pain (CPP) as cyclic or noncyclic pain, emanating from the pelvic area, which has been present for 6 months or more. CPP is not a disease, but a symptom, which rarely reflects a single pathologic process.

ETIOLOGY

Various causes of CPP are listed in **Box 10.2**.

Box 10.2: Causes of chronic pelvic pain

- Gynecological causes:
  - Endometriosis
  - Chocolate cyst of ovary
  - Ovarian adhesions
  - Polycystic ovarian disease
  - Chronic pelvic inflammatory disease
  - Pelvic and tubal adhesions
  - Pelvic tuberculosis
  - Uterine fibroids and adenomyosis
  - Benign or malignant ovarian tumors
- Gastrointestinal causes:
  - Irritable bowel syndrome
  - Chronic intermittent bowel obstruction
  - Diverticulitis, colitis, appendicitis
  - Carcinoma rectum
- Renal causes:
  - Reteric or bladder stones
  - UTI, interstitial cystitis, radiation cystitis
  - Bladder malignancy
- Musculoskeletal disease:
  - Abdominal wall myofasical pain
  - Degenerative joint disease including muscle strains and pain
  - Disc herniation, rupture or spondylosis

Contd...

Contd...

- Psychiatric/neurological cause:
  - Abdominal epilepsy, abdominal migraines
  - Depression, sleep disturbances, somatization
  - Nerve entrapment, neurologic dysfunction
- Miscellaneous causes:
  - Familial Mediterranean fever
  - Herpes zoster
  - Porphyria

DIAGNOSIS

Symptoms

- The pain often localizes to the pelvis, infraumbilical part of anterior abdominal wall, lumbosacral area of the back or buttocks and often leads to functional disability
- It is often associated with symptoms such as premenstrual pain, dysmenorrhea, dyspareunia, exercise related pain or cramping, with or without menstrual exacerbation of sufficient severity to cause functional disability
- The pain may be steady or it may come and go. It can feel like a dull ache, or it can be sharp and may be generalized or localized
- The pain may be mild, or it may be severe enough to negatively affect health related quality of life
- The most common symptoms related to endometriosis are dysmenorrhea, dyspareunia and low back pain which worsen during menses.

Abdominal Examination

The findings on abdominal examination vary with the cause and have been discussed in various fragments.

Pelvic Examination

The findings on pelvic examination vary with the cause and have been discussed in various fragments.

DIFFERENTIAL DIAGNOSIS

The most important causes for CPP in clinical practice include endometriosis, PID, symptomatic leiomyomas, interstitial cystitis and irritable bowel syndrome.

GYNECOLOGICAL MANAGEMENT

- In many women with CPP, treatment begins with identification of source of pain. Treatment should be directed at treating the underlying cause of pelvic pain
- The patient should be given a menstrual calendar to document correlation of pain with menstrual cycle, following which she should be advised to return after 2 months for a follow-up review
- In case of a nongynecological cause of pelvic pain, the patient should be instructed to follow a course of proper bowel hygiene for at least 2 months
- In case of suspected endometriosis as a cause of pelvic pain, diagnostic laparoscopy may be performed.

COMPLICATIONS

Complications related to PID and endometriosis, the two most important gynecological causes of pelvic pain, have been discussed in various fragments.

CLINICAL PEARLS

- Endometriosis and PID are the two most common causes of CPP in women belonging to the reproductive age groups and may be associated with infertility in nearly 30–40% cases
- Endometriosis would be described in details in the next fragment, whereas PID has been described in Chapter 11.

4. ENDOMETRIOSIS

INTRODUCTION

Endometriosis is characterized by occurrence of endometrial stroma and glands outside the uterus in the pelvic cavity, including all the reproductive organs as well as on the bladder, bowel, intestines, colon, appendix and rectum (**Fig. 10.28**). The ectopic endometrial tissues, both the glands and the stroma, are capable of responding to cyclical hormonal stimulation and have the tendency to invade the normal surrounding tissues.

ETIOLOGY

The pathogenesis of endometriosis is yet not clear. Some likely mechanisms for its pathogenesis are as follows:

- *Retrograde menstruation*: Retrograde menstrual flux can be considered as an essential element in the pathogenesis of endometriosis

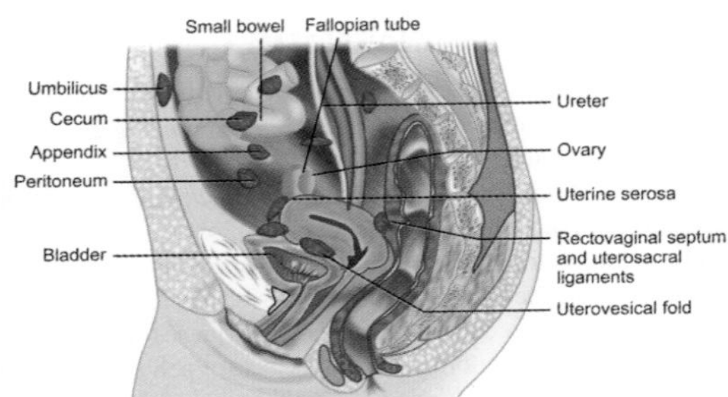

Figure 10.28: Common sites of endometriotic lesions

- *Theory of coelomic metaplasia*: Peritoneal epithelium can get "transformed" into endometrial tissue under the influence of some unknown stimulus
- *Metastatic theory of lymphatic and vascular spread*: Metastatic deposition of endometrial tissues at ectopic sites can occur via lymphatic and vascular routes
- Immunological defects and genetic factors.

DIAGNOSIS

Symptoms

The patients with endometriosis typically present with pain in relation to the menstrual cycles, often in association with menorrhagia and deep dyspareunia.

Abdominal Examination

The abdominal examination can help identify areas of tenderness and the presence of masses or other anatomical findings, which may help in reaching accurate diagnosis. Carnett's sign **(Fig. 10.29)** can be performed to distinguish whether the pain is due to an intra-abdominal pathology or pathology in the anterior abdominal wall.

Bimanual Pelvic Examination

- *Tenderness upon pelvic examination*: This is best detected at the time of menses when the endometrial implants are likely to be largest and most tender. A moistened cotton swab can be used to elicit point

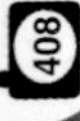

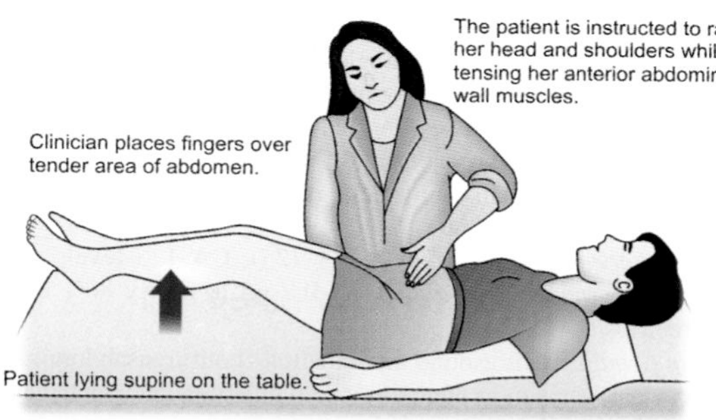

Figure 10.29: Carnett's sign for patients with pelvic pain: a positive test occurs when the pain increases during this maneuver and indicates myofascial cause of the pain. On the other hand, tenderness originating from inside the abdominal cavity usually decreases with this maneuver

tenderness in the vulva and vagina. The bimanual examination may reveal nodularity and thickening of uterosacral ligaments and cul-de-sac, which may be present in moderate to severe cases
- The uterus may be fixed in retroversion, owing to adhesions
- A bluish nodule may be seen in the vagina due to infiltration from the posterior vaginal wall
- Adnexal tenderness with or without enlargement may indicate ovarian endometriosis.

Rectal Examination

A rectal examination may show rectal or posterior uterine masses, presence of nodules in the uterosacral ligaments, cul-de-sac or rectovaginal septum and/or pelvic floor point tenderness.

 DIFFERENTIAL DIAGNOSIS

Other causes of CPP which need to be ruled out are listed in the previous fragment on CPP.

Investigations

Investigations, which may facilitate diagnosis, are:
- *Urine β hCG levels*: This helps in ruling out pregnancy related complications

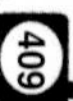

- *Complete blood count*: Elevated leukocyte count points towards infection, whereas reduced hemoglobin level suggests anemia, which could be the result of chronic or acute blood loss
- *Urine analysis/urine culture*: This helps in excluding out the presence of possible urolithiasis, cystitis and UTI
- *Cervical cultures*: This may help in detecting infection such as gonorrhea and Chlamydia
- *Serum cancer antigen 125 test (CA 125)*: CA 125 levels may be increased to values greater than 35 IU/ ml in nearly 80% cases of endometriosis
- *Imaging studies*: Ultrasound examination (both transabdominal and transvaginal) is the most commonly used investigation which may help in revealing the pelvic pathology responsible for producing pain. Imaging investigations such as CT and MRI may be helpful in some cases
- *Diagnostic laparoscopy*: Diagnostic laparoscopy remains the gold standard for diagnosis of pelvic pathology. Laparoscopy can help in identifying the following lesions: endometriotic nodules or lesions having blue-black or a powder burned appearance **(Figs 10.30 and 10.31)**. However, the lesions can be red, white or nonpigmented. Laparoscopy can also detect presence of blood or endometriotic deposits in cul-de-sac and its obliteration. Therapeutic treatment such as adhesiolysis **(Figs 10.32A and B)** and cauterization of endometriotic lesions can be applied in the same sitting.

MANAGEMENT

Management of patients with endometriosis may be expectant or medical or surgical and is usually based on the presenting complaints **(Fig. 10.33)**

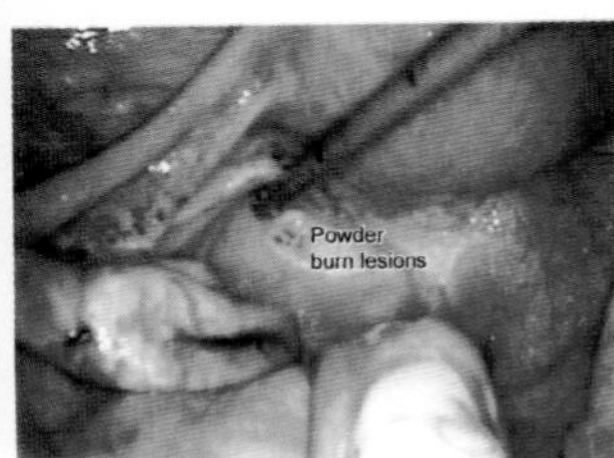

Figure 10.30: Powder burn lesions of endometriosis

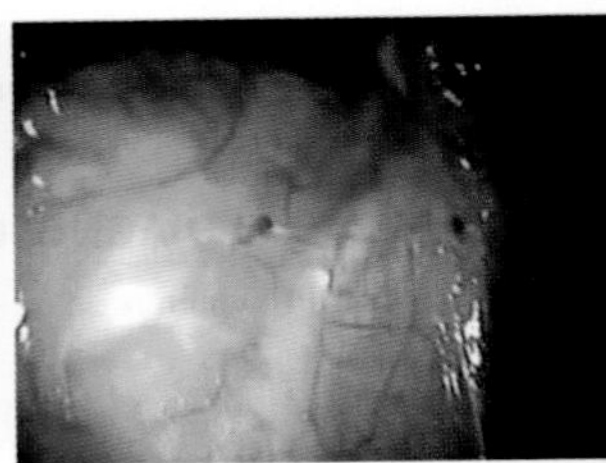

Figure 10.31: Endometriotic nodules

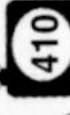

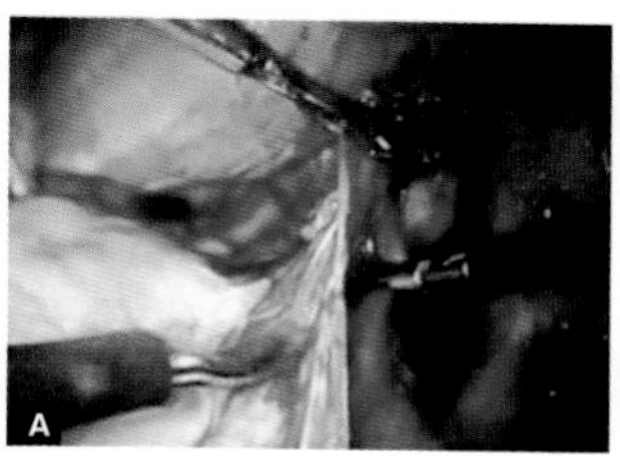

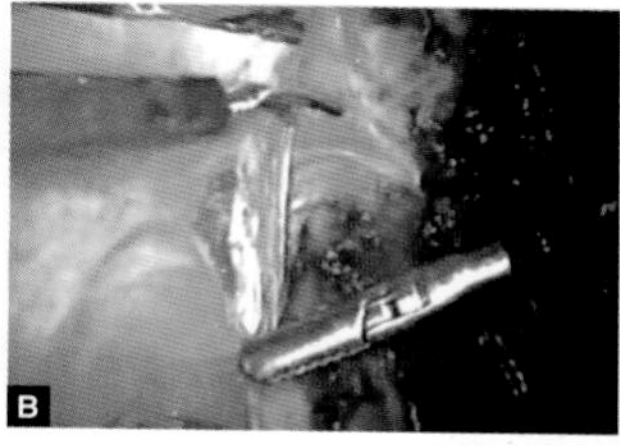

Figures 10.32A and B: Laparoscopic adhesiolysis of the endometriotic lesions

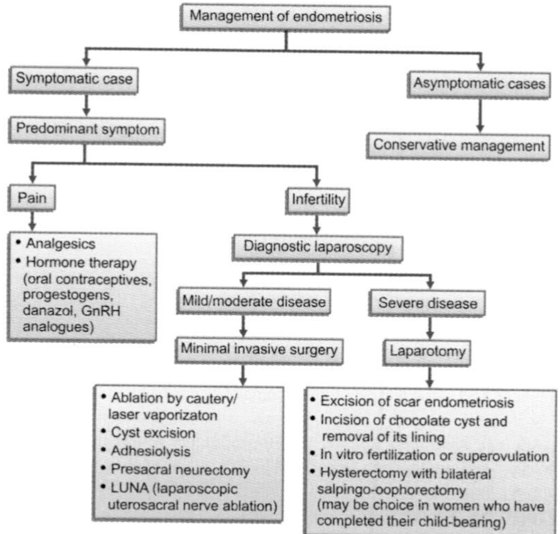

Figure 10.33: Management of endometriosis

and the disease staging **(Table 10.3)**. One of the main criteria which help the gynecologist decide whether to consider medical or surgical management is whether the patient's main complaint is infertility or pelvic pain.

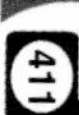

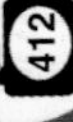

Table 10.5: Revised American Fertility Society classification of endometriosis

	Peritoneum		
Endometriosis lesion	< 1 cm	1–3 cm	> 3 cm
Superficial	1	2	4
Deep	2	4	6
Endometriosis lesion		*Ovary*	
Right superficial	1	2	4
Right deep	4	16	20
Left superficial	1	2	4
Left deep	4	16	20
	Posterior Cul-De-Sac obliteration		
	Partial	*Complete*	
	4	40	
		Ovary	
Adhesions	< 1/3 enclosure	1/3–2/3 enclosure	> 2/3 enclosure
Right filmy	1	2	4
Right dense	4	8	16
Left filmy	1	2	4
Left dense	4	8	16
Adhesions		*Tube*	
Right filmy	1	2	4
Right dense	4*	8*	16
Left filmy	1	2	4
Left dense	4*	8*	16

*If the fimbriated end of the fallopian tube is completely enclosed, the point assignment is changed to 16.

Source: Revised American Society for Reproductive Medicine classification of endometriosis: 1996. Fertil Steril. 1997;67:817-21.

CLINICAL PEARLS

- Endometriosis is an estrogen dependent disease, characterized by the regression of lesions following treatment with drugs that block estradiol synthesis
- The ovary is the most common site for endometriosis. Lesions can vary in size from tiny spots to large endometriomas/chocolate cysts
- Hormone therapy and GnRH agonists help in providing pain relief but they delay fertility

- Both laparoscopy and laparotomy are associated with similar pregnancy rates. However laparoscopy is associated with reduced postoperative morbidity.

5. ADENOMYOSIS

INTRODUCTION

Adenomyosis is a condition in which there is a growth of endometrial cells inside the uterine myometrium (usually > 2.5 mm beneath the basal endometrium) **(Fig. 10.34)**. It is associated with myometrial hypertrophy and may be either diffuse or localized (adenomyoma).

ETIOLOGY

The cause of adenomyosis is unknown. Some likely causes are as follows:

- *Uterine trauma*: Various causes of uterine trauma that may break the barrier between the endometrium and myometrium include cesarean section, tubal ligation, pregnancy and pregnancy termination
- *Estrogen dominance*: Conditions associated with the production of excessive estrogens
- *Abnormal level of various substances*: Increased levels of IL-18 receptor mRNA and the ratio of IL-18 binding protein to IL-18; and dysregulation of leukemia inhibitory factor.

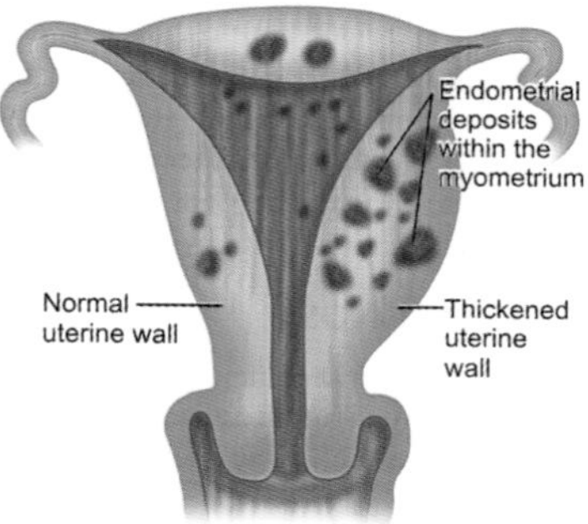

Figure 10.34: Adenomyosis

DIAGNOSIS

Symptoms

Commonly occurring symptoms include menorrhagia (unresponsive to hormonal therapy or uterine curettage) and progressively increasing dysmenorrhea. Other symptoms may include pelvic pain, backache, dyspareunia and subfertility.

Pelvic Examination

Uterus is enlarged to about 12–14 weeks in size and may be tender to touch, soft and boggy. Adenomyosis is associated with uterine fibroids in about 6–20% cases.

Investigations

- *Ultrasound examination*: Upon ultrasound examination, adenomyosis may present with heterogeneous myometrial echotexture, ill-defined, anechoic areas of thickened myometrium, consisting of blood-filled, irregular cystic spaces, or as an area of hyperechoic myometrium with several cysts (hypoechoic lacunae) **(Fig. 10.35)**. Other features include asymmetrical uterine enlargement, indistinct endometrial-myometrial border and subendometrial halo thickening
- *MRI*: This is superior to ultrasound for diagnosis of adenomyosis. The presence of heterotopic endometrial glands and stroma in the myometrium appear as bright foci within the myometrium on T2-weighted MR images **(Fig. 10.36)**. Adjacent smooth muscle hyperplasia may present as areas of reduced signal intensity on MR imaging
- *CA 125*: Level of CA 125 in the peripheral blood may be raised
- *Histopathologic examination*: The final diagnosis is established by histopathological examination of the hysterectomy specimen.

DIFFERENTIAL DIAGNOSIS

Leiomyomas: Adenomyosis is most commonly confused with leiomyomas. Transvaginal ultrasonography is an effective, noninvasive and relatively inexpensive procedure for establishing the diagnosis of adenomyoma preoperatively.

MANAGEMENT

Diagnostic hysteroscopy in combination with curettage helps in management of menorrhagia. Total hysterectomy with or without bilateral

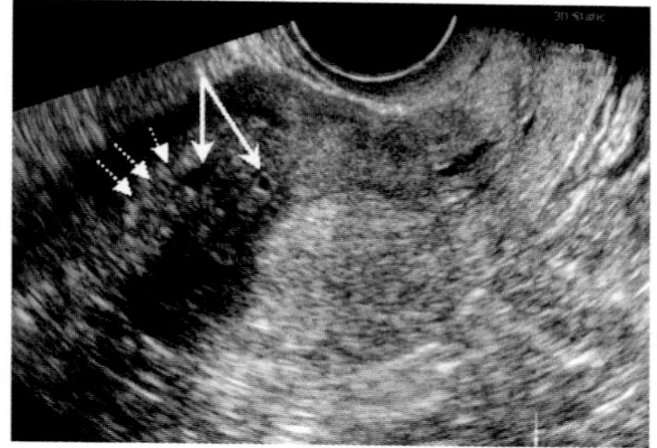

Figure 10.35: Ultrasound showing mottled texture of the myometrium and presence of hypoechoic areas within the hyperechoic area in the fundal region which is suggestive of adenomyosis

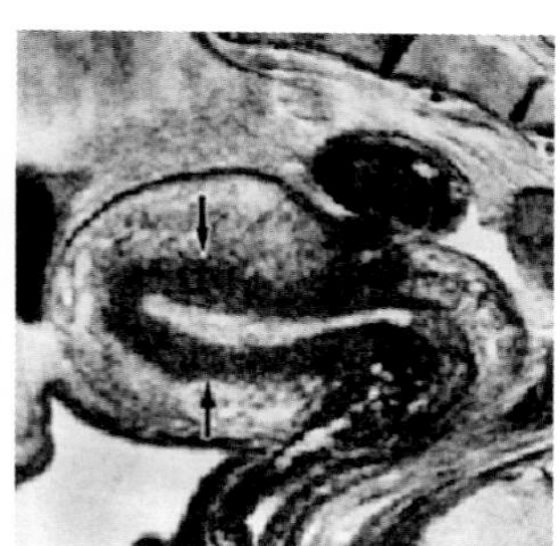

Figure 10.36: Sagittal T2-weighted MR image showing diffuse, even thickening of the junctional zone (as depicted by arrows) which is consistent with the diagnosis of diffuse adenomyosis

salpingo-oophorectomy is the treatment of choice in elderly patients who are past their childbearing age. Conservative resection may be performed in the younger patients. Medical treatment comprises of NSAIDS, hormone therapy, danazol, GnRH agonists and Mirena IUCD. Recently, uterine artery embolization is emerging as an effective and safe method in the treatment of adenomyosis. However the recurrence rate has yet not been evaluated.

COMPLICATIONS

- Adenemosis can be associated with considerable morbidity due to the presence of debilitating symptoms such as menorrhagia, dysmenorrhea, CPP, etc.
- Reduced fertility
- Coexistence of pelvic abnormalities such as uterine fibroids, endometrial hyperplasia and endometrial adenocarcinoma

CLINICAL PEARLS

- Multiparas between the ages of 30 years and 50 years are most commonly affected with this disease
- The diagnosis of adenomyosis can only be confirmed by pathologist
- MRI had a higher specificity than TVS, but similar sensitivity regarding the diagnosis of adenomyosis.

6. UTERINE MALFORMATIONS

INTRODUCTION

Congenital uterine anomalies may arise from malformations at any step of the Müllerian developmental process. The classification of Müllerian abnormalities as proposed by the American Society for Reproductive Medicine is described in **Figure 10.37** and **Table 10.4**. Amongst the various anomalies, septate uterus is the most common structural defect. Three main Müllerian abnormalities, which would be discussed in this fragment, include vaginal agenesis, bicornuate uterus and septate uterus.

Table 10.4: American Society for Reproductive Medicine classification of congenital uterine anomalies

Classification	*Clinical finding*	*Description*
I	Segmental or complete Müllerian agenesis or hypoplasia	• Vaginal • Cervical • Fundal • Tubal • Combined
II	Unicornuate uterus with or without a rudimentary horn	• With a communicating rudimentary horn • With a noncommunicating rudimentary horn

Contd...

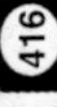

Contd...

Classification	*Clinical finding*	*Description*
III	Didelphys uterus partial duplication of the	Characterized by complete or vagina, cervix and uterus
IV	Complete or partial bicornuate uterus	• Complete • Partial
V	Complete or partial septate uterus	• Complete • Partial
VI	Arcuate uterus	A small septate indentation is present at the fundus
VII	Diethylstilbestrol-related abnormalities	Presence of a T-shaped uterine cavity with or without dilated horns

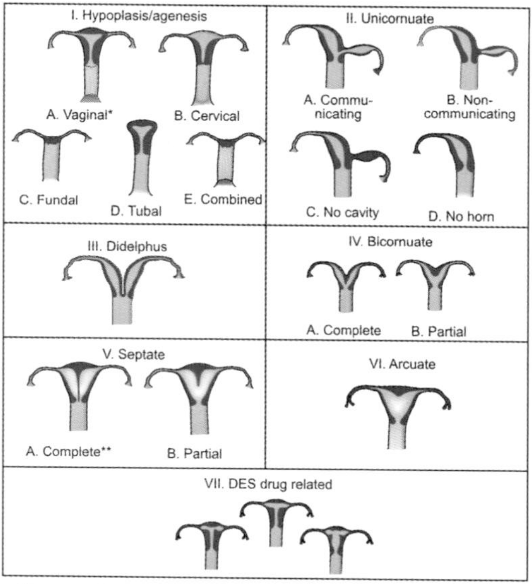

I. Hypoplasis/agenesis
A. Vaginal*
B. Cervical
C. Fundal
D. Tubal
E. Combined
II. Unicornuate
A. Communicating
B. Non-communicating
C. No cavity
D. No horn
III. Didelphus
IV. Bicornuate
A. Complete
B. Partial
V. Septate
A. Complete**
B. Partial
VI. Arcuate
VII. DES drug related

Figure 10.37: Classification of the uterine anomalies

* Uterus may be normal or take a variety of abnormal forms;** May have two distinct cervices.
Source: The American Fertility Society classifications of adnexal adhesions, distal tubal occlusion, tubal occlusion secondary to tubal ligation, tubal pregnancies, Müllerian anomalies and intrauterine adhesions. Fertil Steril. 1988;49(6):944-55.

INDICATIONS

Vaginoplasty

- Complete absence of uterus and vagina [Mayer-Rokitansky-Küster-Hauser (MRKH) syndrome]
- Incomplete absence of uterus and vagina
- Cases of testicular feminization syndrome where the vagina is incompletely developed
- Congenital adrenal hyperplasia having ambiguous genitalia associated with small rudimentary uterus or a partially developed vagina
- Patients with severe stenosis following irradiation therapy.

Metroplasty

- Metroplasty in cases of bicornuate and septate uterus is recommended only for those women who have experienced more than three recurrent spontaneous abortions, midtrimester losses or premature births, and in whom no other etiologic factor for pregnancy wastage has been identified
- Dysmenorrhea in women with septate uteri may be considered an indication for hysteroscopic metroplasty if medical therapy is not effective.

DIAGNOSIS

Symptoms

- Amenorrhea (with Müllerian agenesis)
- Recurrent pregnancy losses.

Per Speculum Examination

- Absent vagina and/or uterus (MRKH syndrome)
- Duplicate cervices/vagina (Uterus didelphys).

Investigations

Initial investigations include hysterosalpingography **(Figs 10.38 and 10.39)** and two-dimensional ultrasound examination. The diagnosis can be confirmed with the help of combined hysteroscopy, laparoscopy and/or three-dimensional ultrasound examination **(Figs 10.40A and B, Fig. 10.41)**.

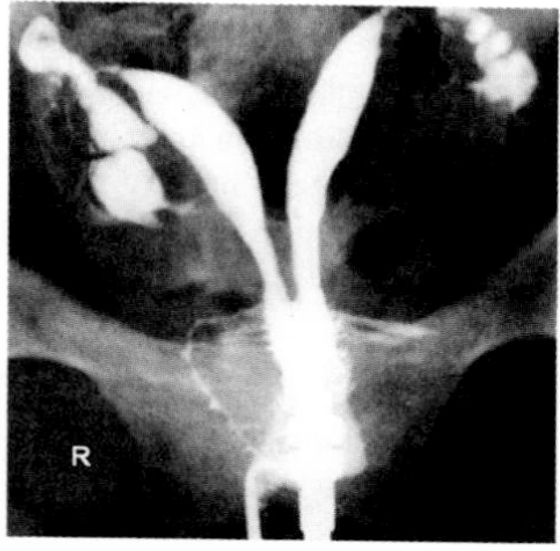

Figure 10.38: HSG showing presence of uterine septum which was confirmed on hysteroscopy

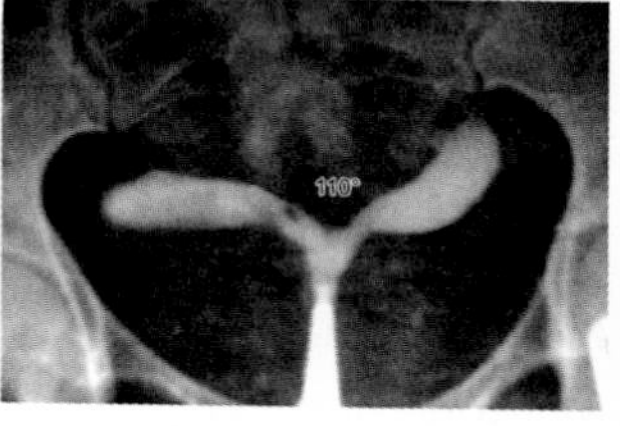

Figure 10.39: HSG showing a single cervical canal and a possible duplication of the uterine horns. Since an angle of greater than 105° was found to be separating the two uterine horns, the diagnosis of bicornuate uterus was made

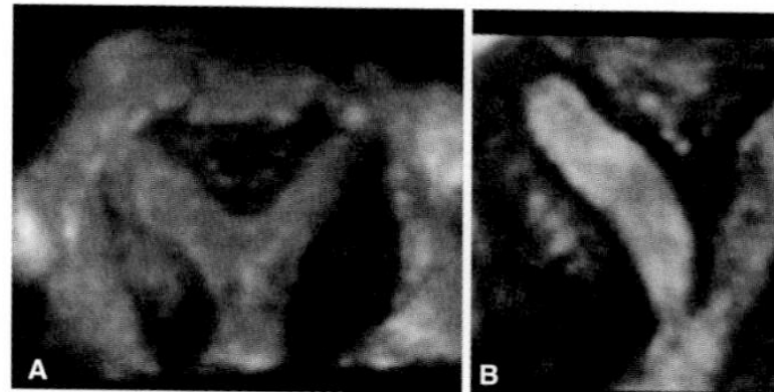

Figures 10.40A and B: Three-dimensional reconstruction of a uterine septum: (A) partial and (B) complete

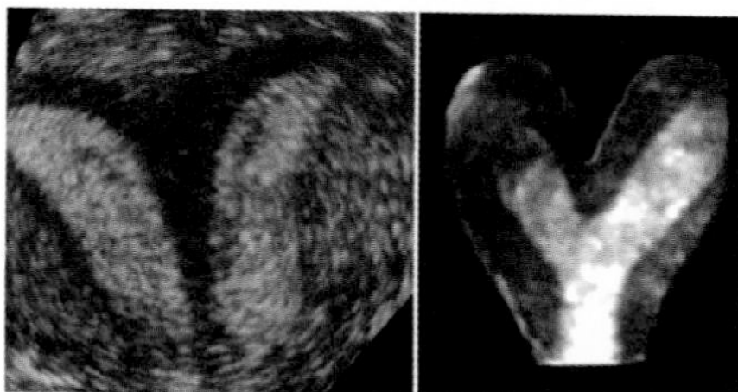

Figure 10.41: Visualization of outer uterine contour with three-dimensional ultrasound showing complete bicornuate uterus. The central myometrial tissue extends up to internal cervical os. (Fundal indentation of > 1 cm is suggestive of bicornuate uterus)

MANAGEMENT

The surgical approach for correction of various Müllerian duct anomalies needs to be individualized, taking into account various factors such as patient's age, desire for future fertility, desire to have healthy sexual relationships and achievement of successful reproductive outcomes.

Preoperative Preparation

Müllerian Agenesis

- *Imaging modalities*: The most commonly used imaging modality for confirmation of diagnosis is ultrasound examination. MRI is another extremely useful but costly investigation
- *Hormone profile*: The hormonal profile in these cases is similar to that of a normal female, having age-appropriate levels of LH, FSH, estradiol and testosterone
- *Other routine preoperative investigations*: These include IVP and renal sonography to exclude presence of urinary tract anomalies.

Bicornuate/Septate Uterus

- *Differentiating between bicornuate and septate uterus*: This is especially important because bicornuate uterus usually does not require surgery and is associated with minimal reproductive problems. The septate uterus on the other hand is associated with a high rate of reproductive failure and therefore requires treatment
- The diagnostic modalities, which are commonly used to establish a definitive diagnosis, include HSG, hysteroscopy and laparoscopy. Ultrasonography and MRI are also useful investigations.

Steps of Surgery

- *Müllerian agenesis*: In patients with Müllerian agenesis, nonsurgical method comprising of vaginal dilatation must be the first line of treatment (**Fig. 10.42**). The McIndoe's vaginoplasty can also be considered as a safe and effective procedure for the surgical creation of a neovagina in cases where simple vaginal dilatation fails to be successful
- *Metroplasty for bicornuate uterus*: The Strassman procedure (**Fig. 10.43**) is surgical treatment of choice for unifying the bicornuate uteri

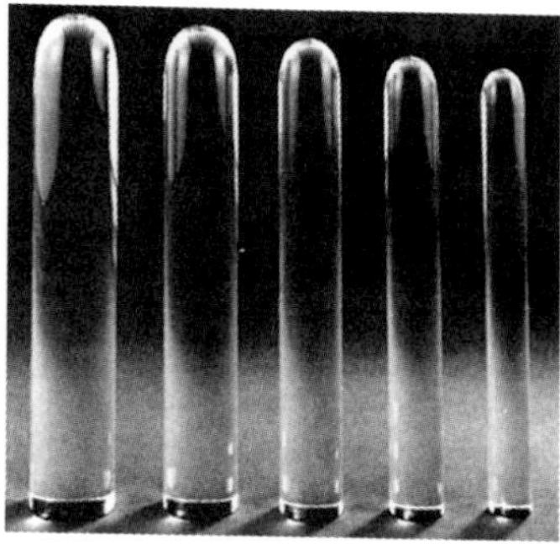

Figure 10.42: Vaginal dilators with progressively increasing size

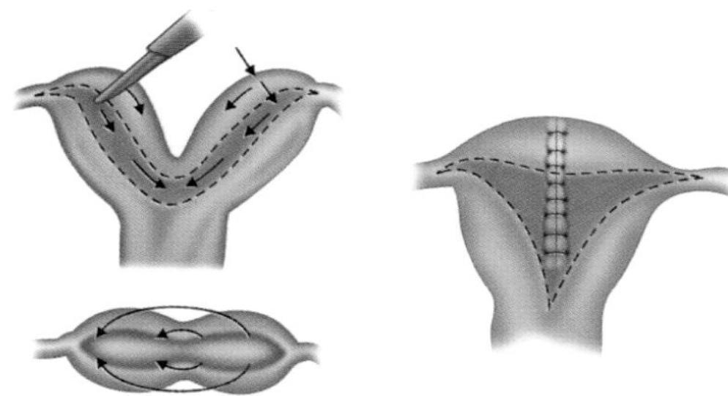

Figure 10.43: Strassman metroplasty

- *Metroplasty for septate uterus*: The surgical procedure of choice for cases of septate uterus is hysteroscopic metroplasty **(Figs 10.44 A to C)** which has been found to be safer than the traditionally performed abdominal metroplasty, using either Jone's **(Figs 10.45A to C)** or Tompkin's technique **(Fig. 10.46)**.

COMPLICATIONS

Vaginoplasty

- These include postoperative infection, hemorrhage, graft failure, development of excessive granulation tissue, vaginal stenosis, postoperative fistula formation and rarely enterocele.

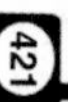

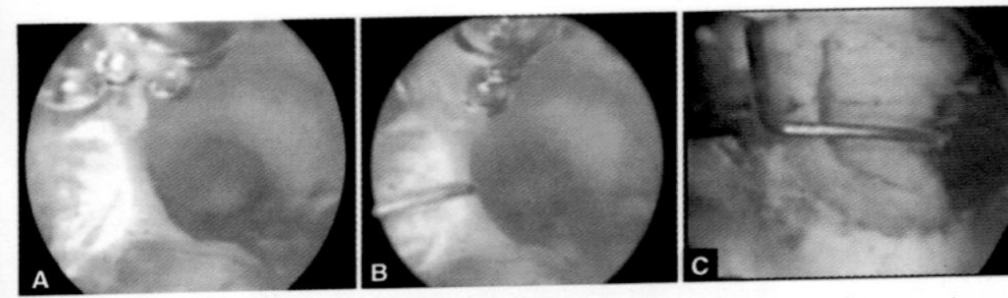

Figures 10.44A to C: Hysteroscopic resection of the uterine septum: (A) hysteroscopic appearance of the uterine septum; (B and C) resectoscope loop transecting the uterine septum

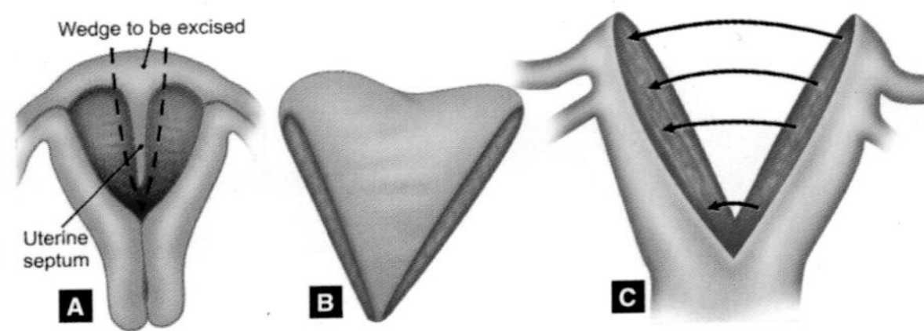

Figures 10.45A to C: Jones metroplasty: (A) wedge shaped incision over the uterine surface inclusive of the septum; (B) separated uterine wedge; (C) suturing of the cut uterine surface

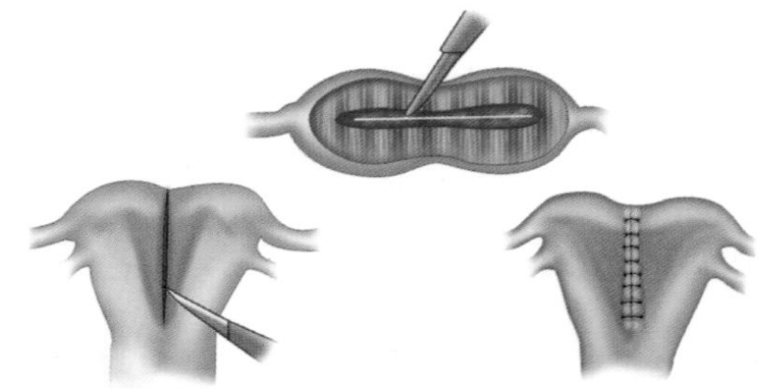

Figure 10.46: Median bivalving technique of Tompkins metroplasty

Metroplasty

- Complications are similar to those found in any other gynecologic surgery such as bleeding, infection, and injury to the bowel and bladder, etc.
- Cervical injuries and uterine perforation may sometimes occur with hysteroscopic metroplasty
- Postoperative hemorrhage and uterine rupture during subsequent pregnancies have also been reported.

CLINICAL PEARLS

- It is important for the gynecologist to establish an accurate diagnosis of each congenital anomaly in order to plan adequate treatment and management strategies
- No surgical intervention is required for the cases with uterine didelphys.

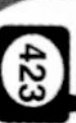

CHAPTER 11

Gynecological Infections

1. SEXUALLY TRANSMITTED DISEASES

1.1. CHLAMYDIAL INFECTION

INTRODUCTION

Chlamydia trachomatis is a gram-negative, aerobic, intracellular pathogen which is typically coccoid or rod shaped. However, it is different from other bacteria because it requires growing cells in order to remain viable. Therefore, it cannot be grown on an artificial medium because it cannot synthesize its own ATP molecules. *C. trachomatis* can be considered as one of the most common causes for sexually transmitted diseases (STDs) worldwide, in association with blindness and infertility. Chlamydia has a very unique life cycle (**Fig. 11.1**), which alternates between a non-replicating, infectious elementary body and a replicating, noninfectious reticulate body.

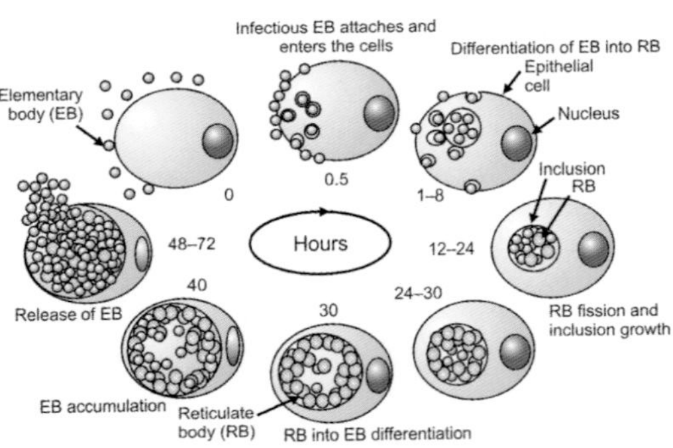

Figure 11.1: Life cycle of *C. trachomatis*

DIAGNOSIS

Clinical Presentation

- Most women with chlamydial infection remain asymptomatic
- Some women may develop symptoms such as vaginal discharge, dysuria, abdominal pain, increased urinary frequency, urgency, urethritis and cervicitis
- Infection of the urethra is often associated with chlamydial infection of the cervix
- Chlamydia is very destructive to the fallopian tubes. If left untreated, nearly 30% of women with chlamydia may develop PID
- Pelvic infection often results in symptoms such as fever, pelvic cramping, abdominal pain or dyspareunia.

Investigations

- *Direct immunofluorescence test*: Fluorescein-conjugated monoclonal antibodies can be used on smears prepared from urethral and cervical swabs for detecting chlamydial antigens
- *Enzyme-linked immunosorbent assay (ELISA)*: Can help in detecting the chlamydial antigen
- *Polymerase and ligase chain reactions*: Newer tests such as polymerase and ligase chain reactions, DNA probe and DNA amplification are also being used.

MEDICAL MANAGEMENT

- Treatment of chlamydia involves the use of broad-spectrum antibiotics, with the most commonly used antibiotic being azithromycin in a single-dosage of 1 gram per orally. Alternatively, doxycycline can be used orally in the dosage of 100 mg BID for 7 days
- The combination of cefoxitin and ceftriaxone with doxycycline or tetracycline also proves to be useful
- Erythromycin or amoxicillin in TID or QID dosage may also be given during pregnancy.

COMPLICATIONS

- Pelvic infection can often lead to infertility or even absolute sterility
- Tubal destruction due to chlamydial infection may also result in an increased incidence of tubal pregnancy

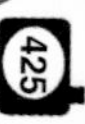

- Chlamydial infection is associated with an increased incidence of premature births and may cause serious eye damage or pneumonia in the infant.

CLINICAL PEARLS

- Gonorrhea and chlamydia are bacterial STDs, which are frequently found together
- All newborns born to women infected with *C. trachomatis* must be treated with eye drops containing tetracycline in order to prevent the occurrence of complications
- Use of protective barrier, such as condoms, often help prevent the spread of the infection.

1.2. GENITAL HERPES

INTRODUCTION

Genital herpes is a viral infection caused by the *herpes simplex virus* (most commonly HSV-II), which is transmitted through sexual contact.

ETIOLOGY

Genital herpes spreads only by direct person-to-person contact. The virus enters through the mucous membrane of the genital tract via microscopic tears. From there the virus travels to the nerve roots near the spinal cord and settles down permanently.

DIAGNOSIS

Symptoms

- The primary infection may be associated with constitutional symptoms like fever, malaise, vulval paresthesia, itching or tingling sensation on the vulva and vagina followed by redness of skin
- Eventually, there is formation of blisters and vesicles on the vulva, vagina, cervix, perianal area **(Fig. 11.2)** or inner thigh, which ultimately develop into shallow and painful ulcers within a period of 2–6 weeks. They are frequently accompanied by itching and mucoid vaginal discharge.

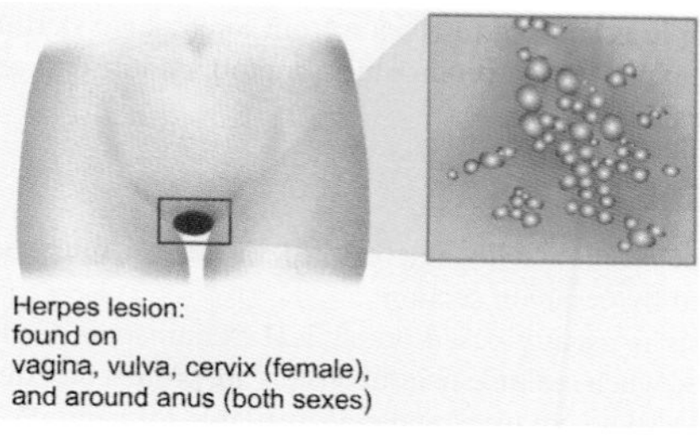

Figure 11.2: Herpetic lesions in women

Investigations

- *Cytological tests*: The blister fluid may be sent to the laboratory for culturing the virus. However, it is associated with a high false negative rate of nearly 50%
- *Immunological tests*: These tests are specific for HSV-I or HSV-II and may be able to demonstrate that a person has been infected at some point in time with the virus
- *Other diagnostic tests*: These include tests such as polymerase chain reaction and rapid fluorescent antibody screening tests
- *Biopsy*: The Tzanck smear is a rapid, fairly sensitive and inexpensive method for diagnosing HSV infection. Smears are preferably prepared from the base of the lesions and stained with 1% aqueous solution of toluidine blue "O" for 15 seconds. Positive smear is indicated by the presence of multinucleated giant cells with faceted nuclei and homogeneously stained "ground glass" chromatin (Tzanck cells).

MEDICAL MANAGEMENT

- Oral antiviral medications, such as acyclovir, (Zovirax), famciclovir (Famvir) or valacyclovir (Valtrex), which prevent the multiplication of the virus, are commonly used
- For the treatment of primary outbreaks, oral acyclovir is prescribed in the dosage of 200 mg five times a day for 5 days
- Local application of acyclovir provides local relief and accelerates the process of healing
- In severe cases, acyclovir can be administered intravenously in the dosage of 5 mg/kg body weight every 8 hourly for 5 days

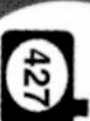

- The couple is advised to abstain from intercourse starting right from time of experiencing prodromal symptoms until total repithelization of the lesions occurs.

CLINICAL PEARLS

- Pregnant women with active herpetic lesion must be preferably delivered by cesarean section
- Diagnosis is usually based on clinical examination. Genital herpes is suspected when multiple painful blisters are present on external genitalia
- There is still no curative medicine available for genital herpes and the antiviral drugs only help in reducing the severity of symptoms and duration of outbreaks
- Herpes can be spread from one part of the body to another during an outbreak. Thorough hand washing is a must during outbreaks in order to prevent the spread of infection
- Couples who want to minimize the risk of transmission should always use condoms if a partner is infected. Such couples must be instructed to avoid all kinds of sexual activity, including kissing, during an outbreak of herpes.

1.3. GONORRHEA

INTRODUCTION

Gonorrhea is a STD, which is derived from the Greek words *gonos* (seed) and *rhoia* (flow) implying "flow of seeds" and is caused by the bacterium *Neisseria gonorrheae*. The disease is characterized by adhesion of the gonococci to the surface of urethra or other mucosal surfaces.

ETIOLOGY

Gonorrhea spreads through contact with the penis, vagina, mouth or anus. Gonorrhea can also be spread from mother to baby at the time of delivery.

DIAGNOSIS

Symptoms

- The commonest clinical presentation of the disease in men is acute urethritis resulting in dysuria and a purulent penile discharge
- Symptomatic women commonly experience vaginal discharge, dysuria and abdominal pain

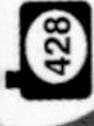

- The infection, if untreated, may extend to Bartholin's glands, endometrium and fallopian tubes. The gonococci can typically ascend to the fallopian tubes at the time of menstruation or after instrumentation (for MTP) giving rise to acute salpingitis. Lesions due to gonorrhea are summarized in **Figure 11.3**.

Investigations

- Culture and sensitivity
- DNA probes.

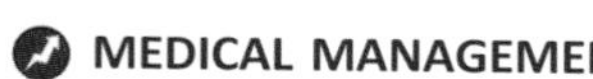

MEDICAL MANAGEMENT

Treatment comprises of using the following antibiotics: Ceftriaxone 125 mg IM or Cefixime 400 mg or Ciprofloxacin 500 mg PO or Ofloxacin 400 mg PO. Doxycycline 100 mg BID × 7 days or Azithromycin 1 gm PO (single dose).

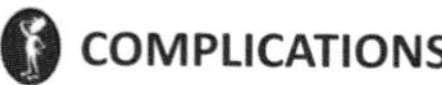

COMPLICATIONS

- The infection may extend along the urethra to the prostate, seminal vesicles and epididymis, resulting in complications such as epididymitis, prostatitis, periurethral abscesses and chronic urethritis
- The infection may spread to the periurethral tissues, resulting in formation of abscesses and multiple discharging sinuses ("watercan perineum")
- Acute salpingitis may be followed by PID. This may be associated with a high probability of sterility if not treated adequately
- Peritoneal spread occasionally occurs and may produce a perihepatic inflammation, resulting in Fitz-Hugh-Curtis syndrome.

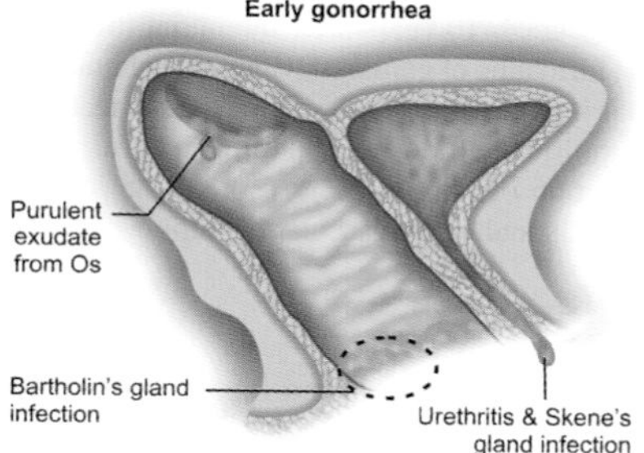

Figure 11.3: Lesions due to gonorrhea

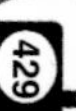

1.4. SYPHILIS

INTRODUCTION

Syphilis is a STD caused by the spirochete *Treponema pallidum*. Though the route of transmission of syphilis is almost always through sexual contact, sometimes congenital syphilis can occur via transmission from mother to child in utero.

DIAGNOSIS

Symptoms

- The disease is typically characterized by three stages: primary; secondary and tertiary
- Primary lesion, also known as a chancre, often appears at the point of contact, usually the external genitalia. The "hard chancre" of syphilis is a firm, painless, relatively avascular, circumscribed, indurated, superficially ulcerated lesion, which usually persists for about 4–6 weeks before healing spontaneously **(Fig. 11.4)**
- In most patients, a painless regional lymphadenopathy develops within 1–2 weeks after the appearance of the chancre. As a result, the regional lymph nodes often become swollen, discrete, rubbery and nontender
- Secondary syphilis is typically characterized by a "flu-like" syndrome, lymphadenopathy and the appearance of symmetrical reddish-pink nonitchy rashes on the trunk and extremities. In moist areas of the body, such as the anus and vagina, the rash often develops into flat, broad, whitish lesions known as condylomata lata. Mucous patches may also appear on the genitals or in the mouth
- Other common symptoms of this stage include fever, malaise, sore throat, weight loss, headache, enlarged lymph nodes, etc.
- Tertiary syphilis usually occurs 1–10 years after the initial infection and is characterized by the formation of gummas, which are soft, tumor-like balls of granulomatous inflammation. Other characteristic features of untreated tertiary syphilis include neuropathic joint disease (characterized by degeneration of joint surfaces resulting in loss of proprioception), neurosyphilis and cardiovascular syphilis.

Investigations

- Dark-field microscopy
- Nontreponemal tests: Kahn test, rapid plasma regain (RPR) and venereal disease research laboratory (VDRL)

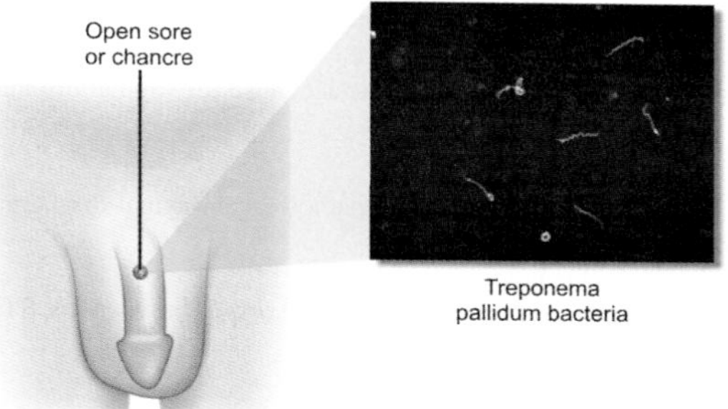

Figure 11.4: Hard chancre due to syphilis on the shaft of penis in males

- Treponemal tests: *Treponema pallidum* microhemagglutination assay (MHA-TP), fluorescent treponemal antibody assay (FTA-ABS).

MEDICAL MANAGEMENT

Primary, secondary and early latent stages of syphilis can generally be treated with a single-dose intramuscular injection of 2.4 million units benzathine penicillin G.

CLINICAL PEARLS

- The chancre of syphilis is often termed as "hard chancre" in order to distinguish it from the "soft sore" caused by *Hemophilus ducreyi*
- All of the lesions of secondary stage are infectious and harbor active treponema organisms and therefore patients in this stage are most contagious
- The rash of secondary syphilis can involve the palms of the hands and the soles of feet.

2. VAGINAL DISCHARGE

INTRODUCTION

Vaginal discharge is one of the most common presenting complaints faced by the gynecologists in clinical practice, which can be caused by physiological or pathological causes. The most important challenge for the

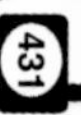

gynecologist is to differentiate between the pathological and physiological causes of discharge. If a pathological cause of discharge is suspected, the gynecologist needs to diagnose the exact cause for vaginal discharge.

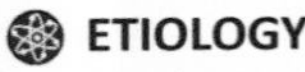

ETIOLOGY

Some common infective causes of pathological vaginal discharge are as follows:

- Vulvovaginal candidiasis (VVC)
- Vaginitis caused by *Trichomonas vaginalis, C. trachomatis,* STDs (*e.g. N. gonorrheae)*
- Bacterial vaginosis
- Acute PID
- Postoperative pelvic infection
- Postabortal/postpartum sepsis.

Various non-infective causes for vaginal discharge are as follows:

- Vault granulation tissue
- Vesicovaginal fistula
- Rectovaginal fistula
- Neoplasia (cervical, vulvar, vaginal or endometrial)
- Retained tampon or condom
- Chemical irritation
- Allergic responses
- Atrophic vaginitis
- Ectropion
- Endocervical polyp
- Intrauterine device
- Atrophic changes
- Physical trauma.

Vulvovaginitis can be considered as one of the most common causes for pathological vaginal discharge, irritation and itching in women. Vulvovaginitis commonly results due to inflammation of the vagina and vulva, and is most often caused by bacterial, fungal or parasitic infection.

DIAGNOSIS

Diagnostic features of the most common causes of vaginitis have been described in **Table 11.1**.

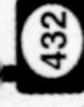

Table 11.1: Diagnostic features of the most common causes of vaginitis

Basis of diagnosis	*Bacterial vaginosis*	*Vulvovaginal candidiasis*	*Trichomoniasis*
Signs and symptoms	Thin, grayish to off-white colored discharge; unpleasant "fishy" odor especially increasing after sexual intercourse. The discharge is usually homogeneous and adheres to vaginal walls	Thick, white ("curd like") discharge with no odor	Copious, malodorous, yellow-green (or discolored) discharge, pruritus and vaginal irritation, dysuria, asymptomatic in many cases
Physical examination	Normal appearance of vaginal tissues; grayish white colored discharge may be adherent to the vaginal walls	Vulvar and vaginal erythema, edema and fissures; thick white discharge that adheres to the vaginal walls **(Fig. 11.5)**	Vulvar and vaginal edema and erythema, "strawberry" cervix in up to 25% of affected women; frothy, purulent discharge **(Fig. 11.6)**
Vaginal pH	Elevated (> 4.5)	Normal	Elevated (> 4.5)
Microscopic examination of wet-mount and KOH preparations of the vaginal discharge	"Clue cells" (vaginal epithelial cells coated with coccobacilli **(Fig. 11.7)**, few lactobacilli, occasional motile, curved rods, belonging to preparations of *Mobiluncus* species	Pseudohyphae, mycelial tangles or budding yeast cells **(Fig. 11.8)**	Motile trichomonads, many polymorphonuclear cells
"Whiff" test (Normal = no odor)	Positive	Negative	Can be positive

Contd...

Contd...

Additional tests	Amsel's criteria **(Box 11.1)** is positive in nearly 90% of affected women with bacterial vaginosis	KOH microscopy, gram stain, culture	DNA probe tests: sensitivity of 90% and specificity of 99.8% Culture: sensitivity of 98% and specificity of 100%

Source: 1. Carr PL, Felsenstein D, Friedman RH. Evaluation and management of vaginitis. J Gen Intern Med. 1998;13:335-46.
2. Sobel JD. Vaginitis. N Engl J Med. 1997;337:1896-903.

Box 11.1: Amsel's diagnostic criteria for bacterial vaginosis

- Thin, homogeneous discharge
- Positive "Whiff" test
- Presence of "clue cells" on microscopic examination
- Vaginal pH > 4.5

DIFFERENTIAL DIAGNOSIS

Various causes of vaginal discharge have been described in "Etiology" pat of this fragment.

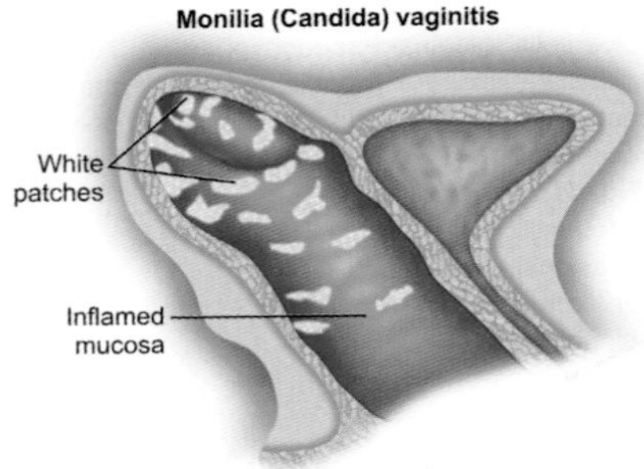

Figure 11.5: Appearance of vulva and vagina in vulvovaginal candidiasis

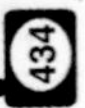

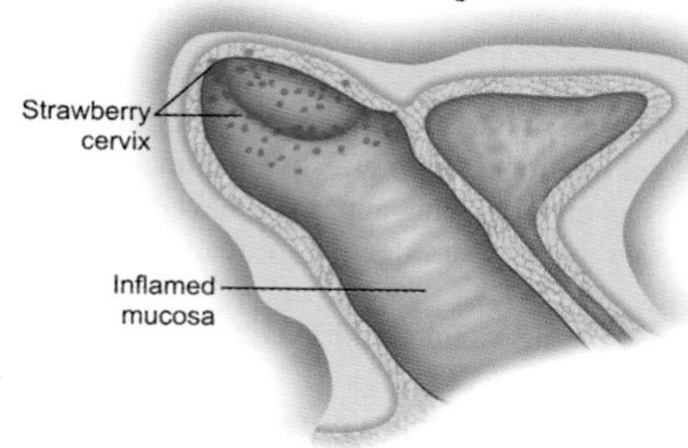

Figure 11.6: Appearance of vulva and vagina in trichomoniasis

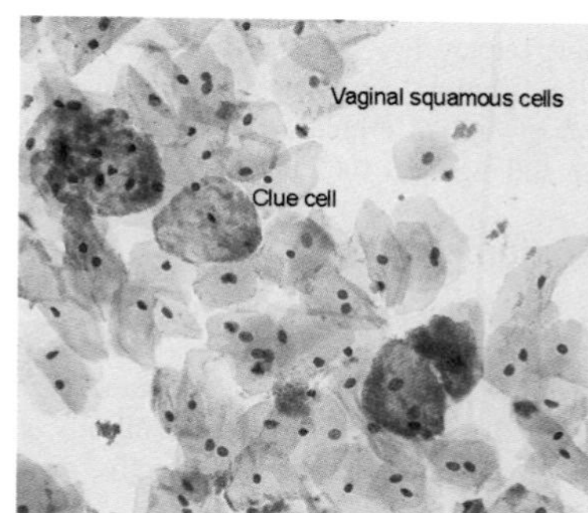

Figure 11.7: Clue cells observed in bacterial vaginosis

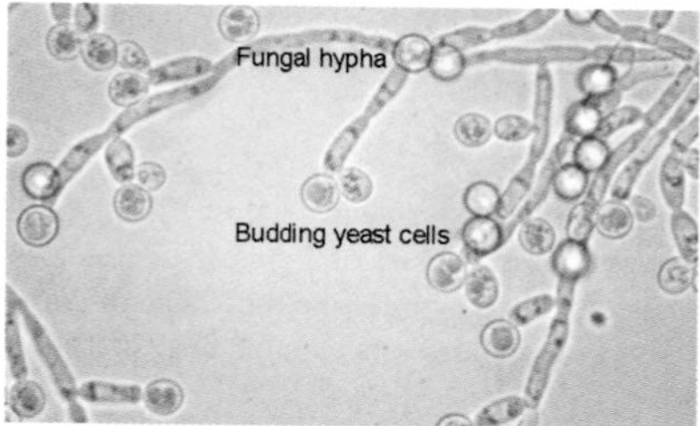

Figure 11.8: Wet mount preparation of *Candida albicans*

MANAGEMENT

Bacterial Vaginosis

- *Metronidazole*: A 7-day course of oral metronidazole, 400 mg TDS or vaginal metronidazole gel (metrogel) is an effective treatment
- *Tinidazole*: Tinidazole is an antibiotic that appears to have fewer side effects than metronidazole and is also effective in treating bacterial vaginosis
- *Ornidazole*: Ornidazole, 500 mg vaginal tablet daily for 7 days, is another effective option
- *Ampicillin*: Ampicillin 500 mg TDS or cephalosporin 500 mg BID for 7 days is also effective
- *Tetracyclines*: Tetracycline 500 mg, four times a day or doxycycline 100 mg twice daily for 7 days may also be used
- *Lincosamides*: Vaginal clindamycin cream 2% (cleocin) or oral clindamycin 300 mg daily for 7 days is also effective.

Candidal Infection

- *Antifungals*: Imidazoles and triazoles are presently the most extensively used antifungal drugs for treatment of VVC. Imidazoles can be used in form of creams and pessaries and include butoconazole, clotrimazole and miconazole. Trizole agents include systemically acting agents such as fluconazole, which has shown to be effective in a single oral dose of 150 mg in most of the cases
- *Antiseptics*: Boric acid suppositories are often used for the treatment of VVC
- *Corticosteroids*: Topical corticosteroids are commonly prescribed to alleviate symptoms such as itchiness and redness.

Vaginal Trichomoniasis

- *Nitroimidazoles*: Metronidazole in the dose of 200 mg TDS or 375 mg BID for 7 days or a single dose of 2 gm can be used. An alternative to metronidazole could be to prescribe tinidazole in the dose of 300 mg BD for 7 days or secnidazole in a single dose of 1000 mg daily for 2 days.

COMPLICATIONS

Some complications related to bacterial vaginosis are as follows:

- Pelvic inflammatory disease
- There may be an increased frequency of endometritis, abnormal Pap smears, abdominal pain, uterine bleeding and uterine or adnexal tenderness
- Development of vaginal cuff cellulitis, PID and endometritis in case of an invasive gynecological procedure
- Bacterial vaginosis during pregnancy can result in complications like premature labor, preterm birth, chorioamnionitis, postpartum endometritis, ectopic pregnancy and postcesarean section wound infections.

CLINICAL PEARLS

- The physiological vaginal discharge is formed by sloughing epithelial cells, normal bacteria and vaginal transudate. The quality and quantity of this physiological vaginal discharge may vary even in the same woman over different phases of menstrual cycle
- In case of VVC and trichomoniasis, ideally, both the partners should be treated and be advised to avoid intercourse or use a condom during the course of therapy
- Topical formulations of imidazole and triazole antifungals can be used during pregnancy for treatment of VVC. Topical nystatin can be recommended in the dose of 100,000 units intravaginally once daily for 2 weeks
- For treatment of vaginal trichomoniasis, use of metronidazole is contraindicated during pregnancy and lactation. During early pregnancy, vinegar douches to lower the vaginal pH, trichofuran suppositories and Betadine® gel can be used.

3. PELVIC INFLAMMATORY DISEASES

INTRODUCTION

PID represents a spectrum of infections and inflammatory disorders of the uterus, fallopian tubes and adjacent pelvic structures. This spectrum includes infections such as endometritis, salpingitis (discussed in details in the Chapter 13), tubo-ovarian abscess (TOA) and oophoritis. Five stages of PID as described by Gainesville are shown in the **Table 11.2**.

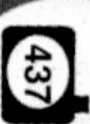

Table 11.2: Stages of PID

Disease stage	*Description*
I	Acute salpingitis without peritonitis
II	Acute salpingitis with peritonitis
III	Acute salpingitis with superimposed tubal occlusion or TOA
IV	Ruptured TOA
V	Tubercular salpingitis

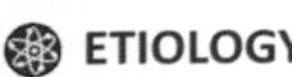

ETIOLOGY

PID occurs as a result of spread of microorganisms from the cervix upwards to the superior portion of genital tract such as fallopian tubes, ovaries and other adjacent structures. *C. trachomatis* is responsible for approximately 25–50% cases of PID, whereas *N. gonorrhoeae* is responsible for about 10–20% cases. Mixed infection with both aerobic and anaerobic microorganisms (*bacteroides, peptostreptococcus, peptococcus*, etc.) may be also responsible. Risk factors for occurrence of PID include sexual activity with multiple sexual partners, young age, procedures requiring cervical and uterine instrumentation such as intrauterine device insertion, endometrial biopsy, and D and C.

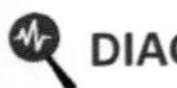

DIAGNOSIS

Symptoms

- Lower abdominal pain or tenderness
- Fever, nausea, vomiting and malaise
- Back pain
- Abnormal uterine bleeding
- Unusual or foul smelling vaginal discharge
- Dysuria and dyspareunia.

Physical Examination

- *Pulse rate*: This may be increased due to fever
- *Temperature*: The body temperature may be elevated to more than 101°F (> 38.3°C).

Pelvic Examination

- There may be cervical, uterine or adnexal tenderness on pelvic examination

- Uterus may be retroverted and immobile
- The appendages may be thickened and tender to touch.

Investigations

- *Blood investigations*: This must include a CBC along with DLC and hematocrit. Blood culture may be required in cases of bacteremia. Blood urea, serum electrolytes and levels of CRP may also be done
- Culdocentesis may be required to rule out ectopic pregnancy or to establish the diagnosis of ectopic pregnancy
- Laparoscopic examination is not routinely required in cases of PID
- *Urine investigations*: This must include urine pregnancy test in order to rule out pregnancy amongst the women of child-bearing age group. A routine urine analysis is also required to rule out infection
- *Cervical culture*: This is required to rule out gonorrhea and Chlamydia infection
- *Imaging studies such as ultrasound, CT and MRI*: A pelvic ultrasound may help in diagnosing complications such as ovarian cysts, TOAs, hydrosalpinx, pyosalpinx, ovarian torsion, ectopic pregnancy, etc. **(Figs 11.9 to 11.11)**. TOA appears as a complex cystic adnexal mass with thick irregular walls and septations.

DIFFERENTIAL DIAGNOSIS

- Appendicitis, ectopic pregnancy
- Hemorrhagic ovarian cysts, ovarian torsion
- Endometriosis, urinary tract infection
- Irritable bowel disease, cholecystitis, neprolithiasis.

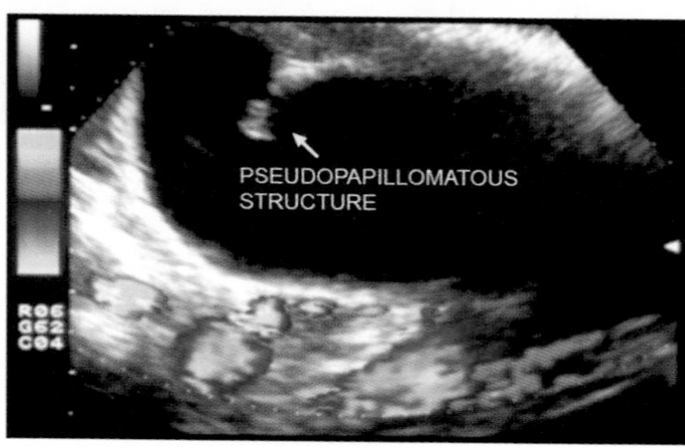

Figure 11.9: Chronic hydrosalpinx: dilated fallopian tube with thin-walled incomplete septations

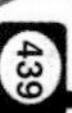

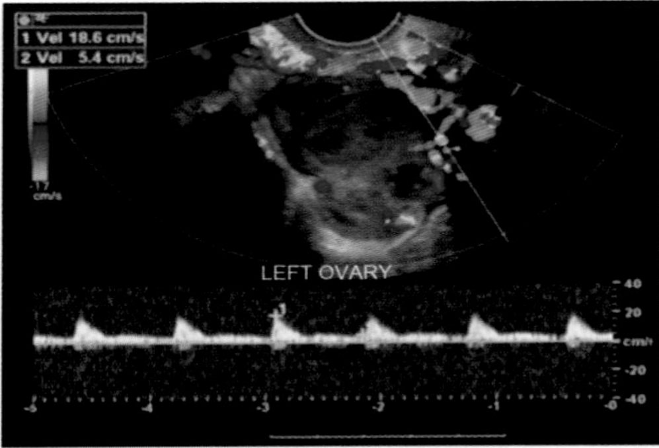

Figure 11.10: Tubo-ovarian mass: complex cystic solid structure showing prominent vascular perfusion with low-moderate vascular impedence on color flow Doppler

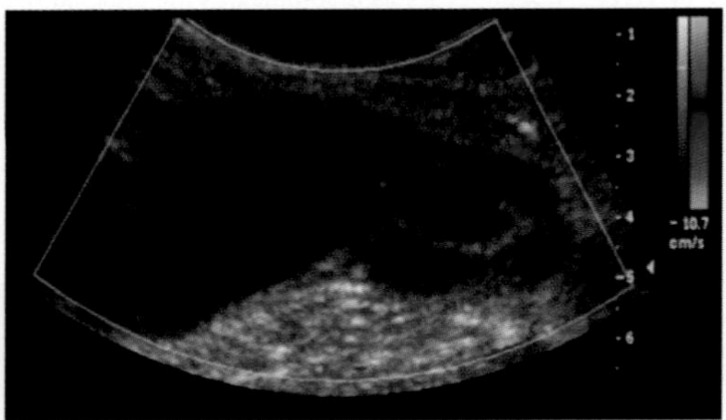

Figure 11.11: Retort-shaped tubal mass suggestive of hydrosalpinx

MEDICAL MANAGEMENT

Medical treatment mainly comprises of using antibiotics, pain-killers and IV fluids.

The CDC (2010) recommended outpatient antibiotic regimens (both inpatient and outpatient) for treatment of PID are shown in **Box 11.2**.

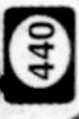

Box 11.2: Recommended antibiotic regimens for PID

Recommended outpatient regimen

Ceftriaxone 250 mg IM in a single dose
Plus
Doxycycline 100 mg orally twice a day for 14 days
With or *Without*
Metronidazole 500 mg orally twice a day for 14 days
Or
Cefoxitin 2 g IM in a single dose and Probenecid, 1 g orally administered concurrently in a single dose
Plus
Doxycycline 100 mg orally twice a day for 14 days
With or *Without*
Metronidazole 500 mg orally twice a day for 14 days
Or
Other parenteral third-generation cephalosporin (e.g., ceftizoxime or cefotaxime)
Plus
Doxycycline 100 mg orally twice a day for 14 days
With or *Without*
Metronidazole 500 mg orally twice a day for 14 days

Recommended inpatient regimens

Parenteral Regimen A
Cefotetan 2 g IV every 12 hr
Or
Cefoxitin 2 g IV every 6 hr
Plus
Doxycycline 100 mg orally or IV every 12 hr*

Parenteral Regimen B
Clindamycin 900 mg IV every 8 hr
Plus
Gentamicin loading dose IV or IM (2 mg/kg of body weight), followed by a maintenance dose (1.5 mg/kg) every 8 hr. This can be substituted with a single daily dosing (3–5 mg/kg)

Cefoxitin must be discontinued 24 hours after improvement in the patient's symptoms and doxycycline must be continued in the dosage of 100 mg PO bid for a total of 14 days. If TOA is present, clindamycin or metronidazole can be added for better anaerobic coverage.

Source: Centers for Disease Control and Prevention. (2011). CDC website [online] Available from *http://www.cdc.gov/std/treatment/2010/pid.htm* [Accessed September 2011].

SURGICAL MANAGEMENT

Indications for surgery in cases of PID are enumerated in **Box 11.3**.

Box 11.3: Indications for surgery in cases of PID

- Drainage of a pelvic abscess
- Acute spreading peritonitis resistant to medical treatment
- Presence of a pyoperitoneum
- Intestinal obstruction
- Ruptured TOA
- Suspected intestinal injury
- Removal of septic products of conception from the uterine cavity

Drainage of a TOA can be done through minimal invasive surgery or posterior colpotomy **(Fig. 11.12)**.

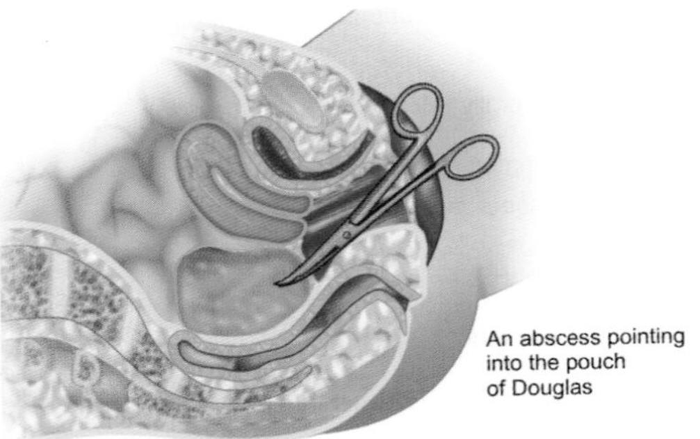

Figure 11.12: Posterior colpotomy for drainage of tubo-ovarian abscess

COMPLICATIONS

- Ectopic pregnancy
- Infertility
- Chronic pelvic pain
- Tubo-ovarian abscess
- Pelvic adhesions.

CLINICAL PEARLS

- PID almost exclusively occurs in sexually active women and amongst adolescents
- Symptoms related to PID are usually worse at the end of a menstrual period and for a few days afterwards
- TOA can be defined as the collection of pus involving the tubes and the ovary
- The major clinical significance of a hydrosalpinx is its adverse effect on fertility, thereby resulting in a reduced pregnancy rate
- A hydrosalpinx, although sterile, can be reinfected at a later date leading to a pyosalpinx.

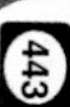

CHAPTER 12

Infertility

1. AMENORRHEA

INTRODUCTION

Amenorrhea or absence of menstrual periods can be of two types: primary (woman has never experienced menstrual cycles) and secondary (woman had experienced menstrual bleeding previously before experiencing cessation for at least 6 months). Primary amenorrhea can be defined as follows:

- Absence of menses by age of 14 years with the absence of growth or development of secondary sexual characteristics or
- Absence of menses by the age of 16 years with normal development of secondary sexual characteristics.

ETIOLOGY

The causes of primary amenorrhea are related to defects in either of the four compartments as shown in **Figure 12.1** and **Box 12.1**.

Box 12.1: Causes of primary amenorrhea

Defects in compartment I (outflow tract and uterus)

- Müllerian agenesis (Mayer-Rokitansky-Küster Hauser syndrome)
- Androgen insensitivity syndrome
- 5-alpha reductase deficiency
- Asherman's syndrome
- Imperforate hymen.

Defects in compartment II (ovulation)

- Gonadal dysgenesis (Turner's syndrome)
- Premature ovarian failure
- Polycystic ovarian syndrome (PCOS)
- Post-pill amenorrhea.

Contd...

Contd...

Defects in compartment III (disorders of anterior pituitary)

- Hyperprolactinemia
- Gonadotropin deficiency, e.g. Kallman's syndrome
- Tumors of the hypothalamus or pituitary
- Hypopituitarism.

Defects in compartment IV (hypothalamus)

- Anorexia nervosa
- Chronic illness, anorexia, weight loss, stress
- Hyperprolactinemia.

DIAGNOSIS

Clinical Presentation

- Absence of periods
- *Body mass index (BMI)*: Increased BMI could be associated with polycystic ovarian disease (PCOD)
- *Anthropomorphic measurements and growth chart*: These measurements may detect abnormalities, such as constitutional delay of growth and puberty

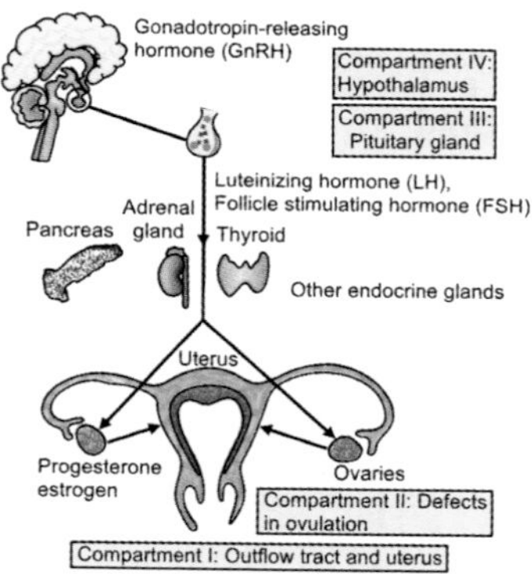

Figure 12.1: Causes of primary amenorrhea related to defects in either of four compartments

- *Signs of androgen excess*: Signs such as hirsutism or acne could be associated with polycystic ovary syndrome
- *Signs of virilization*: Signs such as deep voice, clitoromegaly, etc. could be related to the presence of androgen-secreting tumors
- *Clitoral measurement*: A clitoral index greater than 35 mm^2 is an evidence of increased androgen effect
- *Dysmorphic features*: Such as webbed neck, short stature and widely spaced nipples could be suggestive of Turner's syndrome
- *Symptoms suggestive of Cushing's disease*: These include features, such as striae, buffalo hump, central obesity, easy bruising, hypertension or proximal muscle weakness
- *Thyroid examination*: This is especially essential because thyroid diseases serve as an important cause of amenorrhea and menstrual irregularities
- *Breast examination*: This helps in ruling out galactorrhea
- *Fundoscopy and assessment of visual fields*: This must be done if there is suspicion of pituitary tumor
- *Pubertal development*: Tanner stage of development of breast and pubic hair has been described in **Figures 12.2A and B** respectively.

Per Speculum Examination

- Detection of outflow tract abnormalities, such as transverse vaginal septum, imperforate hymen, etc.
- Distribution of pubic hair pattern.

Pelvic Examination

Rudimentary or absent uterus can be detected on bimanual examination.

Investigations

- *Karyotyping*: This is important for identifying the patient's genetic sex
- *Serum testosterone/androgen level*: May be mildly raised in women with PCOS or may be highly raised in women with androgen-secreting tumors of the ovary or adrenal gland
- *Gonadotropin levels*: Low level of gonadotropins is associated with hypogonadotropic hypogonadism, while high level of gonadotropins is associated with hypergonadotropic hypogonadism
- *Serum prolactin levels*: This may be raised in women with prolactinomas
- *Thyroid function tests*: These may be indicative of thyroid dysfunction, as a possible cause of amenorrhea.

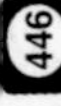

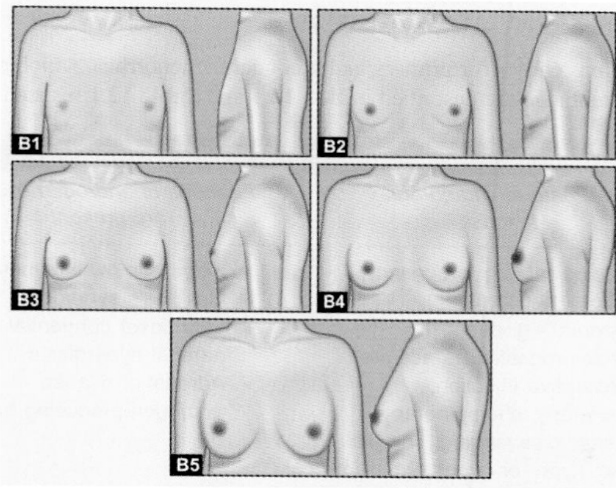

Figure 12.2A: Tanner staging for breast development

B-1: Pre-pubertal; B-2: Breast bud; B-3: Enlargement of breast and areola with no separation of the contour; B-4: Projection of areola and papilla to form a secondary mound above the level of the breast; B-5: Recession of the areola to the general contour of the breast with projection of the papilla only

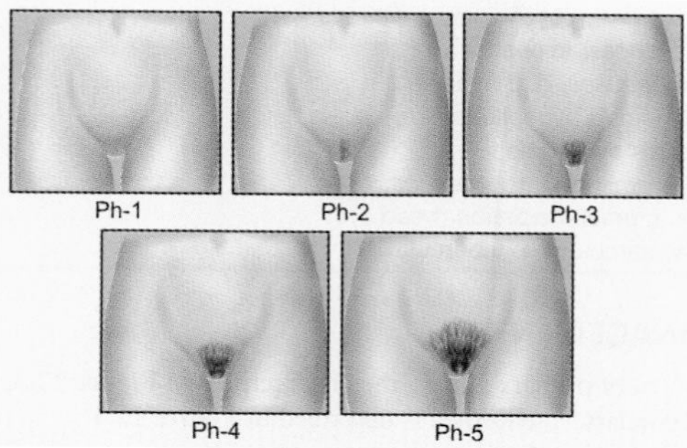

Figure 12.2B: Tanner staging for development of pubic hair in females

Ph-1: pre-pubertal; Ph-2: sparse growth of long slightly pigmented hair usually slightly curly mainly along the labia; Ph-3: the hair is darker, coarser and curlier and spreads over the junction of the pubes; Ph-4: the hair spreads covering the pubes; Ph-5 the hair extends to the medial surface of the thighs and is distributed as an inverse triangle

DIFFERENTIAL DIAGNOSIS

The various causes for primary and secondary amenorrhea, which need to be differentiated are described in **Box 12.1** and **Table 12.1** respectively.

Table 12.1: Various causes of secondary amenorrhea

No features of androgen excess	*Features of androgen excess are present*
• *Physiological*, e.g. pregnancy, lactation, menopause • *Iatrogenic*, e.g. depot medroxyprogesterone acetate contraceptive injection, radiotherapy, chemotherapy • *Systemic disease*, e.g. chronic illness, hypo- or hyperthyroidism • *Uterine causes*, e.g. cervical stenosis, Asherman's syndrome • *Ovarian causes*, e.g. premature ovarian failure, resistant ovary syndrome • *Hypothalamic causes*, e.g. weight-loss, exercise, psychological distress, chronic illness, idiopathic • *Pituitary causes*, e.g. hyper-prolactinemia, hypopituitarism, Sheehan's syndrome • *Hypothalamic/pituitary damage*, e.g. tumors, cranial irradiation, head injuries, sarcoidosis, tuberculosis	• Polycystic ovary syndrome • Cushing's syndrome • Late-onset congenital adrenal hyperplasia • Adrenal or ovarian androgen-producing tumor

MANAGEMENT

Management of primary amenorrhea is described in **Figure 12.3**, whereas that of secondary amenorrhea is described in **Figure 12.4**.

The treatment of primary and secondary amenorrhea is based on the causative factor. Human menopausal gonadotropin (hMG) is the treatment of choice for patients with primary amenorrhea due to hypopituitarism.

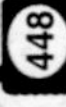

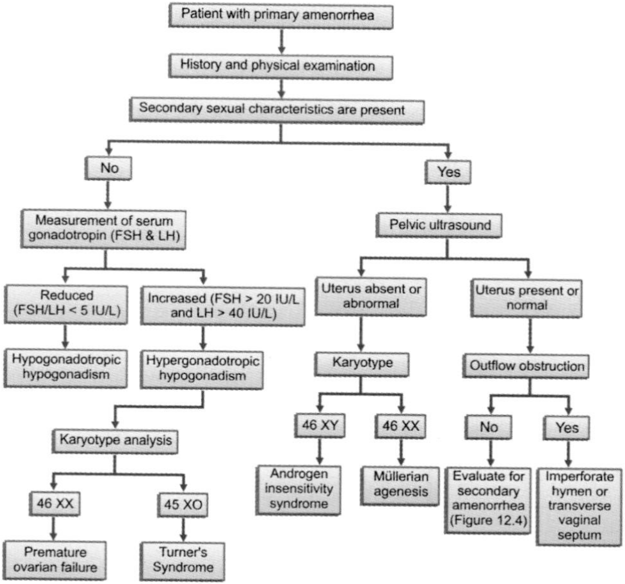

- Patient with primary amenorrhea
  - History and physical examination
    - Secondary sexual characteristics are present
      - No
        - Measurement of serum gonadotropin (FSH & LH)
          - Reduced (FSH/LH < 5 IU/L)
            - Hypogonadotropic hypogonadism
          - Increased (FSH > 20 IU/L and LH > 40 IU/L)
            - Hypergonadotropic hypogonadism
              - Karyotype analysis
                - 46 XX
                  - Premature ovarian failure
                - 45 XO
                  - Turner's Syndrome
      - Yes
        - Pelvic ultrasound
          - Uterus absent or abnormal
            - Karyotype
              - 46 XY
                - Androgen insensitivity syndrome
              - 46 XX
                - Müllerian agenesis
          - Uterus present or normal
            - Outflow obstruction
              - No
                - Evaluate for secondary amenorrhea (Figure 12.4)
              - Yes
                - Imperforate hymen or transverse vaginal septum

Figure 12.3: Management of cases with primary amenorrhea

COMPLICATIONS

- *Osteoporosis*: Use of HRT, calcium and vitamin D preparations may prove to be useful in these patients
- *Cardiovascular disease*: Young women having amenorrhea associated with estrogen deficiency may also be at an increased risk of developing cardiovascular disease, hypertension and Type 2 diabetes in future
- *Endometrial hyperplasia*: Women with amenorrhea having unopposed estrogen secretion are at an increased risk of developing endometrial hyperplasia and endometrial carcinoma in future
- *Infertility*: Women with amenorrhea generally do not ovulate and are usually infertile

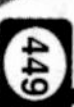

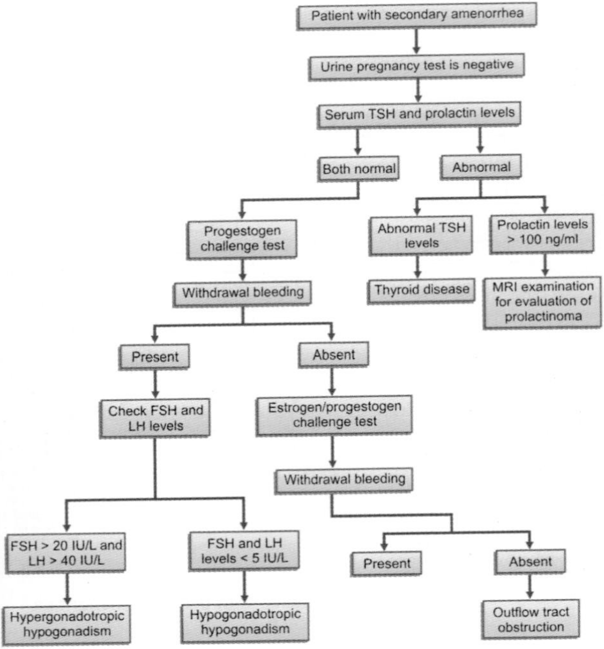

Patient with secondary amenorrhea
→ Urine pregnancy test is negative
→ Serum TSH and prolactin levels
- Both normal
  - Progestogen challenge test
    - Withdrawal bleeding
      - Present
        - Check FSH and LH levels
          - FSH > 20 IU/L and LH > 40 IU/L → Hypergonadotropic hypogonadism
          - FSH and LH levels < 5 IU/L → Hypogonadotropic hypogonadism
      - Absent
        - Estrogen/progestogen challenge test
          - Withdrawal bleeding
            - Present
            - Absent → Outflow tract obstruction
- Abnormal
  - Abnormal TSH levels → Thyroid disease
  - Prolactin levels > 100 ng/ml → MRI examination for evaluation of prolactinoma

Figure 12.4: Management plan of a patient with secondary amenorrhea

- *Psychological distress*: Amenorrhea may cause women to start having concerns regarding the loss of fertility or loss of femininity, thereby resulting in anxiety.

CLINICAL PEARLS

- Treatment goals in these cases include prevention of complications, such as osteoporosis, endometrial hyperplasia, heart disease, etc., preservation of fertility and, in case of primary amenorrhea, progression of normal pubertal development

- In cases of androgen insensitivity syndrome, due to high incidence of malignancy in the gonads with Y chromosomes, the testes must be removed at the age of 16–18 years, once full development has been attained after puberty.

2. MALE INFERTILITY

INTRODUCTION

Infertility is defined as the inability to conceive even after trying with unprotected intercourse for a period of 1 year for couples in which the woman is under 35 years and 6 months of trying for couples in which the woman is over 35 years of age. In nearly 30% of cases, the cause can be attributed to the male partner, which would be primarily discussed in this fragment.

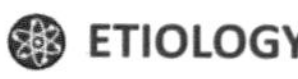

ETIOLOGY

Some of the important causes of male infertility are described in **Box 12.2**.

Box 12.2: Causes of male infertility

Idiopathic: No obvious cause of infertility can be found

Varicocele

Infections

- *STDs*: Chlamydia, gonorrhea and syphilis
- *Acute systemic infections*: Smallpox, mumps, other viral infections, etc.
- *Chronic systemic infections*: TB, leprosy, filariasis, prostatitis, renal, hepatic diseases, diabetic neuropathy
- *Undescended testes* (cryptorchidism)
- *Genetic and endocrine disorders*: Klinefelter's syndrome, androgen insensitivity syndrome, disorders of pituitary and adrenal glands, adrenal hyperplasia, etc.
- *Substance abuse* (excessive intake of alcohol and/or drugs)
- *Testicular factors*: Torsion, undescended testes, damage to the testis due to exercise or heat, tumors (seminoma), hydrocele, etc.
- *Long term use of drugs*: Antihypertensive drugs such, as reserpine, methyldopa, guanethidine, cimetidine, spironolactone, propranolol, corticosteroids, anabolic steroids, antipsychotics and certain anticancer drugs
- *Environmental factors*: Eexposure to chemicals, such as lead, nickel, mercury, anesthetic agents, pesticides, tobacco smoking, excessive alcohol intake, etc.
- *Previous surgery*: Inguinal, scrotal, retroperitoneal, bladd vasectomy, hernia repair
- Sexual dysfunctions, ejaculatory disturbances, impotence, et

DIAGNOSIS

General Physical Examination

These include examination of the patient for development of male secondary sex characteristics, gynecomastia or hirsutism. The complete physical examination also includes a digital rectal examination.

Examination of Male External Genitalia

- *Scrotum*: This must be evaluated for the presence of congenital abnormalities, such as hypospadias, cryptorchidism, absence of vas deferens (unilateral or bilateral), etc.
- *Testis*: This involves assessment of testicular size, presence of tenderness on palpation of testicles and presence of any associated mass, such as an inguinal hernia or varicocele (bag of worms appearance).

Investigations

- *Semen* analysis: The primary values that are evaluated at the time of semen analysis include the volume of the ejaculate, sperm motility, total sperm concentration, sperm morphology, motility and viability **(Table 12.2)**.

Table 12.2: World Health Organization reference values for semen analysis

Parameter	*Normal range*
Volume	2–5 mL
Liquefaction time	Within 60 min.
pH level	7.2–7.8
Sperm concentration	20 million or greater
Total sperm count	40 million spermatozoa per ejaculate or more
Motility	50%, forward progression; 50% or more motile (Grades a* and b**) or 25% or more with progressive motility (grade a) within 60 min. of ejaculation
Morphology	Normal sperms (> 4%)
Vitality	75% or more live
White blood cells	Fewer than 1 million cells/µL

* Grade a: Rapid progressive motility (sperm moving swiftly, usually in a straight line).
** Grade b: Slow or sluggish progressive motility (sperms may be less linear in their progression).

- *Serum testosterone levels*: Testicular function can be assessed by levels of male hormones in the blood (total testosterone, free testosterone, LH, FSH, etc.)
- *Other investigations*: These may include investigations, such as semen culture, anti-sperm antibody estimation, scrotal ultrasound, hormonal assays, karyotyping, vasography, etc.

MANAGEMENT

- *Life style modification*: The patient must be advised to discontinue smoking, stop consumption of excessive alcohol and/or intake of drugs, such as body-building steroids and illicit drugs, wear loose fitting underwear and cool clothes and avoid high temperature baths like saunas, etc. Coital frequency should be increased in order to improve the chances of conception
- *Medical therapy*: Some of these include clomiphene citrate, tamoxifen, gonadotropins, antibiotics (for treatment of infection), steroids, etc. Vitamin E can help counter oxidative stress, which is associated with sperm DNA damage. A hormone-antioxidant combination may improve sperm count and motility. Phosphodiesterase Type 5 inhibitors, e.g., sildenafil, can be used in the patients with ejaculatory sexual dysfunction
- *Surgical therapy*: Surgery may be employed for treatment of conditions, such as duct obstruction, varicoceles, undescended testes, etc. Modern microsurgical techniques can also prove to be useful for procedures such as vasectomy reversal and tubal recanalization
- *Assisted reproductive techniques*: This includes procedures, such as sperm washing/capacitation, intrauterine insemination, gamete intrafallopian transfer, in vitro fertilization and micromanipulation [intracytoplasmic sperm injection (ICSI)]
- *Incurable cases*: In cases where none of the treatment modalities seem to work, the only options may be donor insemination or adoption.

CLINICAL PEARLS

- The first test in the evaluation of the infertile couple is the semen analysis. A perfectly normal semen analysis report generally precludes a significant male factor component. Therefore treatment should be more appropriately targeted towards the woman
- Ideally, the semen analysis should be performed at least t confirm results

- Low sperm count is termed as oligospermia, whereas complete absence of sperms in the ejaculate is termed as azoospermia. Severely reduced sperm motility is termed as asthenospermia.

3. FEMALE INFERTILITY

INTRODUCTION

In nearly 30% of the cases, the cause of infertility may be attributed to the female partner, which would be primarily discussed in this fragment.

ETIOLOGY

Various causes of female infertility are illustrated in **Figure 12.5**.

DIAGNOSIS

General physical examination: See the fragment on amenorrhea.

Abdominal examination: Masses felt in the hypogastrium could be arising from the pelvic region.

Per speculum examination: This involves inspection of the following:

- The distribution of hair pattern on the external genitalia
- Inspection of the vaginal mucosa to detect abnormalities, such as deficiency of estrogen or the presence of infection
- Cervical abnormalities, e.g. cervical stenosis

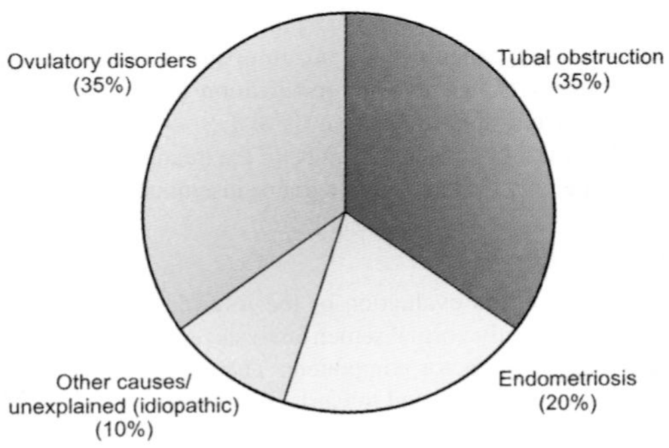

Figure 12.5: Female causes of infertility

Pelvic examination: Various pelvic pathologies, such as fibroids, adnexal masses, tenderness or pelvic nodules indicative of infection or endometriosis, uterine defects (such as absence of the vagina and uterus, presence of vaginal septum, etc.), can be detected on bimanual examination.

Investigations

- *Routine investigations*: These include thyroid function tests (particularly TSH levels) and serum prolactin levels
- *Evaluation of cervical factor*: This aims at testing the characteristics of the cervical mucus with help of postcoital test (Sim's or Huhner's test)
- *Tests for uterine factor*: The commonly used investigations include HSG, pelvic ultrasonography, SIS and endometrial biopsy or operative procedures, such as laparoscopy and hysteroscopy
- *Tubal and peritoneal factors*: The two most frequent tests used for diagnosis of tubal pathology are laparoscopy and HSG.
- *Ovarian factors*: Assessment of ovarian function can be done with help of tests such as clomiphene citrate challenge test, estimation of serum progesterone levels on day 21, ultrasound examination to confirm follicular rupture or ovulation, and/or establish the diagnosis of PCOD and basal body temperature charting.

DIFFERENTIAL DIAGNOSIS

Female factor infertility can result from various causes (**Box 12.3**).

Box 12.3: Causes of female infertility

Cervical factor infertility

- Abnormalities of the mucus-sperm interaction
- Narrowing of the cervical canal due to cervical stenosis.

Uterine factor infertility

- Total absence of the uterus and vagina (Rokitansky-Küster-Hauser syndrome)
- DES induced uterine malformations
- Asherman's syndrome, endometritis (due to tuberculosis)
- Leiomyomas.

Ovarian factor infertility

- Polycystic ovarian syndrome.

Contd...

Tubal factors

- PID associated with gonorrheal and chlamydial infection.

Peritoneal factors

- Infection
- Adhesions and adnexal masses
- Endometriosis.

MANAGEMENT

A treatment plan should be generated based on the diagnosis established through the findings of laboratory investigations, clinical examination, duration of infertility and the woman's age. Following this, the treatment can comprise of the following:

- *Patient counseling*: The couple must be instructed that for conception to occur, they must have intercourse every 2–3 days
- *Lifestyle changes*: For couples attempting conception, it is recommended that the BMI is achieved between 20 and 25. Alcohol consumption must be limited to one or two units, once or twice a week for women. Women who smoke should be advised to quit smoking
- *Treatment of cervical factors*: Chronic cervicitis may be treated with antibiotics. The most successful treatment option for infertility related to cervical factors is artificial intrauterine insemination (IUI). This can be performed by depositing the sperms at the level of internal cervical os (cervical insemination) or inside the endometrial cavity
- *Treatment of uterine factors*: This involves lysis of uterine septae and uterine synechiae, surgical treatment of uterine anomalies (e.g. bicornuate uterus, etc.), hysteroscopic removal of endometrial polyps, etc. Treatment of fibroids has been described in Chapter 7
- *Treatment of tubal factors of infertility*: This may include microsurgery and laparoscopy. Tubal obstruction due to elective sterilization is usually repaired using microsurgical techniques. Nowadays, laparoscopic surgical approach is widely being used for the treatment of multiple tuboperitoneal pathologies, especially endometriosis, using techniques, such as electrocautery, endocoagulation, lasers, etc. Treatment of endometriosis has been discussed in details in the Chapter 10. For women with proximal tubal obstruction, selective salpingography plus tubal catheterization, or hysteroscopic tubal cannulation, may serve as effective treatment options

- *Treatment of ovarian factors:*
  - Polycystic ovarian disease: Some commonly used treatment options for PCOS include weight loss through diet and exercise, ovulation inducing medicines, such as clomiphene citrate, insulin sensitizing agents (such as glucophage and metformin), dietary changes (low glycemic diet) and surgery (ovarian drilling)
  - Ovulation inducing drugs: These include clomiphene citrate, hMGs and synthetic GnRH analogues
  - Assisted reproductive techniques: If no treatment option seems to work, the last option for the clinician to consider is ARTs, which have been discussed in the next fragment.

CLINICAL PEARLS

- The pregnancy rate following a tubal reanastomosis performed by surgeons skilled in microsurgery varies from 70% to 80%.
- The optimal female age range for achieving a successful IVF treatment is 23–39 years.

4. ASSISTED REPRODUCTIVE TECHNIQUES

INTRODUCTION

In vitro fertilization is one of the most commonly used ART. It consists of retrieving a preovulatory oocyte from the ovary; fertilizing it with sperm in the laboratory, and subsequently transferring the embryo within the endometrial cavity. IVF is now being recognized as an established treatment for infertility.

INDICATIONS

Indications for IVF include the following:

- Uterine malformations (e.g. unicornuate uterus)
- Damage/absence of fallopian tubes
- Severe pelvic adhesions, and/or endometriosis
- Severe oligospermia or a history of obstructive azoospermia in the male partner
- Premature ovarian failure.

MANAGEMENT

The procedure of IVF comprises of the following steps **(Fig. 12.6**

1. *Ovarian stimulation for IVF*: Several protocols are used fo stimulation such as clomiphene citrate protocol; use of cl

citrate with hMGs; use of hMGs only; use of GnRH agonists and antagonists. Following 36–72 hours after oocyte retrieval, the endometrium must be supplemented with progesterone in order to maintain the luteal phase

2. *Follicular aspiration*: Oocytes are aspirated from the ovary 35–36 hours following administration of hCG. Follicular aspirations are commonly performed under ultrasonographic guidance
3. *Sperm preparation and oocyte maturation*: The procedure of sperm preparation involves the removal of certain components of the semen sample (i.e. seminal fluid, excess cellular debris, leukocytes, morphologically abnormal sperms, etc.) along with the retention of the motile fraction of sperms. The sperms are incubated for 60 minutes in an atmosphere of 5% CO_2 in air. Oocyte maturation can be achieved with FSH treatment for 3–6 days, followed by retrieval on days 9–10, or using a single dose of hCG (10,000 IU), 36 hours before retrieval
4. *Fertilization and embryo culture*: Each oocyte is incubated with 50–100 thousand motile sperms for 12–18 hours. The fertilized embryos are then transferred into growth media and placed in the incubator. A 4-cell to 8-cell stage, pre-embryo is observed approximately 36–48 hours after insemination
5. *Embryo transfer*: The procedure of embryo transfer is performed transcervically under guidance of transabdominal ultrasound within 72 hours following fertilization, when the embryo has become approximately 8–16 cells in size.

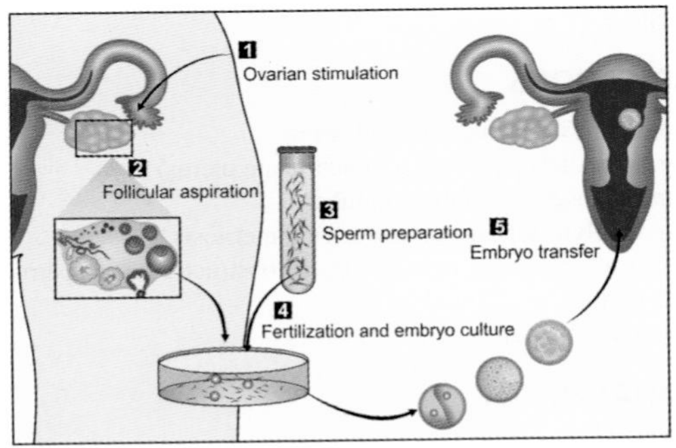

Figure 12.6: Procedure of in vitro fertilization

COMPLICATIONS

- Multiple pregnancies
- Ovarian hyperstimulation syndrome
- Preterm delivery and low birth weight babies
- Probable likelihood of congenital anomalies such as hypospadias, neural tube defects, cleft lip and palate, gastrointestinal malformations, musculoskeletal and chromosomal defects.

CLINICAL PEARLS

- IVF-related procedures such as gamete intrafallopian transfer (GIFT) and zygote intrafallopian transfer (ZIFT) are sometimes used as alternatives to IVF
- Some techniques which help in facilitating fertilization include partial zona dissection (PZD), subzonal sperm injection (SUZI), ICSI and assisted hatching (AH). Currently, only ICSI and AH are being used clinically
- ICSI involves injection of a single live sperm directly into the ovum. ICSI is commonly used in cases of male factor infertility such as obstructive azoospermia
- In order to reduce the chances of multifetal gestation with IVF, the number of embryos transferred has been limited to two at most of the IVF centers.

CHAPTER 13

Disorders of Ovaries and Fallopian Tubes

1. BENIGN OVARIAN TUMORS

INTRODUCTION

Ovarian neoplasms are the most common ovarian masses encountered among women belonging to the reproductive age group. Ovarian cysts (**Fig. 13.1**) can be either neoplastic or non-neoplastic in nature. Of all the ovarian neoplasms, most ovarian tumors (80–85%) are benign and occur in the women between 20 years and 44 years. The classification system devised by WHO for benign and malignant ovarian tumors is shown in **Table 13.1**. Non-neoplastic cysts of ovary are extremely common and can occur at any age (early reproductive age until perimenopause). These cysts are also known as functional cysts and include follicular cysts, corpus luteum cysts and theca lutein cysts.

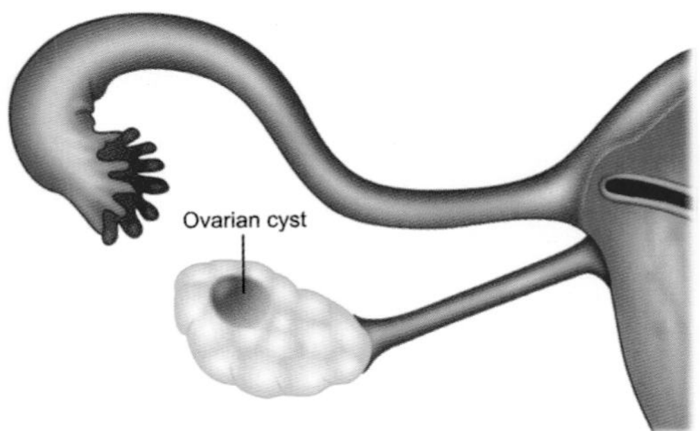

Figure 13.1: An ovarian cyst

Table 13.1: Histological classification of neoplastic ovarian growths

I. Common Epithelial Tumors

A. *Serous Tumors*
   1. Benign
      a. Cystadenoma and papillary cystadenoma
      b. Surface papilloma
      c. Adenofibroma and cystadenofibroma
   2. Of borderline malignancy (carcinomas of low malignant potential)
      a. Cystadenoma and papillary cystadenoma
      b. Surface papilloma
      c. Adenofibroma and cystadenofibroma
   3. Malignant
      a. Adenocarcinoma, papillary adenocarcinoma and papillary cystadenocarcinoma
      b. Surface papillary carcinoma
      c. Malignant adenofibroma and cystadenofibroma

B. *Mucinous Tumors*
   1. Benign
      a. Cystadenoma
      b. Adenofibroma and cystadenofibroma
   2. Of borderline malignancy (carcinomas of low malignant potential)
      a. Cystadenoma
      b. Adenofibroma and cystadenofibroma
   3. Malignant
      a. Adenocarcinoma and cystadenocarcinoma
      b. Malignant adenofibroma and cystadenofibroma

C. *Endometrioid Tumors*
   1. Benign
      a. Adenoma and cystadenoma
      b. Adenofibroma and cystadenofibroma
   2. Of borderline malignancy (carcinomas of low malignant potential)
      a. Adenoma and cystadenoma
      b. Adenofibroma and cystadenofibroma
   3. Malignant
      a. Carcinoma
         i. Adenocarcnoma
         ii. Adenoacanthoma
         iii. Malignant adenofibroma and cystadenofibroma
      b. Endometrioid stromal sarcomas

Contd...

Contd...

   c. Mesodermal (Müllerian) mixed tumors, homologous and heterologous

D. *Clear Cell (Mesonephroid) Tumors*
   1. Benign
   2. Of borderline malignancy (carcinomas of low malignant potential)
   3. Malignant: Carcinoma and adenoma

E. *Brenner Tumors*
   1. Benign
   2. Of borderline malignancy (proliferating)
   3. Malignant

F. *Mixed Epithelial Tumors*
   1. Benign
   2. Of borderline malignancy potential
   3. Malignant

G. *Undifferentiated Carcinoma*

H. *Unclassified Epithelial Tumors*

II. Sex-Cord Stromal Tumors

A. *Granulosa-Stromal Cell Tumors*
   1. Granulosa cell tumor
   2. Tumors in the thecoma-fibroma group
      a. Thecoma
      b. Fibroma
      c. Unclassified

B. *Androblastomas, Sertoli-Leydig Cell Tumors*
   1. Well-differentiated
      a. Tubular androblastoma, Sertoli cell tumor (tubular adenoma of Pick)
      b. Tubular androblastoma with lipid storage, Sertoli cell tumor with lipid storage (folliculome lipidique of Lecene)
      c. Sertoli-Leydig cell tumor (tubular adenoma with Leydig cells)
      d. Leydig cell tumor, hilus cell tumor
   2. Of intermediate differentiation
   3. Poorly differentiated (sarcomatoid)
   4. With heterologous elements

C. *Gynandroblastoma*

D. *Unclassified*

Contd...

Contd...

III. Germ Cell Tumors

A. Dysgerminoma

B. Endodermal Sinus Tumor

C. Embryonal Carcinoma

D. Polyembryoma

E. Choriocarcinoma

F. Teratomas

1. Immature
2. Mature
   a. Solid
   b. Cystic
      i. Dermoid cyst (mature cystic teratoma)
      ii. Dermoid cyst with malignant transformation
3. Monodermal and highly specialized
   a. Struma ovarii
   b. Carcinoid
   c. Struma ovarii and carcinoid
   d. Others G. Mixed Forms

IV. Lipid (Lipoid) Cell Tumors

V. Gonadoblastoma

A. Pure

B. Mixed with dysgerminoma or other form of germ cell tumor

VI. Soft Tissue Tumors Not Specific to Ovary

VII. Unclassified Tumors

VIII. Secondary (Metastatic Tumors)

IX. Tumor Like Conditions

A. Pregnancy Luteoma

B. Hyperplasia of ovarian stroma and hyperthecosis

C. Massive edema

D. Solitary follicle cyst and corpus luteum cyst

E. Multiple follicle cysts (polycystic ovaries)

F. Multiple luteinized follicle cysts and/or corpora lutea

G. Endometriosis

H. Surface-epithelial inclusion cysts (germinal inclusion cysts)

I. Simple cysts

J. Inflammatory lesions

K. Parovarian cysts

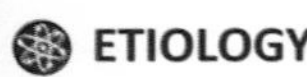

ETIOLOGY

Functional cysts develop due to accumulation of fluid in unruptured Graafian follicles or follicles that have ruptured and sealed.

DIAGNOSIS

Symptoms

- Functional ovarian cysts may be multiple and are usually small in size (1.1–1.5 cm). However, sometimes they can grow up to 3–4 cm in size
- Spontaneous rupture of these cysts can cause pelvic pain and bleeding
- Benign ovarian tumors may sometimes present as massive abdominal swellings (size of a football)
- Menstrual cycles are usually not affected
- Benign ovarian tumors may produce pressure symptoms, such as increased frequency of micturition, dyspnea, palpitations, etc.
- Usually there is no abdominal pain
- Massive tumors may cause abdominal discomfort and distension.

Abdominal Examination

- The upper and lateral limits of the tumor are usually well-defined, but the lower limit of the tumor cannot be identified
- The tumor is not fixed either to the skin or underlying tissues
- Cystic tumors have a tense and cystic consistency. Fluid thrill can be elicited
- Presence of ascites is indicative of underlying malignancy.

Bimanual Examination

- Uterus is felt separate from the tumors in case of small tumors
- With large tumors, it may be difficult to feel the uterus separately

Investigations

Ultrasound: Ultrasonography (both TAS and TVS) is accurate in differentiating tumors of the ovary from other types of tumors of the pelvis in more than 90% of the patients. It also helps in differentiating between benign and malignant lesions of the ovary **(Fig. 13.2)**. In general, benign lesions are likely to be unilateral, unilocular and thin walled with no papillae or solid areas and thin septae. In contrast, malignant lesions are often multilocular with thick walls, thick septae and mixed echogenicity due to the presence of solid areas. Doppler flow studies of the ovarian artery may also help in differentiating between benign and malignant growths.

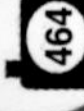

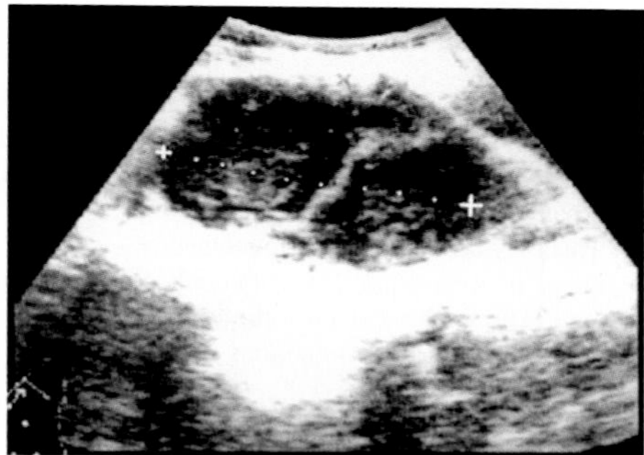

Figure 13.2: TAS showing a multiloculated mass with presence of cystic areas along with a few brightly echogenic areas. Differential diagnosis of mucinous cystadenoma and dermoid cyst were established

DIFFERENTIAL DIAGNOSIS

These include conditions, such as full bladder, pregnancy, myomas, ascites, abdominal tumors, such as hydroneprosis, mesenteric cysts, retroperitoneal tumors and tuberculous peritonitis.

MANAGEMENT

- Most follicular ovarian cysts are likely to disappear spontaneously within a period of few weeks to a few months. Therefore, the first line of management involves close observation of the patient
- Ultrasound-guided cyst aspiration is another option, but is associated with a high recurrence rate
- If the cyst persists for longer than 2 months, possibility of malignancy must be kept in mind and the patient investigated for underlying neoplastic changes
- Laparotomy is required in cases of persistent cysts in order to obtain the specimen for histopathology and for its definitive treatment involving removal. Even a benign ovarian tumor may require removal because of the risk of development of malignancy in the long term
- At the time of laparotomy, various treatment options that can be considered in cases of benign diseases are abdominal hysterectomy with bilateral salpingo-oophorectomy, unilateral ovariotomy, ovarian cystectomy or laparoscopic cystectomy or ovariotomy.

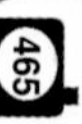

COMPLICATIONS

- *Torsion*: This complication most commonly occurs with parovarian or broad ligament cysts. Torsion causes occlusion of veins in the pedicle resulting in congestion and hemorrhage. This may cause severe abdominal pain and signs of peritoneal irritation
- *Rupture*: This may be traumatic or spontaneous
- *Pseudomyxoma of peritoneum*: This commonly occurs with a mucinous cystadenoma. The peritoneal mesothelium is converted into high columnar cells which secrete mucinous material into the peritoneal cavity
- *Infection*.

CLINICAL PEARLS

- Most follicular ovarian masses resolve spontaneously in 4–8 weeks
- Persistence of an ovarian lesion for more than 6–12 weeks is an important sign indicating the presence of neoplastic ovarian masses
- The most common histological type of nonmalignant ovarian neoplasm is papillary serous cystadenoma
- Torsion most commonly occurs with a mucinous cystadenoma

2. POLYCYSTIC OVARIAN DISEASE

INTRODUCTION

The condition, polycystic ovarian syndrome, also known as PCOS, is a relatively common endocrine disorder amongst women of reproductive age group. It is characterized by the presence of many minute cysts in the ovaries and excessive production of androgens. According to the American Society of Reproductive Medicine (ASRM) and the European Society of Human Reproduction and Embryology (ESHRE) joint consensus meeting in November 2003, the diagnosis of PCOS should be made, when two of the following three criteria are met:

1. Infrequent or absent ovulation
2. Clinical or biochemical features of hyperandrogenism, such as excessive hair growth, acne, raised LH and raised androgen levels
3. Morphologically there is bilateral enlargement, thickened ovarian capsule, multiple follicular cysts (usually ranging between 2 mm to 8 mm in diameter) and an increased amount of stroma.

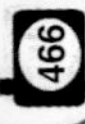

ETIOLOGY

Despite of many years of research, the pathophysiology of PCOS has not been completely understood. Common endocrine abnormalities in PCOS include chronically high levels of LH, thereby resulting in an elevated LH/FSH ratio (usually 2.5 or greater), hyperandrogenism, hyperinsulinemia, insulin resistance and dyslipidemia. These endocrine disturbances interfere with ovarian folliculogenesis and result in anovulation. Moreover, these endocrine disturbances are likely to constitute towards an increased risk for development of cardiovascular diseases and diabetes.

DIAGNOSIS

Symptoms

Symptoms such as obesity, features of androgen excess such as hirsutism, oligomenorrhea or amenorrhea, infrequent or absent ovulation, miscarriage and infertility are commonly present.

Investigations

- *Blood hormone levels*: FSH levels are low or normal and LH levels are often raised, resulting in a raised LH/FSH ratio. The levels of androgens and testosterone may also be raised
- *Ultrasound examination*: Features of polycystic ovarian morphology on ultrasound scan are as follows **(Fig. 13.3)**:
  - Greater than 12 follicles measuring between 2 mm and 9 mm in diameter, located peripherally, resulting in a pearl necklace appearance
  - Increased echogenity of ovarian stroma and/or ovarian volume greater than 10 mL.

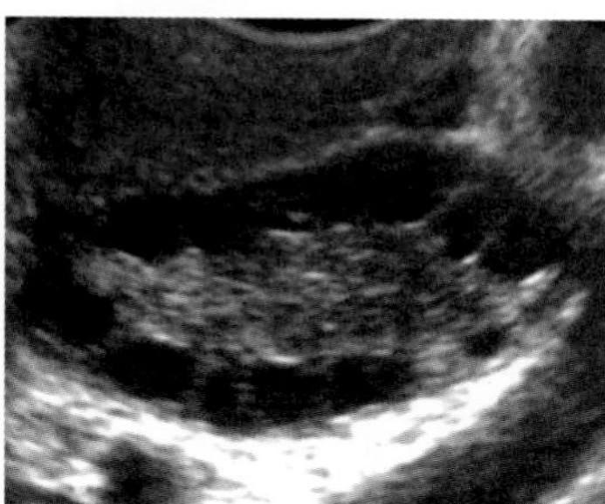

Figure 13.3: Ultrasound features of polycystic ovarian morphology

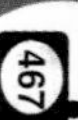

MEDICAL MANAGEMENT

- *Life style changes*: Exercise to maintain a normal BMI
- *Ovulation induction drugs*: The treatment of choice in patients with PCOS is ovulation induction with clomiphene citrate, which is associated with nearly 70% rate of ovulation after the first treatment cycle
- *Metformin*: Metformin has now become the first line of management in cases of clomiphene citrate resistant women with PCOS.

SURGICAL MANAGEMENT

Laparoscopic ovarian drilling (LOD) is sometimes used for women with PCOS, who do not respond to first line treatment options, such as weight loss and use of medicines. In LOD, different techniques, such as electrocauterization, laser, electrocoagulation, biopsy, etc. are used for destroying ovarian follicles. The procedure of LOB is demonstrated in **Figures 13.4A to D**.

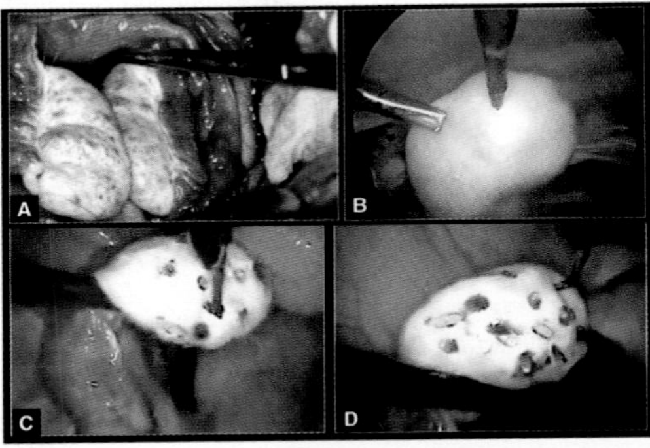

Figures 13.4A to D: (A) Laparoscopic visualization of the pelvis in an effort to locate the ovaries; (B) lifting the ovaries out of the ovarian fossa and placing them over the cervicouterine junction; (C) the procedure of LOD using electrocauterization; Cauterization is performed by utilizing pure cutting current equivalent to 40 watts. Number of holes varying from 4 to 20 are usually made in each ovary; (D) appearance of ovary following the procedure

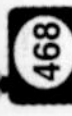

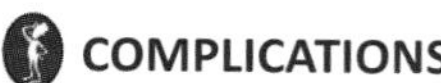

COMPLICATIONS

- Accidental injury to internal organs or major blood vessels from laparoscope or other surgical instruments
- Internal bleeding
- Pain after the procedure as a result of pneumoperitoneum
- Problems caused by anesthesia
- *Adhesions*: LOD has a small but definite potential for causing tubal adhesions
- *Atrophy*: Ovarian atrophy and failure is a rare complication of LOD
- The use of gonadotropins may be associated with complications, such as polyfollicular response, risk of ovarian hyperstimulation syndrome, multiple pregnancy, etc.

CLINICAL PEARLS

- Usually, the surgical approach (LOD) is chosen when a patient has already failed to ovulate on clomiphene citrate at maximal doses and has not responded to insulin sensitizing agents
- LOD is a minimally invasive, safe and cost-effective procedure, which is associated with a low complication rate, such as postoperative adhesions.

3. DISORDERS OF FALLOPIAN TUBES

3.1. SALPINGITIS

INTRODUCTION

Salpingitis is the inflammation of the fallopian tube, which is most commonly caused by an infection (see the fragment on PID in Chapter 11). The tubes become swollen, hyperemic and edematous. Some discharge of seropurulent fluid may occur from the fimbrial end of the tube. Initially, as the fimbrial end of the tube is open, pus discharge pours out into the pelvic cavity resulting in the formation of pelvic abscess. Eventually with the sealing of fimbrial end by fibrinous exudates, there is accumulation of pus in the tubal lumen, resulting in the formation of pyosalpinx. Involvement of ovaries, along with the tubes and presence of adhesions results in the development of TOA.

ETIOLOGY

STDs such as *Neisseria gonorrhoeae* and *Chlamydia trachomatis* are the most common causes of acute salpingitis.

Multiple organisms which may be involved include *Gardnerella vaginalis*, *Escherichia coli*, *Haemophilus influenzae*, Group B beta-hemolytic streptococci, nonhemolytic streptococci, *Prevotella bivia*, *Bacteroides* species, *Peptostreptococcus* species, *Mycoplasma hominis*, etc.

Risk factors for development of salpingitis are same as that described in the fragment on PID.

DIAGNOSIS

Clinical Presentation

- The clinical presentation of salpingitis may range from asymptomatic to severe pelvic pain and diffuse peritonitis to, rarely, life-threatening illness
- The classic clinical triad of fever, elevated ESR and adnexal tenderness or mass may not be observed in all the cases.

Other symptoms: Lower abdominal pain, vaginal discharge, irregular bleeding, urinary symptoms, vomiting, proctitis and marked tenderness on bimanual examination.

General physical examination: The findings on general physical examination and pelvic examination are same as that described in the fragment on PID.

Investigations

These are same as those described in the fragment on PID.

MANAGEMENT

Medical and surgical management is same as that described in the fragment on PID.

COMPLICATIONS

- Long-term sequelae include chronic pelvic pain, TOA, hydrosalpinx, tubal infertility and ectopic pregnancy
- Distention of ampullary portion more than that of the isthmic portion results in the development of a retort shaped mass called pyosalpinx
- Failure of acute infection to resolve the development of chronic PID, which may result in the formation of hydrosalpinx, pyosalpinx, interstitial salpingitis, TOA, etc.

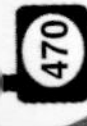

- Rarely, there may be an upwards spread of infection, resulting in the development of peritonitis, paralytic ileus, subdiaphragmatic and perinephric abscess.

CLINICAL PEARLS

- Untreated cases may be associated with irreversible damage to the fallopian tubes
- Recurrent pelvic infection commonly occurs due to tubercular infection.

3.2. ECTOPIC PREGNANCY

INTRODUCTION

Ectopic means "out of place". In an ectopic pregnancy, the fertilized ovum gets implanted outside the uterus as a result of which the pregnancy occurs outside the uterine cavity **(Fig. 13.5)**. Most commonly, i.e. in nearly 95% of cases, the fertilized ovum gets implanted inside the fallopian tube. Other extrauterine locations where an ectopic pregnancy can get implanted include the ovary, abdomen or the cervix. Since none of these locations have been equipped by nature to support a growing pregnancy, with continuing growth of fetus, the gestational sac and the organ containing it burst open **(Figs 13.6A to D)**. This can result in severe bleeding, sometimes even endangering the woman's life.

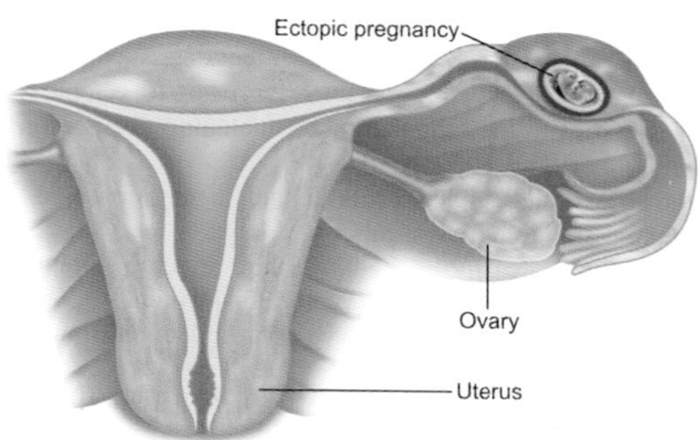

Figure 13.5: Ectopic pregnancy

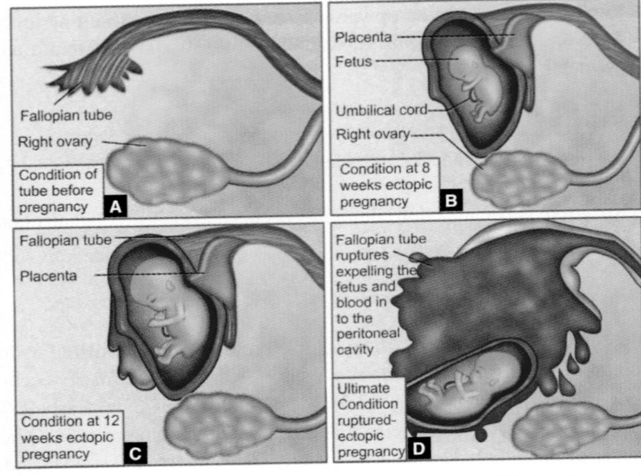

Figures 13.6A to D: Course of ectopic pregnancy with the increasing gestational age

ETIOLOGY

The major cause of ectopic pregnancy is acute salpingitis, accounting for 50% of cases. In nearly 40% of cases, the cause remains unknown. The risk factors for ectopic pregnancy are as follows:

- Prior history of an ectopic pregnancy
- Pelvic infections: History of pelvic infections, such as PID, STD, salpingitis and tuberculosis, is an important cause for ectopic pregnancy
- Prior surgeries to the fallopian tubes, including tubal reconstructive surgery, tubectomy, etc.
- Endometriosis and pelvic scar tissue (pelvic adhesions)
- Congenital abnormalities of tubes
- Smoking is a risk factor in about one third of ectopic pregnancies
- Patients belonging to the age group of 35–44 years
- Infertility problems and use of ovulation induction drugs and other assisted reproductive techniques
- Use of progestin-only pills or progesterone-releasing IUD
- Salpingitis isthmica nodosa (SIN)
- History of in utero exposure to diethylstilbestrol.

DIAGNOSIS

Symptoms

- Initial symptoms are very much similar to those of a normal early pregnancy, e.g. missed periods, breast tenderness, nausea, vomiting or frequent urination
- The typical triad on history for ectopic pregnancy includes bleeding, abdominal pain and a positive urine pregnancy test. These symptoms typically occur 6–8 weeks after the last normal menstrual period. Acute blood loss in some cases may result in the development of dizziness or fainting and hypotension
- Many women with ectopic pregnancy may remain asymptomatic.

General Physical Examination

- Normal signs of early pregnancy (e.g. uterine softening)
- Evidence of hemodynamic instability (hypotension, collapse, signs and symptoms of shock).

Abdominal Examination

- Abdominal pain and tenderness
- Signs of peritoneal irritation (abdominal rigidity, guarding, etc.) are indicative of ruptured ectopic pregnancy.

Pelvic Examination

- Vaginal bleeding may be observed on per speculum examination
- Uterine or cervical motion tenderness on vaginal examination may suggest peritoneal inflammation
- The uterus may be slightly enlarged and soft
- An adnexal mass may be palpated (with or without tenderness).

Investigations

- *Blood (ABO and Rh type)*: Rh negative patients must be injected with 50 μg of anti-D immune globulins to prevent the occurrence of hemolytic disease of the newborn
- *Urine or Serum β hCG levels*: Determination of the levels of β hCG in the urine or serum helps in establishing the diagnosis of pregnancy. According to the ACOG recommendations (2008), an increase in serum β hCG levels of less than 53% in 48 hours confirms an abnormal

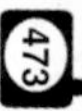

pregnancy. Ectopic pregnancy is suspected if TAS does not show an intrauterine gestational sac and the patient's β hCG level is greater than 6,500 mIU per mL (6,500 IU per L) or if TVS does not show an intrauterine gestational sac and the patient's β hCG level is 1,500 mIU per mL (1,500 IU per L) or greater

- *Imaging studies*: Signs of a definite ectopic pregnancy on TVS examination are as follows:
    - A thick, bright echogenic, ring-like structure, which is located outside the uterus, having a gestational sac containing an obvious fetal pole, yolk sac or both. This usually appears as an intact, well-defined tubal ring (Doughnut or Bagel sign)
    - An empty uterus or presence of a centrally placed pseudogestational sac
    - Cystic or solid adnexal or tubal masses **(Fig. 13.7)** and severe adnexal tenderness with probe palpation are also suggestive of ectopic pregnancy
    - Ruptured ectopic pregnancy: In case of a ruptured ectopic pregnancy, the ultrasonographic findings include presence of free fluid or clotted blood in the cul-de-sac or in the intraperitoneal gutters.

DIFFERENTIAL DIAGNOSIS

Obstetric Causes

- Threatened or incomplete miscarriage or septic abortion
- Early pregnancy with pelvic tumors.

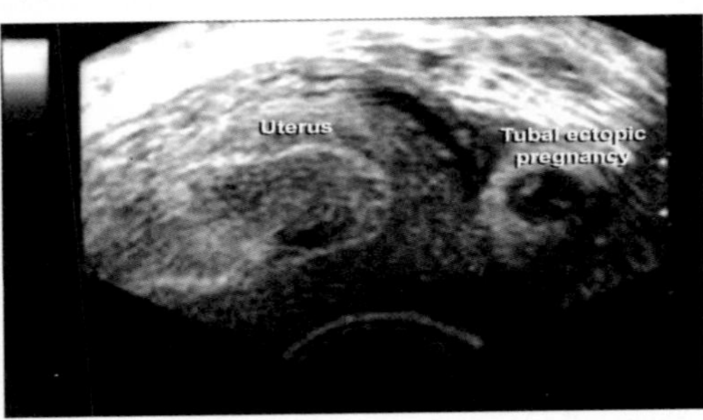

Figure 13.7: Ultrasound showing an ectopic pregnancy of the left tube

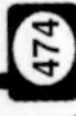

Gynecological Causes

- Pelvic inflammatory disease
- Ruptured or hemorrhagic corpus luteum
- Adnexal torsion
- Degenerating fibroids, DUB, endometriosis.

Non-gynecological Diseases

- Appendicitis, urinary calculi, gastroentritis
- Intraperitoneal hemorrhage, perforated peptic ulcer.

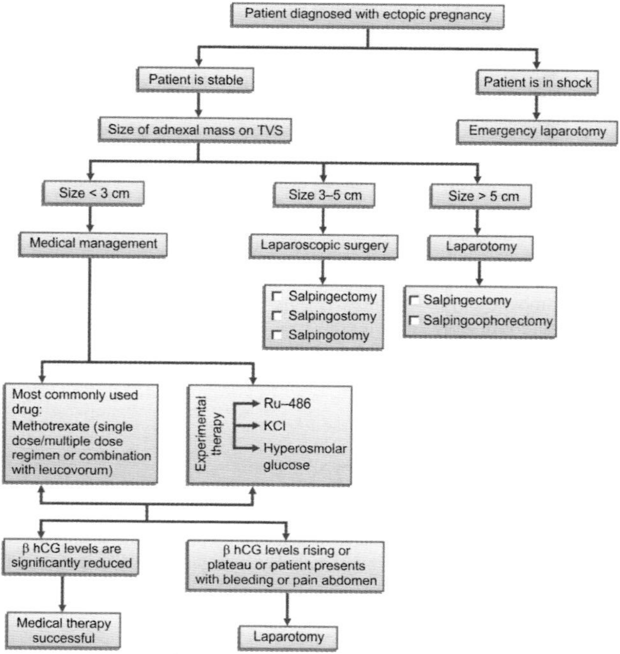

- Patient diagnosed with ectopic pregnancy
  - Patient is stable
    - Size of adnexal mass on TVS
      - Size < 3 cm
        - Medical management
          - Most commonly used drug: Methotrexate (single dose/multiple dose regimen or combination with leucovorum)
          - Experimental therapy
            - Ru–486
            - KCl
            - Hyperosmolar glucose
          - β hCG levels are significantly reduced
            - Medical therapy successful
          - β hCG levels rising or plateau or patient presents with bleeding or pain abdomen
            - Laparotomy
      - Size 3–5 cm
        - Laparoscopic surgery
          - Salpingectomy
          - Salpingostomy
          - Salpingotomy
      - Size > 5 cm
        - Laparotomy
          - Salpingectomy
          - Salpingoophorectomy
  - Patient is in shock
    - Emergency laparotomy

Figure 13.8: Various treatment options in case of an ectopic pregnancy

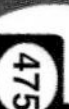

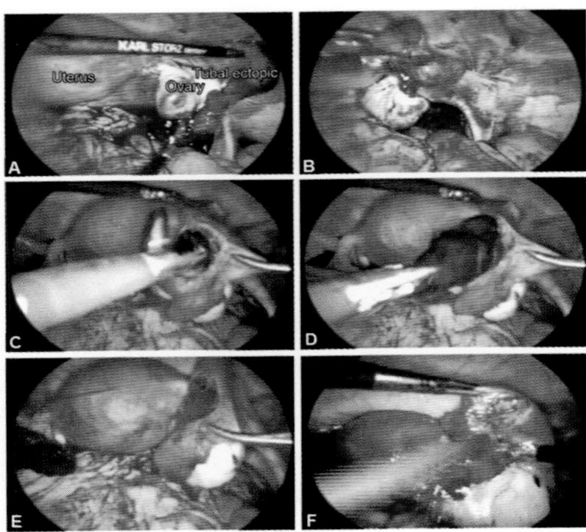

Figures 13.9A to F: Laparoscopic salpingotomy: (A) laproscopic view showing the uterus, adnexa and the tubal ectopic pregnancy; (B) grasping the tube containing ectopic pregnancy, before giving the incision; (C) a small 1 cm incision is given over the tubal ectopic; (D) tubal contents being removed out of the tube; (E) the entire salpingotomy incision is left unstitched, only the bleeding vessels on the incision site are coagulated; (F) irrigation of the area of incision with normal saline before closing the abdomen

MANAGEMENT

Various treatment options in case of an ectopic pregnancy are shown in **Figure 13.8**. Surgical treatment in form of open surgery (laparotomy) or minimal invasive surgery (laparoscopy) is the most commonly used treatment option. The procedures which can be performed at the time of both laparotomy and laparoscopy include salpingectomy or salpingotomy (**Figs 13.9A to F**).

CLINICAL PEARLS

- Ectopic pregnancy can be considered as the leading cause of pregnancy-related deaths during the first trimester

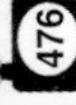

- In a hemodynamically stable patient with ectopic pregnancy, laparoscopic approach is preferable to laparotomy.

4. DISORDERS OF BROAD LIGAMENT AND PARAMETRIUM

4.1. PARAMETRITIS

INTRODUCTION

Parametritis can be defined as cellulitis within the tissues of parametrium. It usually results from an ascending infection, and may be classified under PID.

ETIOLOGY

- Parametritis may follow childbirth or abortion
- Can occur due to infection of parametrium from tears and lacerations of the vaginal portion of the cervix and/or vaginal vault
- Acute infection of uterus and fallopian tubes
- Advanced carcinoma of the cervix.

DIAGNOSIS

Symptoms

- Pain in the hypogastrium and back
- Temperature rise to about 102° F
- Increased pulse rate in proportion to fever
- Rectal symptoms may arise in case of involvement of rectum.

Pelvic Examination

- Development of a large indurated swelling in the pelvis, extending from the uterus to the lateral pelvic wall
- Uterus may be fixed to the pelvis and it may be difficult to separate the swelling from the uterus
- The parametrial effusion may spread upwards, resulting in the development of swelling above the poupart's ligament.

MANAGEMENT

- Bed rest
- Local heat application
- Full course of antibiotics.

COMPLICATIONS

- Scarring of parametrium resulting in chronic pelvic pain
- Kinking of the ureters due to adhesions resulting in hydronephrosis
- Pelvic thrombophlebitis and associated pyemia
- Pulmonary infraction and extension to the lower extremity resulting in white leg.

CLINICAL PEARLS

- Since the effusion is extraperitoneal, symptoms of peritoneal irritation are usually absent.

4.2. BROAD LIGAMENT LEIOMYOMA

INTRODUCTION

Fibroids can sometimes occur at extrauterine locations; amongst the various extrauterine locations, broad ligament fibroids are the most common to occur.

ETIOLOGY

Broad ligament leiomyomas can originate from the uterus and invade the broad ligament or they can originate from the broad ligament itself.

DIAGNOSIS

Symptoms

- Small tumors are usually asymptomatic
- A leiomyoma of significant size, however, can distort the anatomy of the pelvis, pushing the uterus to the contralateral side
- A large tumor can also compress the ureter, resulting in hydronephrosis.

Abdominal Examination

There may be presence of an abdominal lump, which may appear to be arising from the pelvis.

Pelvic Examination

A mass may be felt in the pouch of Douglas.

Investigations

- *Ultrasound examination*
- *Histopathological examination*: This is similar to that of uterine fibroids.

DIFFERENTIAL DIAGNOSIS

Other causes of a pelvic mass, such as ovarian cysts, ovarian cancer, tumors of the retroperitoneum, TOA, etc.

SURGICAL MANAGEMENT

- An incision is made on the anterior or posterior leaf of the broad ligament and the leiomyomas is slowly shelled out in a manner similar to that described in the fragment of fibroids in Chapter 11
- Thorough exposure of ureter and vessels before shelling out of the myoma is required in order to minimize the chances of injury to these structures.

COMPLICATIONS

- Degenerative changes may occur in these extrauterine fibroids
- These fibroids can massively increase in size resulting in an abdominal lump and/or ascites
- Removal of these fibroids may present with difficulties due to risk of injury to ureter and uterine artery at the time of dissection.

CLINICAL PEARLS

- Though the most common solid tumor of the broad ligament is a leiomyoma, other extremely rare primary tumors of the broad ligament include primary leiomyosarcomas, the Ewing sarcoma family of tumors, steroid cell tumor occurring outside the ovary or the adrenal gland and papillary cystadenoma of the broad ligament.

4.3. BROAD LIGAMENT HEMATOMA

INTRODUCTION

- Broad ligament hematoma results from a tear in the upper vagina, cervix or uterus that extends into uterine or vaginal arteries.

ETIOLOGY

- Broad ligament hematoma most commonly occur following operative delivery, trauma or surgery:
  - May occur due to cervical lacerations following spontaneous vaginal delivery
  - May occur due to extraperitoneal rupture of ectopic pregnancy into the broad ligament
  - May occur due to concealed accidental hemorrhage
  - Can occur due to tears during cervical dilatation at the time of D&C or D&E procedures
  - Use of prophylactic or therapeutic anticoagulants in postoperative period can result in the development of a hematoma.

DIAGNOSIS

Clinical Symptoms

- Most patients complain of back pain, fullness or pressure in the rectoanal area, or an urge to push
- Extreme cases may experience tachycardia, hypotension, complaints of dizziness and hemorrhagic shock. This may be a potentially life-threatening condition.

Abdominal Examination

Sometimes the hematoma may spread extraperitoneally and move upwards resulting in the development of swelling above the poupart's ligament. It may sometimes also spread to the perinephric regions, resulting in the development of swelling there.

Pelvic Examination

A rectovaginal examination should be performed to rule out the presence of clots in the vagina or the possibility of an expanding vaginal hematoma.

Investigations

- *Ultrasound examination*
- *Pelvic MRI*: This should be used to evaluate patients with persistent postpartum localized pelvic pain, fullness or discomfort, or a sudden drop in hematocrit level with no apparent source of bleeding.

MANAGEMENT

- *Conservative management*: Small cases of broad ligament hematoma may respond to conservative management comprising of observation, blood transfusion and fluid resuscitation
- *Surgical exploration and evacuation*: Larger hematomas may require hematoma drainage and ligation of the bleeder.

COMPLICATIONS

- Hemorrhagic shock.

CLINICAL PEARLS

- Some cases of broad ligament hematoma have been treated using uterine artery embolization
- These can be dangerous as they may be silent and not cause obvious vaginal bleeding.

CHAPTER 14

Urogynecology

1. GENITOURINARY FISTULAE

INTRODUCTION

Urogenital fistulas (UGFs) can be defined as abnormal communication tracts (lined with epithelium) between the genital tract and the urinary tract or the alimentary tract or both. UGFs can be classified as follows **(Fig. 14.1)**:

- Urethrovaginal
- Vesical fistula [vesicovaginal fistula (VVF) or vesicocervical]
- Ureterovaginal
- Rectovaginal.

VVF is an abnormal fistulous tract extending between the bladder and the vagina that allows the continuous involuntary discharge of urine into the vaginal vault.

ETIOLOGY

- Most common cause in developing countries is obstructed labor **(Fig. 14.2)**

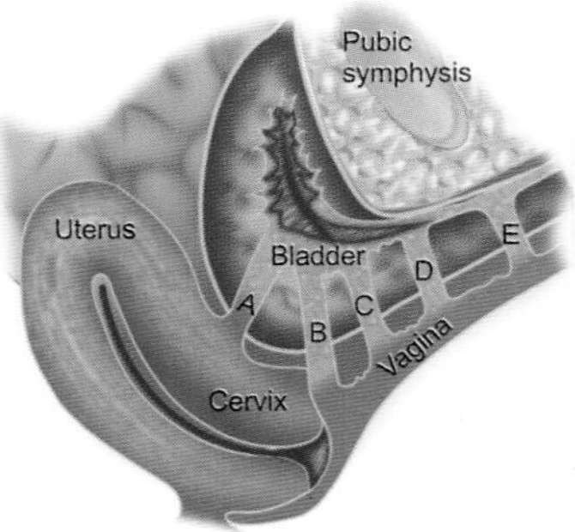

Figure 14.1: Types of genitourinary fistulas: (A) uterovesical fistula; (B) cervicovesical fistula; (C) midvaginal VVF; (D) VVF involving the bladder neck; (E) urethrovaginal fistula

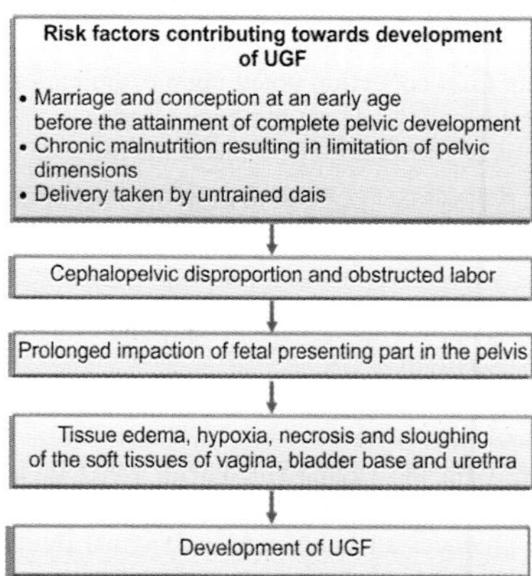

Figure 14.2: Development of UGF as a result of obstructed labor

- Other obstetric causes include difficult forceps or cesarean delivery
- The majority of UGFs in developed countries are a result of gynecological surgery (pelvic surgery, surgery for gynecological malignancy, hysterectomy, urologic and gastrointestinal surgery)
- Radiotherapy and surgery for malignant gynecologic disease is also responsible for a minority of cases.

DIAGNOSIS

Symptoms

- The uncontrolled continuous leakage of urine into the vagina is the hallmark symptom of patients with UGFs
- Patients may complain of urinary incontinence or an increase in vaginal discharge
- Constant wetness in the genital areas can lead to the excoriation of the vagina, vulva, perineum and thighs
- Presence of recurrent cystitis or pyelonephritis, abnormal urinary stream and hematuria following surgery may point towards an underlying UGF.

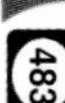

Per Speculum Examination

Evaluation of the fluid collection noted upon examination of the vaginal vault must be performed to rule out presence of urine or vaginal discharge. Once the diagnosis of urine discharge is made, the clinician needs to identify its source.

Investigations

- Complete blood count
- *Urine investigations*: This includes urine routine, microscopy and urine culture and sensitivity
- *Renal function tests*: This includes estimation of serum urea, uric acid, creatinine and electrolytes
- *Cystoscopy*: With the vagina filled with water or isotonic sodium chloride solution, the infusion of gas through the urethra through a cystoscope produces air bubbles in the vaginal fluid at the site of a UGF (Flat tire sign)
- *Methylene blue three-swab test*: With the vaginal cavity packed with three sterile swabs, a catheter is introduced into the bladder through the urethra. Approximately 50–100 mL of methylene blue dye is injected into the bladder via the catheter. In case of VVF, dye stains the upper most swab. The lower most swab gets stained if the leakage is from urethra. If none of the swabs get stained, but get wet from urine, leakage is from the ureter
- *Ultrasonography*: Sonography of the kidney, ureter and bladder must be performed
- *Methylene blue dye test*: The bladder can be filled with sterile milk or methylene blue in retrograde fashion using a small transurethral catheter to identify the site of leakage.

DIFFERENTIAL DIAGNOSIS

The various types of fistulas, which need to be differentiated include vesicovaginal, vesicocervical, urethrovaginal, ureterovaginal and rectovaginal fistulas.

CONSERVATIVE MANAGEMENT

Conservative management can be considered for small fistulas (< 1 cm), and comprises of using an indwelling catheter to ensure continuous drainage of urine and antibiotic therapy.

SURGICAL MANAGEMENT

Preoperative Preparation

- *Timing of repair*: A waiting period for an 8-week to 12-week interval is required for the healing of the tissues to occur
- *Estrogen treatment*: Treatment with estrogen vaginal cream is recommended for patients with VVFs who are hypoestrogenic
- *Patient positioning*: The most commonly followed position for proximal urethral and bladder neck fistulas is Lawson position in which the patient is placed in a prone position with the knees spread and ankles raised in the air and supported by stirrups.

Steps of Surgery

The vaginal approach for surgery includes the following procedures:

Latzko's partial colpocleisis procedure: This involves denuding the vaginal epithelium all around the edge of the fistula and then approximating the wide raw surfaces with rows of absorbable sutures (**Figs 14.3A to C**). The vesical edges of the fistula are not denuded. The posterior vaginal wall becomes the posterior bladder wall and reepithelializes with transitional epithelium.

Flap-splitting technique: This technique is described in **Figures 14.4A to E**. Other points to be noted are:

- In case of extensive fibrosis, application of omental grafts or interpositioning of maritus or gracilis muscle graft between the bladder and vaginal muscles promotes healing
- If the first attempt at the fistula repair fails, the second must be undertaken only after a period of 3 months

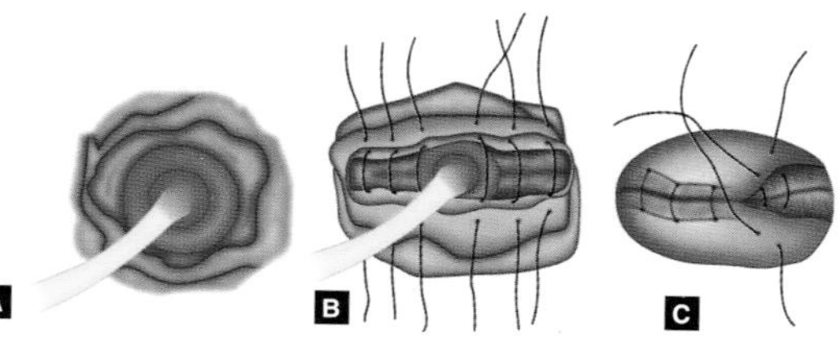

Figures 14.3A to C: Steps of Latzko's partial colpocleisis

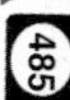

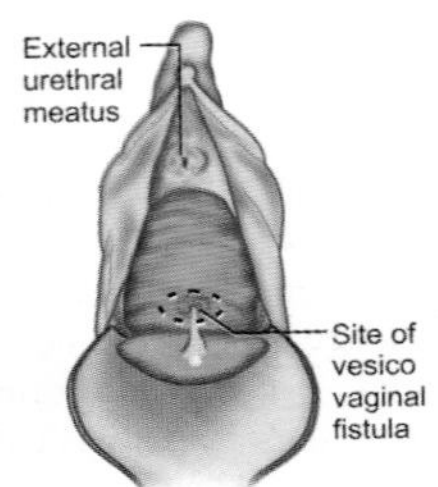

Figure 14.4A: Vesicovaginal fistula located on the posterior wall of the bladder

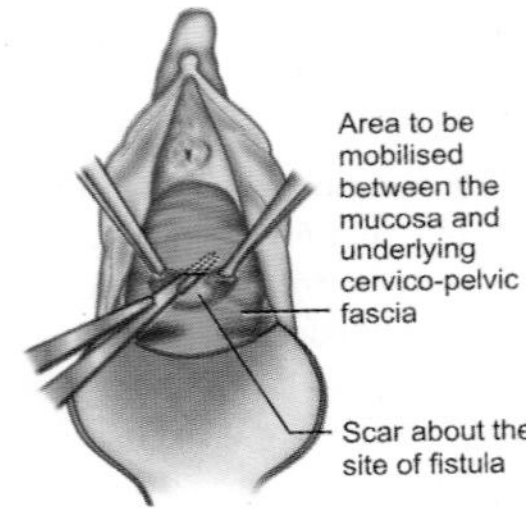

Figure 14.4B: An incision is made about the fistula opening, which is extended into a transverse vaginal incision. The vagina is dissected from the bladder to allow mobilization of tissues and subsequently reduced tension on the suture lines

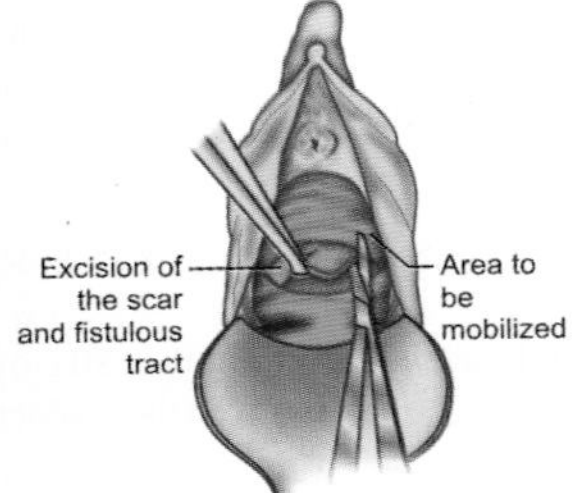

Figure 14.4C: The fistula scar is excised converting the opening into fresh injury

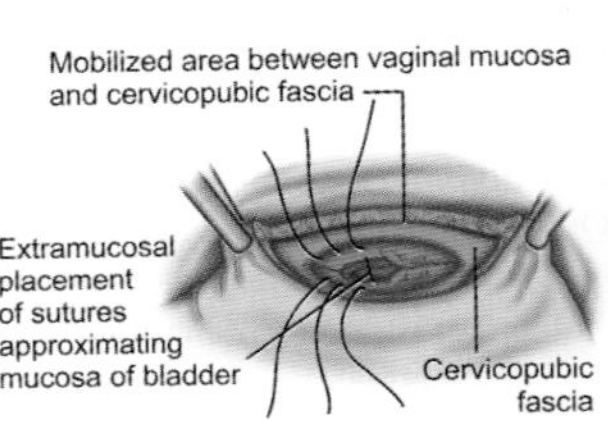

Figure 14.4D: Closure performed with the initial suture layer of 4-0 delayed absorbable sutures placed in an extramucosal fashion

Figure 14.4E: The initial suture line is inverted with similar suture. Each suture line inverting the previous suture line is placed 3–4 mm lateral to the initially closed suture line

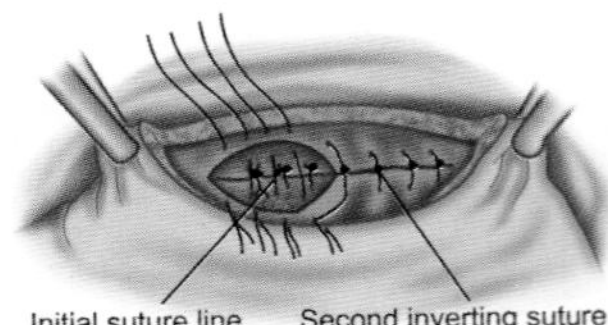

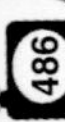

- Urinary diversion procedures (e.g. implantation of ureters into the sigmoid colon, creating an ileal loop bladder or a rectal bladder) can be considered in cases where there is extensive loss of bladder tissue, previous failed attempts at fistula closure or fistula formation due to radiation injury.

Postoperative Care

- *Bladder drainage*: Continuous bladder drainage postoperatively is vital for successful UGF repair
- *Antibiotics*: Treatment with antibiotics helps in eradication of infection
- *Acidification of urine*: This helps in reducing the risk of complications such as cystitis, mucus production and formation of bladder calculi. Vitamin C in the dosage of 500 mg orally 3 times per day may be used to acidify urine
- *Pelvic rest*: Pelvic and speculum examinations of the vagina must be avoided during the first 4–6 weeks postoperatively because during this time, the tissue is fragile and delicate. Sexual intercourse and tampon use must also be prohibited.

COMPLICATIONS

- Risks of infection, hemorrhage, thromboembolism and even death
- Injury to other organs, particularly the ureters
- Possible new fistula formation
- Sexual dysfunction or dissatisfaction, new-onset incontinence, and/or worsening of the previously present incontinence
- Requirement for cesarean delivery during subsequent pregnancies.

CLINICAL PEARLS

- The most common type of fistula in the developing countries is VVF at the bladder neck region following difficult childbirth. Such a woman is often short statured with a contracted pelvis
- Prior to undertaking surgery, urine sample must be collected by catheterization and must be submitted for culture and sensitivity. Any infection must be treated prior to surgery
- At the time of surgery, routine excision of the fistula tract is not mandatory
- Successful fistula repair requires adequate dissection and mobilization of tissues, meticulous hemostasis and reapproximation under minimal tension.

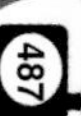

2. URINARY INCONTINENCE

INTRODUCTION

Urinary incontinence can be defined as an involuntary loss of urine which is a social or hygienic problem and can be demonstrated with objective means. There are two main types of urinary incontinence **(Figs 14.5A and B)**: stress incontinence and urge incontinence.

ETIOLOGY

Urinary incontinence usually has a multifactorial etiology and includes the following:

- Structural and functional disorders involving the bladder, urethra, ureters and surrounding connective tissues
- Disorders of the spinal cord or CNS (stroke, multiple sclerosis and Parkinson disease)
- Some cases of urinary incontinence may be pharmacologically induced (e.g. sedatives, anticholinergic drugs, antispasmodics, alpha adrenergic agonists, alpha blockers, calcium channel blockers, etc.)
- Weakening of pelvic connective tissues due to repeated child births (especially vaginal deliveries with episiotomy)
- Genitourinary atrophy due to hypoestrogenism (especially in relation to menopause).

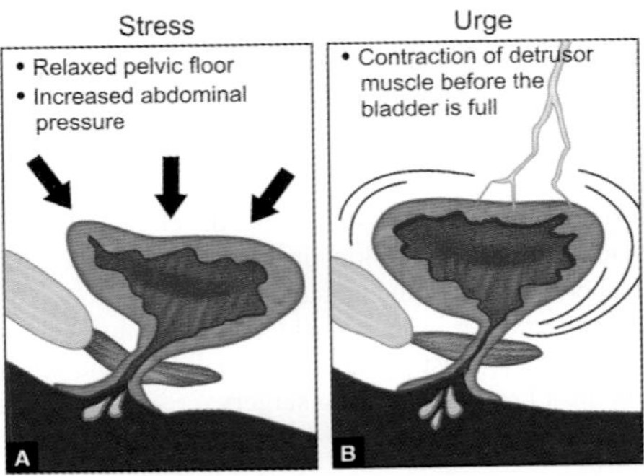

Figures 14.5A and B: Types of incontinence: (A) stress incontinence; (B) urge incontinence

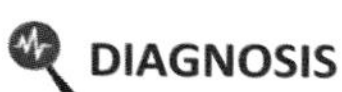

DIAGNOSIS

Clinical Presentation

- Involuntary loss of urine (either triggered by stress or associated with urgency). This may present as a social and/or hygienic problem
- The complaints may be minor and situational or severe, constant and debilitating
- There may be concomitant symptoms of fecal incontinence or pelvic organ prolapse
- *General physical examination*: The examination is tailored based on each specific case history. The following parameters must be recorded for each patient: height; weight; blood pressure and pulse. The grading system for urinary incontinence as devised by Stamey (1970) is described in **Table 14.1**

Table 14.1: Grading system for urinary incontinence

Grade	*Definition*
0	Continent
1	Loss of urine with sudden increase in abdominal pressure, not in bed at night
2	Incontinence worsens with lesser degree of physical stress
3	Incontinence with walking, standing erect from sitting position or sitting up in bed
4	Total incontinence occurs and urine is lost without relation to physical activity or position

- *Pelvic examination*: This is important for ruling out the coexisting pelvic floor relaxation.

Investigations

- Urinalysis and culture to rule out infection
- Urine cytology to rule out malignancy
- Hypermobility of the urethra as determined by the cotton swab test
- Frequency/volume bladder chart
- Measurement of postvoid residual urine
- Cystometry/urodynamic studies: To rule out detrusor over-activity
- Cough stress testing: Described in the fragment on stress incontinence
- Presence of UGF must be ruled out as described in the previous fragment.

MANAGEMENT

Management has been discussed in details in the fragments of stress and urge incontinence.

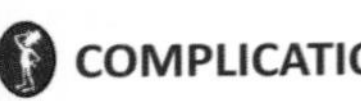

COMPLICATIONS

- The patients should be prepared for the possibility of postoperative complications, procedure failure, and prolonged catheterization or intermittent self-catheterization
- Complications related to surgery are described in the fragment on stress incontinence.

2.1. STRESS URINARY INCONTINENCE

INTRODUCTION

Stress urinary incontinence (SUI) can be defined as involuntary leakage of urine during conditions causing an increase in intra-abdominal pressure (exertion, sneezing, coughing or exercise) which causes the intravesical pressure to rise higher than that which the urethral closure mechanisms can withstand (in the absence of detrusor contractions).

ETIOLOGY

Two separate etiologies can be considered for stress incontinence. These include:

- Anatomic hypermobility of the urethra
- Intrinsic sphincter deficiency/weakness.

Damage to the nerves, muscle and connective tissue of the pelvic floor is important in the genesis of stress incontinence. Intrapartum injury during childbirth probably is the most important mechanism.

DIAGNOSIS

Symptoms

Involuntary loss of urine in presence of conditions associated with an increased intra-abdominal pressure.

Investigations

Stress testing: Stress testing should be performed with a full bladder, with the patient in both lithotomy and standing positions. In either case, the

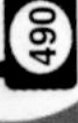

clinician must directly visualize the urethra. The patient then is asked to cough forcefully and repetitively or to perform a strong Valsalva maneuver. Loss of urine directly observed from the urethral meatus, coincident with the peak of increase in intra-abdominal pressure is strongly suggestive of stress incontinence.

MEDICAL MANAGEMENT

Medical therapy of SUI can include pharmacotherapy, behavioral therapy, biofeedback, pelvic floor rehabilitation, bladder training, use of pessaries or occlusive devices, lifestyle modification, intermittent self-catheterization, etc.

- *Pharmacotherapy*: These may include alpha adrenergic drugs (imipramine, ephedrine, pseudoephedrine, etc.); estrogen therapy (in cases of urogenital atrophy) and electric stimulation
- *Pelvic floor rehabilitation*: Kegel exercises have been shown to improve the strength and tone of the muscles of the pelvic floor. Use of weighted vaginal cones is likely to increase the strength of pelvic floor muscles. Biofeedback in form of visual or auditory signals may be an effective method of exercising the pelvic floor
- *Behavioral approaches*: Under this approach, the patient is asked to follow a timed, frequent voiding schedule, which helps to minimize incontinence.

SURGICAL MANAGEMENT

Surgery forms the mainstay of treatment for cases of stress incontinence. Various procedures for stress incontinence share the common goal of stabilizing the bladder neck and proximal urethra.

Preoperative Preparation

- Estrogen replacement therapy may enhance urethral, bladder and vaginal tissue integrity
- Treatment of various underlying medical disorders such as asthma, COPD, diabetes, chronic constipation, etc.
- Good nutrition helps to maximize tissue integrity and to support good healing
- *Patient counseling*: This must comprise of thorough discussion of risks, benefits, anticipated success rates and potential common complications related to the procedure.

Intraoperative Details

Various procedures available for urinary incontinence are as follows:

Retropubic Bladder Neck Suspension Procedures

All these procedures are performed through lower abdominal incision and involve the attachment of periurethral and perivesical endopelvic fascia to some other supporting structure in the anterior pelvis (**Table 14.2 and Fig. 14.6**). Nowadays, some of these procedures are performed through laparoscopic and robotic surgery.

Table 14.2: Various supporting structures in different types of retropubic procedures

Name of surgical procedure	*Supporting structure in the anterior pelvis*
Paravaginal procedure	Arcus tendineus
Modified Marshall-Marchetti-Krantz procedure	Back of pubic symphysis
Burch colposuspension	Iliopectineal ligament (Cooper's ligament)
Turner-Warwick vaginal obturator shelf procedure	Fascia over obturator internus

Transvaginal Urethropexies/Needle Suspension Procedures/ Pereyra's Procedure

This involves passage of sutures between the vagina and anterior abdominal wall using a especially designed long needle carrier, which is inserted through the vaginal incision made at the level of bladder neck. The other end of the suture passes through a small abdominal incision which is made transversely just above the pubic bone and is carried down to the rectus fascia (**Fig. 14.7**).

Suburethral Sling Procedures and Periurethral Injections

These methods are used for stress incontinence resulting from intrinsic sphincteric damage or weakness. Both these methods work by compressing the urethral lumen at the level of bladder neck to compensate for a faulty urethral closure mechanism. Various materials have been used for making slings such as synthetic materials, cadaveric donor fascia, endogenous rectus fascia, fascia lata, etc. Sling operations can be performed using a combined vaginal and abdominal approach and involve midurethral placement of mesh.

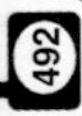

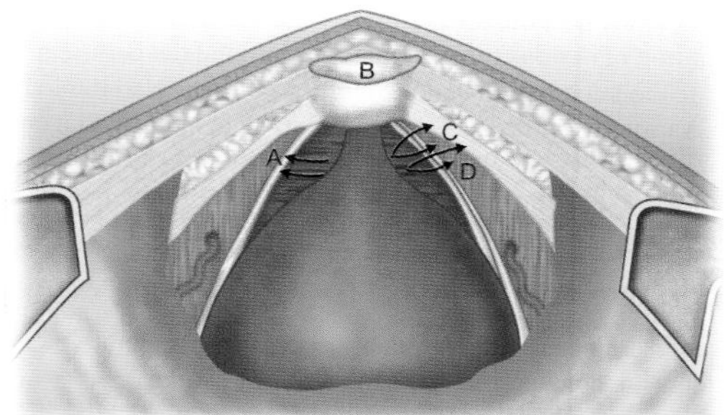

Figure 14.6: Point of attachment of endopelvic fascia during bladder neck suspension procedures: (A) arcus tendinous; (B) periosteum of the pubic symphysis; (C) iliopectineal ligaments (Cooper's ligaments); (D) obturator internus fascia

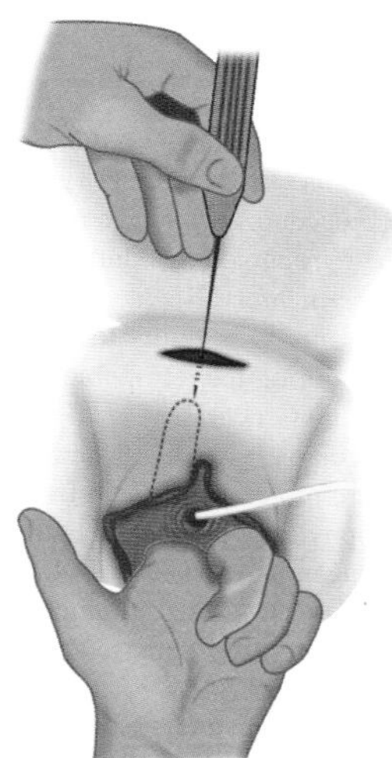

Figure 14.7: Guiding a long needle through the Retzius space using the index finger

Periurethral injections are performed under local anesthesia and involve administration of various types of materials around the periurethral tissues to facilitate their coaptation under conditions of increased intra-abdominal pressure. Various bulking agents have been used including collagen; carbon-coated zirconium; ethylene vinyl alcohol; polydimethylsiloxane; polytetraflouroethylene and glutaraldehyde cross-linked bovine collagen (contigen).

Postoperative Care

- Bladder drainage is an essential aspect of postoperative care. Most patients are able to void spontaneously in 3–7 days
- Measures must be taken to control chronic cough and to avoid or treat constipation
- The patient should avoid lifting anything heavier than 10 pounds for 12 weeks
- The patient must be instructed to avoid smoking and other activities that may repetitively stress the pelvic floor, resulting in long-term failure of the procedure.

COMPLICATIONS

- *Hemorrhage*: Bleeding is usually from the perivesical venous plexus. Needle suspension procedures may have higher rates of hemorrhage in comparison to the retropubic procedures (5–7% vs 2%)
- *Urinary tract and visceral injury*: Bladder injuries can commonly occur with the laparoscopic approach. Injury to the ureter can occur due to kinking or angulation during the retropubic procedures. Injury to the bowel can also sometimes occur
- *UTI*: These are especially associated with postoperative voiding difficulties resulting in prolonged catheterization
- *Wound infection*: Prophylactic antibiotics in the form of a single dose of a broad-spectrum agent are usually effective
- *Osteitis pubis*: This is a self-limited inflammation of the pubic bone related to placement of foreign body material such as sutures, etc. Osteomyelitis can rarely occur
- *Urogenital fistula*: This is also a rare complication
- *Nerve injuries*: Injuries to various nerves such as common peroneal, sciatic, obturator, femoral, saphenous and ilioinguinal nerves have been reported

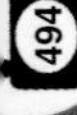

- *Voiding dysfunction*: This may be manifest in form of slow or poor urinary stream or in the inability to void
- *Detrusor overactivity*: De novo detrusor overactivity may at times develop postoperatively
- *Pelvic organ prolapse*: Enterocele formation may be as high as 8% following surgery. Rates of rectocele formation also may be increased
- *Other complications*: These may include complications such as dyspareunia, chronic suprapubic pain, sinus tract formation, etc.

CLINICAL PEARLS

- SUI is the most common form of urinary incontinence
- Urodynamic diagnosis of stress incontinence is termed as genuine stress incontinence
- Some researchers have used microwave energy to heat the connective tissue lateral to the bladder neck and proximal urethra, resulting in shrinkage of the tissue, which provides better support to the bladder neck.

2.2. URGE INCONTINENCE

INTRODUCTION

Urge urinary incontinence can be defined as involuntary leakage of urine accompanied by or immediately preceded by urgency. The corresponding urodynamic term is detrusor overactivity, which is evident in form of involuntary detrusor contractions at the time of filling cystometry.

ETIOLOGY

Urge incontinence is caused by uninhibited contractions of the detrusor muscle.

DIAGNOSIS

Clinical Presentation

See introduction.

MANAGEMENT OF DETRUSOR OVERACTIVITY

Medical Treatment

Management options for urge incontinence include pharmacologic, behavioral therapy and electrical stimulation. These include:

- *Anticholinergic agents*: Propantheline bromide is an anticholinergic agent which is commonly prescribed in the dosage of 15–30 mg every 4–6 hours

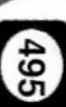

- *Tricyclic antidepressants*: They possess both central and peripheral anticholinergic effect as well as alpha-adrenergic agonist effect and central sedative effect. The resultant clinical effect is bladder muscle relaxation and increased urethral sphincter tone
- *Musculotropic relaxants*: The main smooth muscle relaxant used in these cases is oxybutynin in the dosage of 5 mg, 2–4 times per day
- *Behavior modification*: Behavioral interventions help in establishing or reestablishing cortical control over a hyperactive micturition reflex
- *Intermittent catheterization*: This type of management is most appropriate for patients with detrusor hyperreflexia and functional obstruction
- *Vaginal prosthetic devices*: A disposable vaginal device made of polyurethane has been found moderately effective in patients with detrusor overactivity.

Surgical Treatment

Surgical therapy should be considered only in severe and refractory cases of urge incontinence and include bladder augmentation procedures; denervation procedures; urinary diversion; sacral neuromodulation, etc.

COMPLICATIONS

- Recovery can be difficult, and long-term or permanent disability can occur
- Medications can result in anticholinergic side effects such as dryness of mouth, eyes, blurring of vision, constipation, headaches, etc.

CLINICAL PEARLS

- Urodynamic studies for evaluation of detrusor overactivity include uroflowmetry, filling cystometry, pressure-flow voiding studies, urethral pressure profilometry and determination of leak-point pressure
- Intravesical pharmacotherapy with naturally occurring pungent substances such as capsaicin, resiniferatoxin, etc. may be helpful in cases of urge incontinence.

CHAPTER 15

Contraception

INTRODUCTION

The goal of family planning is to enable couples and individuals to freely choose how many children to have and when to have them. This can best be done if the obstetrician provides them with a full range of safe and effective contraceptive methods and give them sufficient information to ensure they are able to make informed choices. Various contraceptive methods are based on three general strategies: prevention of ovulation; prevention of fertilization or prevention of implantation. Various methods for contraception are described in **Box 15.1**.

Box 15.1: Various methods of contraception

Temporary methods

- Natural regulation of fertility
- Barrier methods
- Hormonal contraception:
  - Combined hormonal contraception:
    1. Combined oral contraceptive pills (COCPs):
       a. Monophasic pills (each tablet containing a fixed amount of estrogen and progestogen)
       b. Biphasic pills (each tablet containing a fixed amount of estrogen, while the amount of progestogen increases in the luteal phase of the cycle)
       c. Triphasic pills (the amount of estrogen may be fixed or variable, while the amount of progestogen increases over three equally divided phases of the cycle)
  - Progestogen only contraception:
    1. Progestin only pill (POP)
    2. Injections (Depo-Provera)
    3. Implants (Norplant I and II)
    4. Patches
    5. Vaginal rings
- Intrauterine contraceptive devices
- Emergency (postcoital) contraception

Permanent methods

- Sterilization
  - Female sterilization
  - Vasectomy

INDICATIONS

Contraception may be required for following conditions:

- Postponement of first pregnancy
- Birth spacing and control
- Prevention of pregnancy.

MANAGEMENT

The detailed use of each contraceptive has been described in each individual fragment. The WHO eligibility criteria for the use of various contraceptive methods have been described in **Table 15.1**.

Table 15.1: World Health Organization eligibility criteria for the use of various contraceptive methods

Category	*Description*
1	A condition where there is no restriction for the use of the contraceptive method
2	A condition where the advantages of using the method generally outweigh the theoretical or proven risks
3	A condition where the theoretical or proven risks usually outweigh the advantages of using the method
4	A condition that represents an unacceptable health risk if the contraceptive method is used

COMPLICATIONS

The specific complications associated with different types of contraceptives have been described in individual fragments.

CLINICAL PEARLS

- The prescription of a contraceptive device must be individualized
- The type of contraception, which must be prescribed to a particular patient, is the one that provides effective contraception, acceptable cycle control and is associated with least side effects.

1. HORMONAL METHOD OF CONTRACEPTION

1.1. COMBINED HORMONAL CONTRACEPTION (ORAL CONTRACEPTIVE PILLS)

INTRODUCTION

There are two main types of hormonal contraception, one being the combined hormonal contraception (containing both estrogen and progestogen), commonly available as combined oral contraceptive pills (COCPs) and the other being formulations containing progestogen only.

Three types of COCPs formulations are available: monophasic pills; biphasic pills and triphasic pills. Most COCPs are contained in a compact package of 21 active pills and 7 inactive pills. However, some 21-day packages may not contain any inactive pills.

ETIOLOGY

COCPs act through following mechanisms:

- Prevention of ovulation
- Thickening of mucus at the cervix so that sperms cannot pass through
- Changing the environment of the uterus and fallopian tubes to prevent fertilization and/or implantation.

MANAGEMENT

Prior to Prescription of COCPs

- Patient assessment: Before prescription of COCPs, a thorough history should be taken, including potential contraindications, smoking history and medications. The physical examination should include a blood pressure measurement
- A pelvic examination is not mandatory before prescription
- Adequate counseling prior to initiation of COCPs may help to improve compliance and adherence.

Prescription

- Conventionally, the COCPs must be started during the first 5 days of the menstrual cycle
- Once a woman has started taking a COCPs, it is important for her to be consistent and take the pill regularly at the same time each day

- Women who use a 21-day preparation need to take the pills for 21 days followed by a 7-day pill-free interval. She should be cautioned not to exceed the 7-day pill-free interval between packs
- If the woman forgets to take a tablet, she should take two tablets the following day
- Backup method of contraception (e.g. condoms, foam) may be required in case the woman exceeds the pill-free interval of 7 days; misses more than one tablet in a cycle; experiences a serious adverse effect or requires protection from STDs.

Follow-up

Follow-up visit after 6 weeks is required to check patient compliance and well-being.

COMPLICATIONS

Minor side effects: These include clinical features such as irregular bleeding, breast tenderness, nausea**,** weight gain and mood changes.

Major risks: These include side effects such as venous thromboembolism, myocardial infarction, stroke, gallbladder disease, breast cancer, cervical cancer, etc.

The patient should be counseled to report any adverse effects related to the use of COCPs, which can be remembered with the mnemonic ACHES:

- A—Abdominal pain (severe)
- C—Chest pain (severe), cough, shortness of breath or sharp pain upon breathing
- H—Headache (severe), dizziness, weakness or numbness (especially one-sided)
- E—Eye problems (complete loss of or blurring of vision)
- S—Severe leg pain (calf or thigh).

CLINICAL PEARLS

- The use of COCPs provides a protective effect against the development of ovarian and endometrial cancer and probably even colorectal cancer
- There is no evidence that the COCPs cause teratogenic effects if taken inadvertently during pregnancy
- Use of COCPs is a highly effective method of reversible contraception, with the failure rate being approximately 0.1 per 100 women years of use

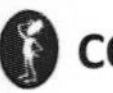

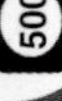

- COCPs do not provide any protection against STD or HIV infection
- Normal menstrual cycles are likely to occur in 99% of the women within 6 months of stopping the pills. However, return of fertility may be slightly late due to delayed return of ovulation.

1.2. PROGESTOGEN ONLY CONTRACEPTION (PROGESTOGEN ONLY PILL)

INTRODUCTION

Progestogen only containing contraceptive methods is available in various formulations:

- Progestogen only pill (POP) or minipill
- Subdermal contraceptive implants (Norplant I, II and implanon)
- Progestogen only injectables (POI), e.g. depot-medroxyprogesterone acetate (DMPA)
- Intrauterine system (Mirena and progestasert).

This fragment will describe POPs; other progestogen only containing contraceptive methods would be described in the subsequent fragments. The POPs may contain 350 µg of norethisterone or 75 µg of norgestrel or 30 µg of levonorgestrel.

ETIOLOGY

POP act through the following mechanisms:

- Inhibition of follicular development and ovulation
- Thickening of cervical mucus, thereby reducing sperm viability and penetration
- Making the endometrium unfavorable to implantation.

MANAGEMENT

Prescription

POPs must be started within 5–7 days of menstruation. Unlike the COCPs, these pills must be taken on a continuous basis without any breaks between packets. These must be consumed in accordance with a strict time schedule everyday (within 3 hours vs 12 hours for COCPs). A backup method should be used for 2 days if a woman is more than 3 hours late taking a dose. Backup contraception should be considered during the 1st month when the woman first starts taking minipills and then at midcycle every month thereafter (the time when ovulation is likely to occur).

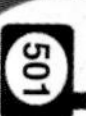

COMPLICATIONS

- Irregular bleeding, spotting, break through bleeding, etc.
- Depression, headache, migraine
- Weight gain and ectopic pregnancy
- Mastalgia (breast tenderness)
- Mood swings
- Abdominal cramps.

CLINICAL PEARLS

- Unlike the COCPs, minipills are not associated with an increased risk of complications such as DVT or heart disease
- Minipills are recommended over COCPs in women who are breastfeeding because they do not affect milk production
- POPs have lower effectiveness than COCPs (pregnancy rate of 2–3 per 100 women years of use)
- Cerazette is an estrogen-free, progestogen-only oral contraceptive pill containing 75 μg of desogestrel.

1.3. INJECTABLE CONTRACEPTIVES

INTRODUCTION

These comprise of delivering certain hormonal drugs in form of deep intramuscular injections into the muscles of arms or buttocks. Two types of injectable contraceptives are available: progestogen-only formulations and combined formulations (**Table 15.2**). The POIs contain only the hormone, progestogen. Two main types of POIs are depot medroxyprogesterone acetate (DMPA) and norethisterone enanthate (NET-EN). Combined formulations (e.g. Mesigyna, Cyclofem, etc.) on the other hand, contain both progestogen and estrogen.

ETIOLOGY

The mechanism of action of injectable progestogens is similar to that of POPs as described in the previous fragment.

MANAGEMENT

Prescription

The medicine must be injected into the thigh, buttocks or deltoid muscle four times a year (every 11–13 weeks) and provides pregnancy protection

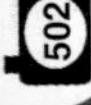

Table 15.2: Different types of injectable contraceptives

Name	*Active ingredients*	*Duration of effect*
Progestogen only injectables (POIs)		
DMPA (progestogen-only) Available as depo-Provera	150 mg medroxyprogesterone acetate in an aqueous micro-crystalline suspension	90 days
DMPA (progestogen-only)	300 mg	180 days
NET-EN(progestogen-only) Available as Noristerat	200 mg norethisterone enanthate in an oily preparation	60 days
Combined injectable contraceptives (CICs)		
Mesigyna	50 mg norethisterone enanthate and 5 mg estradiol valerate	30 days
Cyclofem	25 mg DMPA and 5 mg of estradiol cypionate	
Marvelon	150 µg of desogestrel and 30 µg of ethinyl estradiol	
Femovon	75 µg of gestodene and 35 µg of ethinyl estradiol	

starting a week after the first injection. The injection site should not be massaged afterwards, since this may accelerate absorption of the drug.

Since DMPA is an aqueous suspension, a DMPA vial must be shaken vigorously, before it is loaded into the syringe, to resuspend any active ingredient in the bottom of the vial. The syringe should then be checked to ensure that it contains the correct dosage. Any leakage from the syringe should be checked and kept under control.

COMPLICATIONS

- *Menstrual irregularities*: Disruptions of the menstrual cycle including amenorrhea, prolonged menses, spotting between periods, and heavy or prolonged bleeding
- *Other side effects*: These include adverse effects such as weight gain, headache, dizziness and low bone mass.

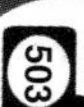

CLINICAL PEARLS

- Injectable contraceptive provide women with safe, highly effective, and reversible contraceptive protection, with the failure rate being 0.1–0.4%
- They overcome the inconvenience of daily compliance required with POPs or COCP
- This is a suitable method for women in whom estrogens present health risks
- POIs can be used by breastfeeding women at 6 weeks postpartum without adverse effects on nursing infants
- Fertility is not impaired after discontinuation of DMPA or NET-EN, although its return may be delayed
- They do not provide protection against HIV and STDs.

1.4. SUBDERMAL IMPLANTS

INTRODUCTION

Contraceptive implant is a method of birth control, where the device is inserted under the skin. Available subdermal implants are as follows:

- Norplant I and Jadelle (Norplant II)
- Implanon
- Sino-implant II marketed as Zarin, Femplant and Trust.

These implants ensure slow, sustained release of progestogens. It is long acting form of contraception, which is associated with minimal side effects.

Norplant I: This contains six silastic capsules made up of siloxane of the size 34 mm × 2.4 mm, with each containing about 36 mg of levonorgestrel **(Fig. 15.1)**. Its effects last for approximately 5 years. The implants release 85 mg of levonorgestrel/day in the first 3 months; 50 mg/day for next 18 months and then gradually levels to about 30 mg/day.

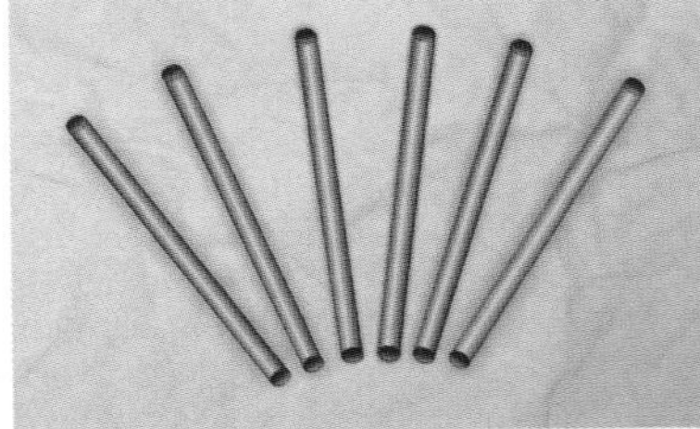

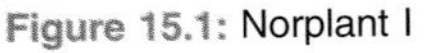

Figure 15.1: Norplant I

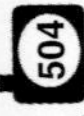

Norplant II: This comprises of two rods, each containing about 70 mg of levonorgestrel. The daily release of hormone is about 50 mg and it provides protection for 3–5 years.

Implanon: This is a single-rod, having dimensions 4 cm by 2 mm, containing 67 mg of a progestogen, desogestrel and usually remains effective for a period of 3 years. Approximately 30 μg of hormone is released daily.

ETIOLOGY

Mechanism of action of subdermal implants is as follows:

- Thickening of cervical mucus making it difficult for sperm to pass through
- Inhibition of ovulation.

MANAGEMENT

The implants are inserted on first day of the menstrual cycle. Following application of a local anesthetic over the upper arm, a needle-like applicator is used to insert the norplant capsules under the skin **(Fig. 15.2)**. They are inserted subdermally on the medial aspect of upper arm. Since the capsules are nonbiodegradable, they need removal at the end of use or earlier if the side effects are intolerable. Both insertion and removal of these implants requires local anesthesia and a small incision.

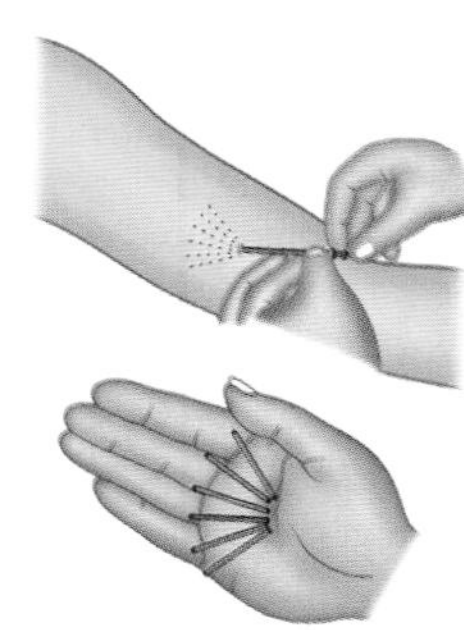

Figure 15.2: Subdermal insertion of Norplant I

COMPLICATIONS

- Side effect profile is similar to those related to POIs, described in the previous fragment
- The main disadvantage associated with this form of contraception is that the woman cannot start or stop using this method on her own. Capsules must be inserted and removed in by a specially trained practitioner
- Some amount of discomfort may be present for several hours following insertion
- Removal is sometimes painful and often more difficult than insertion
- Ectopic pregnancy can occur in approximately 1.3% patients
- Pregnancy rate varies from 0.2 to 1.3 per 100 women years
- This is an expensive form of contraception.

CLINICAL PEARLS

- Return of fertility is almost immediate, following the removal of capsules
- It does not harm the quality and quantity of the breast milk and can be used by nursing mothers starting 6 weeks after childbirth
- These capsules do not provide protection against STDs.

2. INTRAUTERINE DEVICES

INTRODUCTION

Intrauterine devices (IUDs) are flexible plastic devices made up of polyethylene, which are inserted inside the uterine cavity for the purpose of contraception. Each device has a nylon thread, which protrudes through the cervical canal into the vagina, where it can be felt by the patient or the doctor. Initially, biologically inert devices such as lippes loop and saf-T-coil were introduced, which have now been withdrawn from the market. Newer devices are medicated and contain substances such as copper, progestogens, etc. Copper carrying devices include copper T 200, copper 7, multiload, copper 250, copper T 380, copper T 220 and nova T. Their effective life varies from 3 years to 5 years (**Fig. 15.3**). IUDs containing progestogen include progestasert, levonova and Mirena. Mirena is a type of progestogen containing IUCD, having 52 mg of levonorgestrel, which is released at the rate of 20 μg/day. The effects of Mirena last for about 5 years. It is sometimes also know as levonorgestrel-intrauterine system (LNG-IUS).

ETIOLOGY

The possible mechanisms of action of IUD are as follows:

- Copper IUD acts as a foreign body in the uterine cavity, which makes migration of spermatozoa difficult
- Increased release of prostaglandins provokes uterine contractility. This causes the fertilized egg to be rapidly propelled along the fallopian tube so that it reaches the uterine cavity before the development of chorionic villi and thus is unable to implant
- Leukocytic infiltration of the endometrium
- Presence of copper results in certain enzymatic and metabolic changes in the endometrial tissues, which may inhibit implantation of the fertilized ovum.

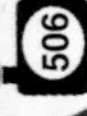

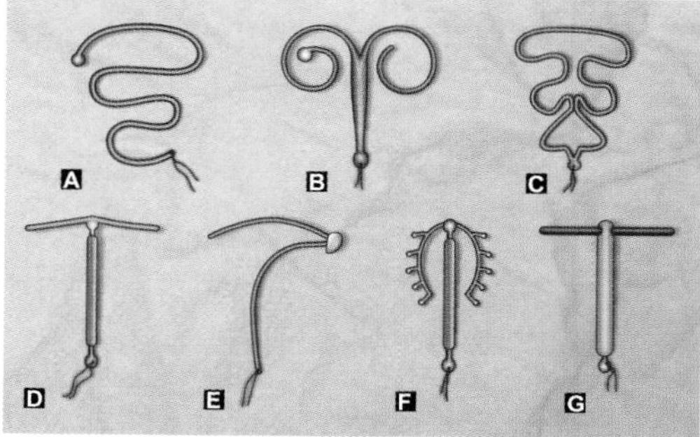

Figure 15.3: Different types of intrauterine contraceptive devices: (A) lippes-Loop; (B) saf-T-Coil; (C) dana-Super; (D) copper-T (Gyne-T) (E) copper-7 (Gravigard); (F) multiload; (G) progesterone IUD

MANAGEMENT

Prior to Insertion

- *Informed consent*: Prior to insertion, informed consent should be obtained and the patient should be aware of the potential side effects, benefits and alternative methods of contraception. It should be emphasized to the patient that the IUD does not provide protection against STIs or HIV
- *Per speculum examination*: The cervix should be carefully inspected for any signs of infection prior to IUD insertion. If there is any evidence of mucopurulent discharge or pelvic tenderness, cervical swabs should be sent for culture and sensitivity and IUD insertion delayed until the infection (if present) has been treated
- *Pelvic examination*: A pelvic examination must be performed prior to the procedure to determine the position and the size of uterus.

Insertion

Various parts of a copper IUCD are shown in **Figure 15.4**, whereas the method for insertion is shown in **Figure 15.5**.

- Cervix is grasped with volsellum or Allis forceps
- Length of the uterine cavity is determined with help of an uterine sound

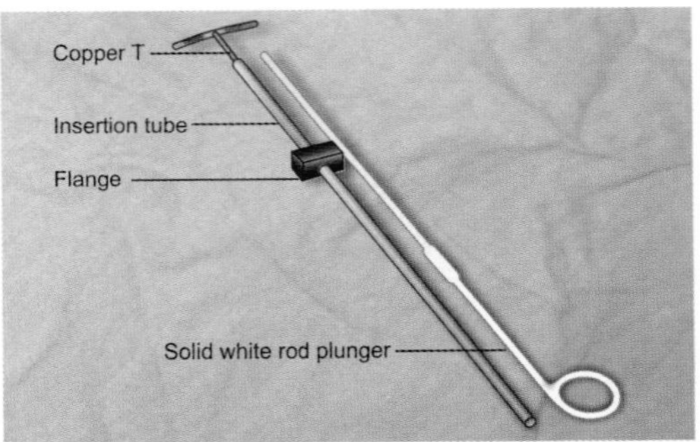

Figure 15.4: Parts of a copper device

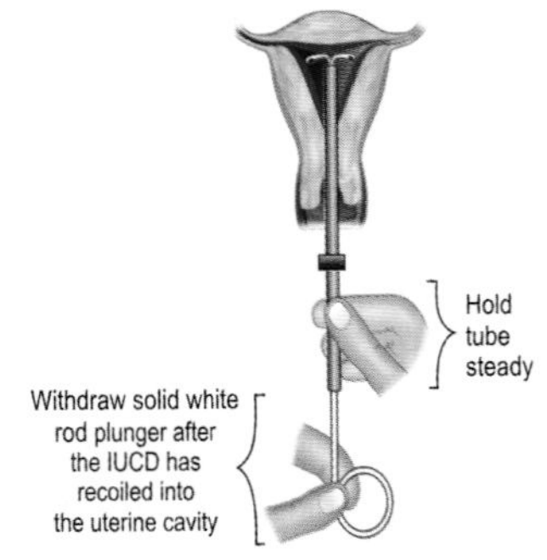

Figure 15.5: Method of insertion of IUCD

- The copper device with an insertion tube is available in presterilized packs. The IUD is mounted into the insertion tube and the flange on the insertion tube is adjusted according to the length of the uterine cavity
- The insertion tube is then passed into the uterine cavity through the cervix
- As the solid white rod plunger is put inside the insertion tube, the IUD recoils within the uterine cavity
- After withdrawing the plunger, insertion tube is removed and the nylon thread is cut to the required length. The speculum and the forceps are then removed.

Postinsertion

- The patient is instructed to examine herself and feel for the thread every week
- A follow-up visit should be scheduled 6 weeks post insertion for the exclusion of presence of infection, an assessment of any abnormal bleeding, and evaluation of the patient and partner satisfaction
- An IUD user should be instructed to contact her health care provider if any of the following occur: IUD's threads cannot be felt; she or her partner can feel the lower end of the IUD; she experiences persistent abdominal pain, fever, dyspareunia and/or unusual vaginal discharge, etc.

COMPLICATIONS

- *Difficulties at the time of insertion*: Immediate difficulties at the time of insertion include vasovagal attack, difficulty in insertion of the copper device and presence of uterine cramps
- *Bleeding*: Irregular menstrual bleeding, spotting, menorrhagia, etc. are the most common side effects of IUDs in the 1st month after insertion. Use of NSAIDs or tranexamic acid may be helpful
- *Pain or dysmenorrhea*: Pain may be a physiological response to the presence of the device, but the possibility of infection, malposition of the device (including perforation) and pregnancy should be excluded. The LNG-IUS has been associated with a reduction in menstrual pain.
- *Systemic hormonal side effects*: These may be typically associated with the LNG-IUS and include side effects such as depression, acne, headache and breast tenderness
- *Functional ovarian cysts*: They may occur in up to 30% of LNG-IUS users and usually resolve spontaneously
- *Uterine perforation*: Uterine perforation is a rare, but serious complication of IUD insertion, occurring at a rate of 0.6–1.6 per 1,000 insertions. This may occur either at the time of insertion or at a later stage due to the embedment of the device into the myometrium and its subsequent migration into the intra-abdominal cavity
- *Infection*: Infection at the time of insertion can result in the development of PID in the long run. To prevent the occurrence of vaginal infection, IUD users should continue to use condoms for protection against STDs. Actinomyosis infection also occurs commonly
- *Expulsion*: Expulsion of the IUD is most common in the 1st year of use (2–10% of users)
- *Ectopic pregnancy*: Ectopic pregnancy can sometime occur with IUCD in situ.

CLINICAL PEARLS

- It is a highly effective method of contraception with the pregnancy rate being 2–6 per 100 women years
- If the IUD strings are not seen in the cervical os, the device may have been expelled or may have perforated the uterine wall. If the IUD strings cannot be found, ultrasound is the preferred method to identify the location of the IUD **(Figs 15.6A and B)**
- If the device is not identified within the uterus or the pelvis, a plain X-ray of the abdomen should be performed to determine whether the device has perforated the uterine wall **(Fig. 15.7)**
- Though IUD is commonly inserted in multiparous women, nulliparity is not a contraindication for IUD use. It can be successfully used in carefully selected nulliparous women
- IUDs per se do not increase the risk of ectopic pregnancy. However, in women who conceive with an IUD in place, the diagnosis of ectopic pregnancy should be excluded
- The copper IUD may decrease the risk of endometrial cancer.

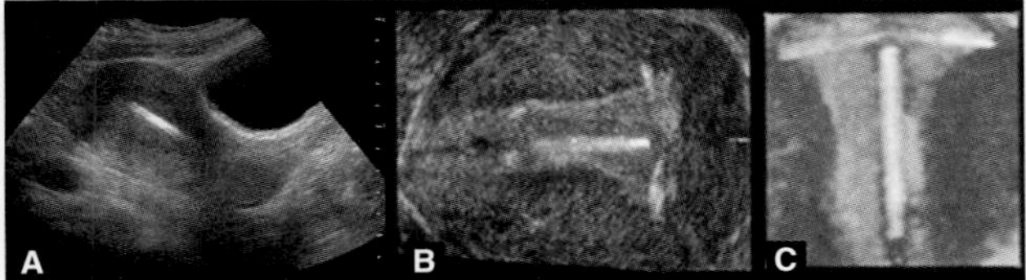

Figures 15.6A and B: (A) Two-dimensional ultrasound showing the presence of copper device in the uterine cavity; (B and C) three-dimensional ultrasound showing the presence of an intrauterine copper device

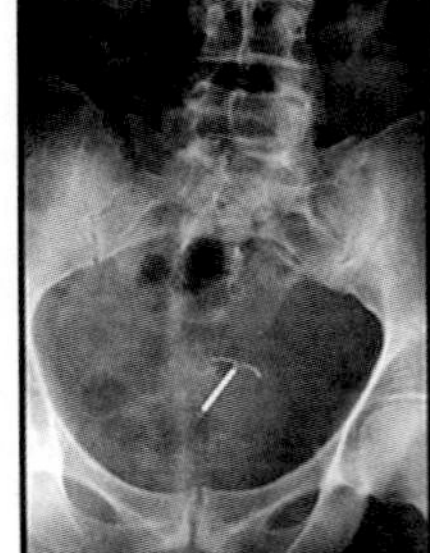

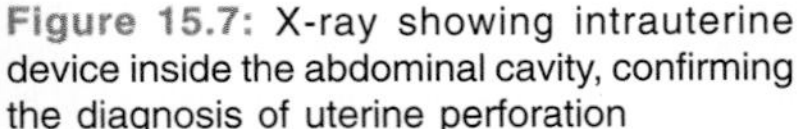

Figure 15.7: X-ray showing intrauterine device inside the abdominal cavity, confirming the diagnosis of uterine perforation

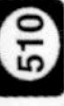

3. NATURAL FAMILY PLANNING METHODS

INTRODUCTION

These methods aim at controlling childbirth by instructing the couple to abstain from sexual intercourse during the fertile period of menstrual cycle. Some of these methods are as follows:

Calendar method: In this method the fertile period is calculated by subtracting 18 days from the shortest cycle and 10 days from the longest cycle. This would give the first and the last day of the fertile period respectively. The couple must be instructed to abstain from sexual relations during this period.

Basal body temperature method: This method is based on the fact that basal body temperature (BBT) increases by 0.2–0.5°C following ovulation due to thermogenic effect of hormone progesterone. The couple must be instructed that the safest way to use BBT for avoiding pregnancy is to avoid intercourse or use a barrier method during at least the first half of the menstrual cycle until 3 days after there has been a rise in BBT.

Ovulation method (cervical mucus or Billings method): This method is based on the fact that as the fertile time approaches, the cervical mucus increases in amount, becomes clearer in color, wetter, stretchy and slippery. Following ovulation, the mucus usually becomes sticky, thicker and pasty in character and reduces in amount **(Fig. 15.8)**. Sexual intercourse is considered safe during the days immediately following the menses until the cervical mucus attains the above-described characteristics. Thereafter, the couple must abstain from having sexual intercourse until the 4th day after the "peak mucus day".

Coitus interruptus (withdrawal): This is a method in which the man takes his penis out of the woman's vagina just before he ejaculates. Ejaculation may or may not take place afterwards.

Symptothermal method: This method includes the combination of calendar method, BBT and cervical mucus method.

COMPLICATIONS

- These methods require a learning period, careful record keeping, periodic abstinence and partner's cooperation
- They do not provide protection against HIV infection and other STDs
- *High failure rate*: Perfect use is associated with a failure rate of 2%, whereas typical use is associated with a failure rate of 20%.

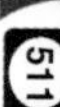

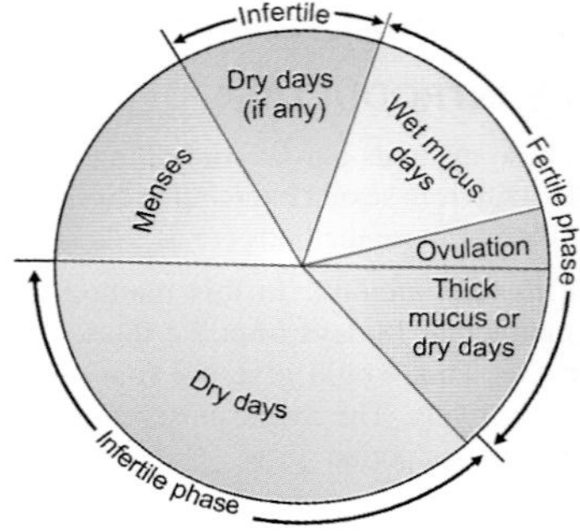

Figure 15.8: Cervical mucus method

CLINICAL PEARLS

- Fertility awareness methods are natural and safe and there are no side effects
- These methods are associated with high failure rates of approximately 20–25 pregnancies per 100 women years of use
- The high failure rate associated with these methods commonly results due to irregular ovulation or irregular menstrual cycles.

4. BARRIER METHOD OF CONTRACEPTION

INTRODUCTION

These methods are moderately effective, but one of the commonly used methods of contraception. These methods aim at creating a type of barrier which prevents the sperm from meeting the ovum. Barrier contraceptives are associated with a failure rate of 9–30 per 100 women years of use. Some of the commonly used barrier methods of contraception include male condom, female condom, diaphragm, cervical cap, vaginal sponge and spermicides.

Male Condom

A male condom is a thin sheath made of latex or other materials **(Fig. 15.9)**. The man puts the condom on his erected penis, while the condom holds the semen. After having sexual intercourse, the man must carefully take off the condom so that it does not leak. Each condom can be used only once.

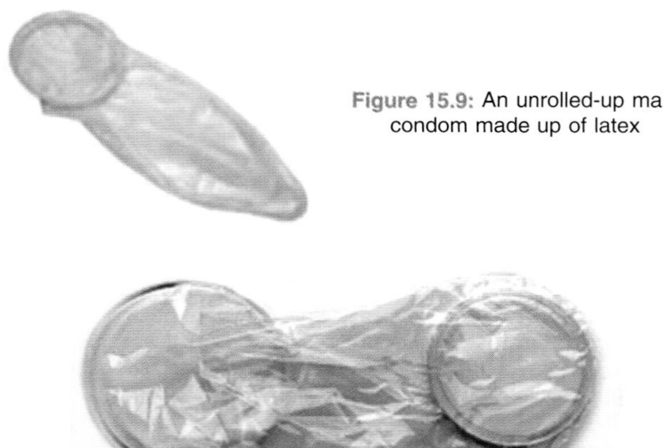

Figure 15.9: An unrolled-up male condom made up of latex

Figure 15.10: Female condom

Female Condom

This comprises of strong, soft, transparent polyurethane sheath, which is inserted in the vagina before sexual intercourse **(Fig. 15.10)**. It is approximately 15 cm in length and 7 cm in diameter. It has two flexible rings, the inner ring and an outer one. The inner ring at the closed end of the condom eases insertion into the vagina, covering the cervix and holding the condom in place.

The outer ring, which is larger than the inner one, stays outside the vagina and covers part of the perineum and labia during intercourse. Female condom is available under the brand names of Reality, Femidom, Dominique, etc.

A Diaphragm

A diaphragm is a shallow rubber dome with a firm flexible rim. It is available in different sizes ranging from 50 mm to 105 mm. It is often used in combination with contraceptive jelly, spermicide, etc. It is immediately effective and reversible method of contraception, which can be inserted up to 6 hours before intercourse.

Cervical Cap

A cervical cap is a soft, deep rubber cup with a firm, round rim that fits snugly over the cervix. The cap provides effective contraception for 48 hours.

Spermicides

Two basic components of spermicides include active spermicidal agents such as surfactants (Nonoxynol-9, Octoxynol-9, Menfegol) and the base (carrier) agent such as foams, jellies, creams, foaming tablet, melting suppositories, aerosols, soluble films or vaginal suppositories. The woman must be instructed to insert the recommended dose of the spermicide deep into vagina to cover the cervix completely, just before sexual intercourse. A second dose of spermicide may be required if more than 1 hour passes before she has sexual intercourse. An additional application of spermicides is needed for each additional act of intercourse.

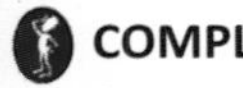

COMPLICATIONS

Male condoms: Some of the complications include:

- Condoms can interrupt with sexual activity, thereby interfering with sexual pleasure
- Condoms may sometimes tear or leak and can cause an allergic reaction.

Female condoms: May be expensive or limited in their availability and may be difficult to insert.

Diaphragm: These include:

- The diaphragm is not an appropriate method if the man or woman has allergy to rubber, latex or spermicide, or if the woman has frequent urinary tract or bladder infections and/or anatomical abnormalities
- May be difficult to insert and remove
- May cause irritation in the vagina.

Cervical cap: These include:

- Toxic shock syndrome
- Unpleasant odor
- Discomfort and awareness of the cap during coitus
- Accidental dislodgment.

Spermicides: These include:

- May cause irritation in the vagina or on the penis, or an allergic reaction
- They cause interruption of sexual activity
- They do not provide protection against STDs.

CLINICAL PEARLS

- Latex condoms provide protection against STDs
- Condoms also provide limited protection against HPV that can cause genital warts, thereby lowering the risk for development of cervical dysplasia and cancer
- To increase the efficacy of condoms, the condoms can be lubricated with contraceptive cream or jelly prior to use
- Condoms are not associated with any medical side effects, are inexpensive and easily accessible
- They are associated with a pregnancy rate of 10–14 per 100 women years of use
- A diaphragm may reduce the risk of cervical cancer
- Spermicides do not require a prescription; may be discontinued at any time and are safe
- While using spermicides, douching should not be allowed for at least 6 hours after coitus.

5. EMERGENCY CONTRACEPTION

INTRODUCTION

Emergency contraception (EC) also known as "postcoital contraception" or the "morning-after pill" is a method of contraception which is used after intercourse and before the potential time of implantation. EC provides women with a safe means of preventing pregnancy following unprotected sexual intercourse or potential contraceptive failure. EC is a backup method for occasional use, and should not be used as a regular method of birth control. There are two methods of EC:

1. *Hormonal methods*: This involves the use of emergency contraceptive pills. The two hormonal preparations which can be used are:
   - *One containing only the progestin levonorgestrel*: The regimen consists of two doses of 750 μg levonorgestrel taken orally 12 hours apart
   - *The other containing a combination of ethinyl estradiol and levonorgestrel (Yuzpe method)*: This method comprises of the oral administration of two doses of 100 μg ethinyl estradiol and 500 μg levonorgestrel taken 12 hours apart
2. *Non-hormonal method*: This comprises of postcoital insertion of a copper containing IUD.

INDICATIONS

Indications for the use of EC are as follows:

- Unwanted pregnancy
- Failure to use a contraceptive method
- Condom breakage or leakage
- Dislodgement of a diaphragm or cervical cap
- Two or more missed birth control pills
- Injection of depo-Provera injection is late by 1 week or more
- Sexual assault when the woman is not using reliable contraception.

MANAGEMENT

A pelvic examination is not a prerequisite to providing EC. There should be no history of recent PID and vaginal or cervical infection.

Hormonal EC should be considered for any woman wishing to avoid pregnancy who presents within 5 days of unprotected or inadequately protected sexual intercourse. Although they have generally been used only up to 72 hours after intercourse, both hormonal methods of EC are effective when taken between 72 hours and 120 hours after unprotected intercourse. A postcoital IUD insertion can be considered up to 7 days after unprotected intercourse. IUDs containing at least 380 mm^2 of copper have the lowest failure rates and should be the first-line choice, particularly if the woman intends to continue the IUD as long-term contraception.

The levonorgestrel EC regimen is more effective and causes fewer side effects than the Yuzpe regimen. One double dose of levonorgestrel EC (1.5 mg) is as effective as the regular two-dose levonorgestrel regimen (0.75 mg each dose), with no difference in side effects.

A barrier method such as the condom can be used for the remainder of the current menstrual cycle, and a regular contraceptive method can be initiated at the beginning of the next cycle if the woman desires.

COMPLICATIONS

- The common side effects of hormonal EC are gastrointestinal and mainly include nausea, vomiting, dizziness and fatigue. Antiemetics such as meclizine can be used for controlling these side effects
- Less common side effects of hormonal methods include headache, bloating, abdominal cramps, and spotting or bleeding
- Possible complications of postcoital IUD insertion include: pelvic pain, abnormal bleeding, pelvic infection, perforation and expulsion.

CLINICAL PEARLS

- EC prevents pregnancy and does not interrupt previously established pregnancy
- ECs are not a good option for providing long-term contraception
- ECs do not protect against STDs
- ECs do not increase the risk of ectopic pregnancy, nor do they affect future fertility
- Presence of pregnancy (either confirmed or suspected) is a contraindication for the use of EC because it would not be effective in these cases.

6. PERMANENT METHOD OF CONTRACEPTION

6.1. TUBAL STERILIZATION

INTRODUCTION

Tubal sterilization causes sterility by blocking a woman's fallopian tubes, thereby preventing the fertilization of sperm with ovum. Dr J Blindell from London was the first to perform tubal ligation in 1823. This procedure can be either performed at the time of delivery or shortly thereafter in the early postpartum period or as an interval procedure (6–12 weeks following delivery or thereafter). The most commonly used approach for performing interval tubal sterilization in nonpregnant women is laparoscopic approach, using application of Falope rings. Periumbilical minilaparotomy, involving the ligation of tubes using Pomeroy's technique, has become the most widely practiced method in women undergoing tubal ligation in the immediate postpartum period.

SURGICAL MANAGEMENT

Preoperative Preparation

- *Complete preoperative workup*: This comprises of adequate history taking and general physical examination
- *Investigations*: Urine analysis, urine pregnancy test and hematocrit with a complete blood count must be done. Other tests such as Papanicolaou test, gonorrhea and chlamydia screening, ultrasonography, etc. may be sometimes required
- *Preoperative counseling*: The procedure being practically irreversible, patients, especially those who are young, require preoperative patient counseling

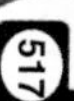

- *Written and informed consent*: After adequate counseling of the patient, written and informed consent from the patient is required in most countries
- *Anesthesia*: Majority of tubal ligation procedures in the United States are performed using general or spinal anesthesia.

Steps of Surgery

- *Incision*: Although subumbilical minilaparotomy is the most common approach worldwide for postpartum procedures, laparoscopy is used most commonly for interval procedures in the United States. In puerperal cases, where the uterus is felt per abdomen, the incision is made approximately 1 inch below the fundus. In interval ligations, the incision is made two finger breadths above the pubic symphysis. This incision could be midline, paramedian or transverse
- *Delivery of the tubes*: In case of laparotomy or minilaparotomy, the index finger is introduced through the incision and is passed across the posterior surface of the uterus and then to the posterior leaf of the broad ligament from where the tube is hooked out
- *Tubal ligation*: Tubal ligation is then performed by one of the following techniques:
    - *Pomeroy's technique*: The technique has been illustrated in **Figures 15.11A to D**. The same procedure is then repeated on the other side and the tubal specimens obtained are submitted for histopathological examination. This technique is highly successful and the failure rate varies between 0.1% and 0.5%
    - *Modified Pomeroy's technique*: Many modifications of the Pomeroy's technique have been described, of which the most commonly performed modification involves double ligation of each tube, thereby reducing the chances of failure
    - *Parkland technique*: The Parkland technique is similar to the Pomeroy technique, except that in this case midsegment resection is performed, involving the excision of 1–2 cm tubal segment, which is then submitted for a histopathological examination
    - *Uchida technique*: In this technique, a relatively long (5 cm) segment of tubal muscularis is pulled out after giving an incision in the mesosalpinx. This portion of the tube is then ligated proximally and distally with No. 0 plain catgut sutures and resected. The serosal edges are then reapproximated, burying the medial exposed tubal end within the leaves of the broad ligament, while the distal end is left exposed

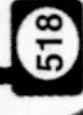

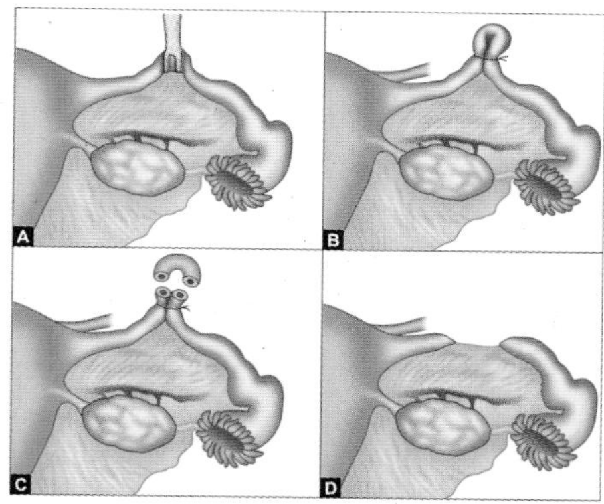

Figures 15.11A to D: Pomeroy's technique of tubal sterilization: (A) the fallopian tube is grasped with Babcock clamp; (B) a loop is created, which is tied with No. 1 plain catgut sutures; (C) excision of the loop; (D) several months later, the ends of the tube get fibrosed, retracting from one another

- *Irving technique*: In this technique, a small portion of the tube, approximately 1–2 cm in length, approximately 4 cm from the uterotubal junction, is doubly ligated with No 0 or 00 absorbable sutures and resected. The medial free end of the tube is then drawn into the myometrial tunnel, following which the sutures are tied
- *Laparoscopic obstruction of tubes*: Laparoscopic tubal ligation can be carried out using techniques such as mechanical blockage of tubes using Falope rings or Filshie clips **(Figs 15.12A to D)**. Electrodessication of tubes using electrosurgery can also be done

- *Closure of incision site*: After performing tubal ligation on both sides, the minilaparotomy incision is closed in layers. The patient is usually discharged within 24–48 hours of surgery.

Postoperative Care

- After undergoing tubal sterilization, the patient must be instructed to come for a follow-up visit at 1–2 weeks postoperatively for examination of the surgical site and removal of nonabsorbable sutures

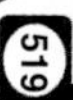

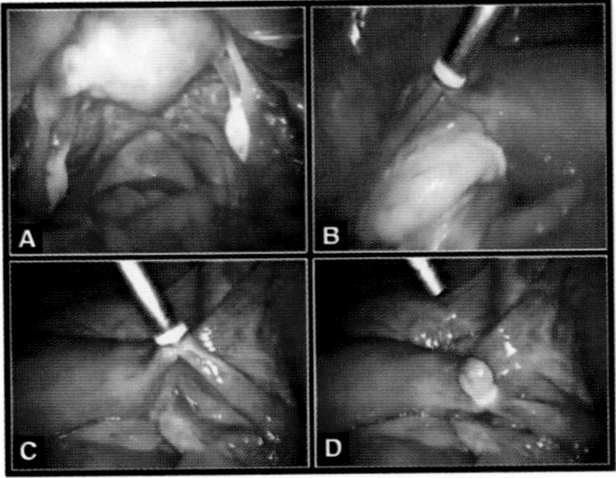

Figures 15.12A to D: Steps of laparoscopic sterilization: (A) laparoscopic visualization of the fallopian tubes of both sides; (B) application of Falope rings; (C) applicator being withdrawn after ring application; (D) ligated tube with the Falope ring in place

- The woman must also be instructed to notify her health care provider in case she has a missed period, develops fever (38°C or 100.4°F), increasing or persistent abdominal pain or bleeding or purulent discharge from the incision site.

COMPLICATIONS

- *Effects of anesthesia*: In cases where general anesthesia is used, the women are at risk of complications inherent to general anesthesia
- *Pain*: After undergoing laparoscopic sterilization, the women may experience some degree of chest and shoulder pain due to pneumoperitoneum, which has been created prior to the insertion of trocar
- *Bleeding and/or infection*: The laparoscopic procedure may be associated with complications such as infection, bleeding, wound infections, hematoma and severe infection, such as PIDs
- *Injury to the body organs*: There is a risk of causing injury to the body organs such as gastrointestinal and genitourinary tract and major vessels, especially when the procedure is performed under laparoscopic guidance

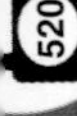

- *Failure of the procedure*: Although sterilization is highly effective and considered the definitive form of pregnancy prevention, it has a failure rate of 0.1–0.8% during the 1st year usually due to incomplete closure of the tubes. At least one-third of these are ectopic pregnancies
- *Mortality*: The risk of death from tubal sterilization is 1–2 cases per 100,000 procedures; most of these are due to complications of general anesthesia, especially hypoventilation
- *Patient regret*: Sterilization is intended to be permanent, but patient regret can commonly occur
- *Post-tubal ligation syndrome*: This syndrome is a constellation of symptoms including pelvic discomfort, ovarian cystic changes and menorrhagia.

CLINICAL PEARLS

- The isthmic portion of the fallopian tube is the most commonly preferred site for all sterilization procedures because of the relative ease of reanastomosis at this site, should the reversal be required in future
- Both laparoscopic sterilization and minilaparotomy approach are associated with a very low risk of complications, when performed according to the accepted medical standards
- Although the procedure of tubal sterilization is practically irreversible in dire circumstances, the reversal can be attempted using microsurgical techniques
- Hysteroscopic sterilization based on using a new device, "Essure system" has recently gained acceptance by "the Food and Drug Administration"
- One of the major causes of failure of sterilization is the inadvertent ligation of the round ligament, which is mistakenly identified as the fallopian tube.

6.2. VASECTOMY

INTRODUCTION

Vasectomy is a procedure in which the vas deferens (tubes carrying sperms from the testicles and epididymis to the urinary tract and urethra) **(Fig. 15.13)** are surgically blocked to prevent the sperms from passing through and fertilizing the egg at the time of sexual intercourse. For couples who do not want to have any more children, vasectomy is the safest and easiest form of permanent sterilization.

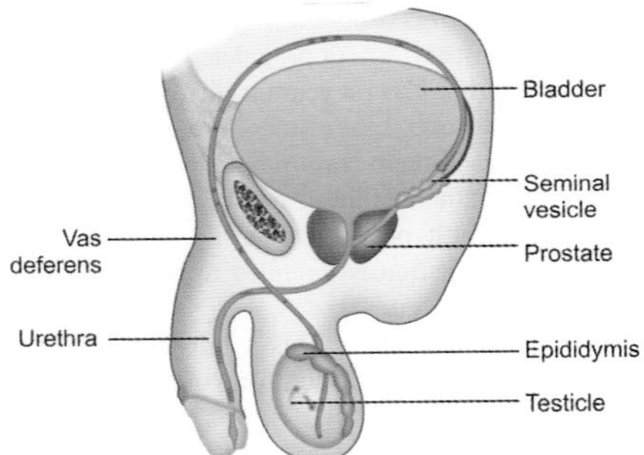

Figure 15.13: Parts of the male reproductive system

SURGICAL MANAGEMENT

Preoperative Preparation

- The person must be instructed to wash meticulously and put on clean, snug underwear or a jock strap (support) before their appointment for surgery
- The front portion of the scrotum may be shaved the night before surgery
- Use of medication such as NSAIDS, aspirin, etc. can increase the risk of bleeding with vasectomy. Therefore the patient must be advised not to use these medicines at least 10 days prior to surgery
- *Informed consent*: The patient must be asked to sign a consent form prior to the procedure
- *Counseling*: This is an essential component because vasectomy is practically a permanent method of contraception
- In order to allow the possibility of reproduction in future via ART after vasectomy, some men opt for cryopreservation of their sperms before sterilization
- The patient is asked to change into a sterile gown and lie on the examination table. The incision site is cleaned and draped taking all aseptic precautions
- Local anesthetic is injected over the scrotal region prior to the procedure.

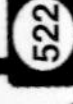

Steps of Surgery

- A scalpel is used to make two small incisions on each side of the scrotum at a location that allows the surgeon to bring out each vas deferens to the surface
- The vas deferentia are cut (sometimes a piece removed), separated and then at least one side is sealed by suture ligation, cauterization or clamping, before being dropped back into the scrotum **(Fig. 15.14)**
- The man must continue to use contraception (such as a condom) until laboratory and microscopic examination of his semen reveals azoospermia. Usually two semen analysis at 3 and 4 months are required to confirm azoospermia.

The no-scalpel vasectomy is less invasive, faster procedure and is associated with fewer complications in comparison to the traditional vasectomy. In contrast to a scalpel (used in the traditional surgery) a sharp hemostat is used for puncturing the scrotal sac, thereby resulting in a smaller "incision" which typically limits infection, bleeding and hematoma formation. No stitches are usually required due to the small size of incision.

Postoperative Care

- The man can be discharged after surgery following 1 hour of observation period at the clinic. However he should be instructed not to drive home by himself. He must be instructed to avoid lifting heavy weights or exercise for at least 1 week following the procedure
- Pain relievers may be used in case of mild discomfort

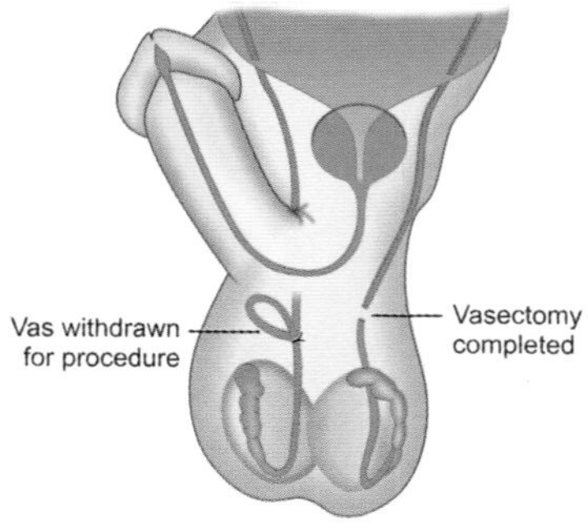

Figure 15.14: The procedure of vasectomy

- In case of soreness over the incision site, the patient can be asked to apply an ice pack (wrapped in towel) to the scrotum for the first 24 hours after the procedure
- The patient must be instructed to wear comfortable cotton briefs or an athletic supporter to help apply pressure and support to the incision site for 1–2 weeks after the procedure.

COMPLICATIONS

Vasectomy is associated with fewer complications in comparison to tubal sterilization. Some of these include:

- Temporary bruising and hematoma formation
- *Postvasectomy pain syndrome*: This is characterized by chronic pain in the scrotal, pelvic and/or lower-abdominal regions and may develop immediately or several years after vasectomy
- Infection
- Sperm granula as a result of sperm leakage
- Epididymitis due to congestion of sperms at the epididymis.

CLINICAL PEARLS

- Vasectomy does not cause loss of masculinity
- Vasectomy is a highly effective, having a failure rate as low as 0.02–0.2%, which is less than that of tubal sterilization. Except for complete abstinence, no method can be considered to be more effective than vasectomy in preventing pregnancy.

Abbreviations

ACOG	American College of Obstetricians and Gynecologists
AFI	Amniotic Fluid Index
AIDS	Acquired Immunodeficiency Syndrome
APGAR	Activity, Pulse, Grimace, Appearance and Respiration
APTT	Activated Partial Thromboplastin Time
ARM	Artificial Rupture of Membranes
ART	Assisted Reproductive Techniques
AUB	Abnormal Uterine Bleeding
BUN	Blood Urea Nitrogen
CAH	Congenital Adrenal Hyperplasia
CBC	Complete Blood Count
CNS	Central Nervous System
COCP	Combined Oral Contraceptive Pill
COPD	Chronic Obstructive Pulmonary Disease
CRP	C-Reactive Protein
CS	Cesarean Section
CT	Computed Tomography
D&C	Dilatation and Curettage
DIC	Disseminated Intravascular Coagulation
DLC	Differential Leukocyte Count
DUB	Dysfunctional Uterine Bleeding
DVT	Deep Vein Thrombosis
EDD	Expected Date of Delivery
ESR	Erythrocyte Sedimentation Rate
FIGO	International Federation of Gynecology and Obstetrics
FHR	Fetal Heart Rate
FHS	Fetal Heart Sounds
FSH	Follicle Stimulating Hormone
GIT	Gastrointestinal Tract
GnRH	Gonadotropin Releasing Hormone
hCG	Human Chorionic Gonadotropin
HELLP	Hemolysis, Elevated Liver Enzymes, Low Platelet Count
HIV	Human Immunodeficiency Virus
HPV	Human Papilloma Virus

HRT	Hormone Replacement Therapy
HSG	Hysterosalpingography
ICSI	Intracytoplasmic Sperm Injection
IUCD	Intrauterine Contraceptive Device
IUD	Intrauterine Death
IUGR	Intrauterine Growth Retardation
IVF-ET	In Vitro Fertilization-Embryo Transfer
IVP	Intravenous Pyelography
LH	Luteinizing Hormone
LMP	Last Menstrual Period
MRI	Magnetic Resonance Imaging
NPO	Nil Per Os
NSAIDS	Nonsteroidal Anti-Inflammatory Drugs
NST	Nonstress Test
OCP	Oral Contraceptive Pill
PAP Smear	Papanicolaou Smear
PCOD	Polycystic Ovarian Disease
PE	Pulmonary Embolism
PID	Pelvic Inflammatory Disease
PIH	Pregnancy Induced Hypertension
PMS	Premenstrual Syndrome
PPH	Postpartum Hemorrhage
PPROM	Preterm Premature Rupture of Membranes
PROM	Premature Rupture of Membranes
PT	Prothrombin Time
PUBS	Percutaneous Umbilical Cord Blood Sampling
ROM	Rupture of Membranes
SIS	Saline Infusion Sonography
STD	Sexually Transmitted Diseases
TAH	Total Abdominal Hysterectomy
TAS	Transabdominal Sonography
TLC	Total Leukocyte Count
TORCH	Toxoplasmosis, Other Infections, Rubella, Cytomegalovirus, Herpes Simplex Virus
TVS	Transvaginal Sonography
UTI	Urinary Tract Infections
VBAC	Vaginal Birth After Cesarean Delivery
VDRL	Venereal Disease Research Laboratory
WHO	World Health Organization

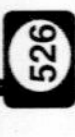

Index

Page numbers followed by *f* refer to figures and *t* refer to tables

A

Abnormal
- postmenopausal
  - bleeding 330
- uterine contractions 248

ABO/RH compatibility 179
Abruption placenta 142, 147, 181, 247, 258
Acute
- hemorrhage 232
- left ventricular failure 144
- salpingitis
  - with peritonitis 438
  - without peritonitis 438

Adenocarcinoma 461
Adenofibroma 461
Adenomyosis 413, 413*f*
Adnexal masses 119
Adolescent and pediatric gynecology 283
Adult circulation 22, 22*f*
Ambiguous genitalia 291, 292
Amenorrhea 418, 444
Amnioinfusion 187
Amniotic fluid 46
- embolism 231*f*, 232*t*

Amsel's diagnostic criteria for bacteria 434
Androblastomas 462
Androgen insensitivity syndrome 444
Anembryonic gestation 173
Anemia 121, 206, 319, 328
Anorexia nervosa 445
Anovulatory DUB 309
Anterior colporrhaphy 393
Antiandrogens 296
Antiphospholipid syndrome 218
Apgar score 248, 248*t*
Application of falope rings 520*f*
Arcuate uterus 417
Arcus tendineus 492, 493
ART 453, 457
Arteries of
- anterolateral abdominal wall 278*f*
- vulva and perineum 275

Asherman's syndrome 169, 444, 448, 455
Asphyxia neonatorum 247
Atonicity of uterus 232
Atrophic vaginitis 311, 315, 432

B

Bacterial vaginosis 432, 434, 436
Baden-Walker halfway system 391*t*
Balby-Webster's operation 404
Barrier method 512
Basal body temperature 8
Benign ovarian tumors 460
Bethesda system 342
Bi-ischial diameter 52
Bituberous diameter 52
Blood
- cellular indices 149
- supply
  - of pelvis 275
  - to uterus 275
  - to vagina 275

Body mass index 445
Bornow's combination therapy 357
Brachial plexus injuries 159
Braxton Hicks contractions 29
Breast 221
- changes during pregnancy 31*f*
- engorgement 223
- tenderness 328

Breastfeeding 206
Breech vaginal delivery 97
Brenner tumors 462
Broad ligament
- hematoma 479
- leiomyoma 478

C

Calendar method 342, 511
Carbon dioxide insufflation 384
Cardiac disease in pregnancy 159
Carnett's sign 409*f*
Caudal regression sequence 159
Cephalohematoma 159
Cephalopelvic disproportion 75, 77, 96
Cervical
- cancer 311, 500
- cap 514
- dystocia 75
- ectropion/erosion 315
- endometriosis 345
- incompetence 127
- punch biopsy 343, 345*f*

Cervicitis 311
Cervicovesical fistula 482*f*
Cesarean delivery 90
Chadwick's sign 30
Cherney's incision 368f
Chest encircling technique 252*f*
Chlamydia trachomatis 424, 469
Chocolate cyst of ovary 405

Chorioamnionitis 76, 147, 248
Choriocarcinoma 175, 463
Chronic
hydrosalpinx 439*f*
intrauterine infection 199
pelvic
inflammatory disease 405
pain 405, 442
CIN 214, 342
Clomiphene citrate 312
Clue cells 435*f*
Coitus interruptus 511
Colposcopy 343
Complete
abortion 164
hydatidiform mole 170, 171*f*
Conjoint twins 77
Conjugated estrogen 300
Contraception 497
Contraceptive injection 448
Contracted pelvis 113
Contraction stress test 46
Coomb's test 191, 206
Copper-7 507*f*
Copper-T 507*f*
Cord prolapse 108, 121, 129
Corpus luteum hematoma 326
Couvelaire uterus 185
Criminal abortion 303
Cryptomenorrhea 285
Cystadenocarcinoma 461
Cystadenoma 461
Cytotrophoblastic shell 18

D

Daily fetal movement count 201
Decubitus ulceration 398
Deep vein thrombosis 226
prophylaxis 384
Delayed puberty 285, 288
Dermoid cyst 463
Dexamethasone suppression test 296
Diameters of fetal skull 56*f*
Didelphys uterus 417
Discoid lupus 205
Dominant follicle 271
Down's syndrome 42
Duplex Doppler ultrasound 227
Duplicate cervices 418
Dysfunctional uterine
bleeding 309
contractions 121
Dysgerminoma 463
Dysmenorrhea 285, 324, 329
Dystocia 248

E

Eclampsia 142, 143, 232
Ectopic pregnancy 305, 307, 308, 310, 315, 442, 471, 471*f*, 475f, 509
Ectropion 432
Ejaculatory disturbances 451
Embryo transfer 458
Emergency contraception 497, 515
Endocrinological changes during pregnancy 4*f*
Endodermal
sinus tumor 463
adenocarcinoma 336*f*
cancer 334, 335f, 390
hyperplasia 302, 449
Endometrioid
stromal sarcomas 461
tumors 461
Endometriosis 369, 403, 405, 407, 456, 463
Endometritis 214, 315
Enterocele 392*f*
Epithelioid trophoblastic tumor 175
Erythroblastosis fetalis 194

F

Fallopian tube 273, 308
False labor pains 131
Fatty liver of pregnancy 121
Fetal
abdominal
circumference 202
acidosis 76
anemia 192
arm prolapse 103
asphyxia 103
blood
lactate sampling 249
pH sampling 249
cardiotocography 201
congenital anomalies 131
descent 64
injury 86
lie 61
macrosomia 119
malposition 83
malpresentation 121
skull 55
trauma 130
Fetus with polyhydramnios 188*f*
Fibroid uterus 369
Fixed retroversion 402
Flap-splitting technique 485
Follicular aspiration 458
Footling breech 96
Foreign bodies in vagina 315
Functional ovarian cysts 509

G

Galactokinesis 37
Gametogenesis 10
Genital
herpes 426
tuberculosis 308
Genitourinary
disorders 195
fistulae 482
Germ cell tumors 462
Gestational
diabetes 155, 190
trophoblastic disease 170, 195

Glucose challenge test 156
Godell's sign 30
Gonadoblastoma 463
Gonadotropin 287
deficiency 445
releasing hormone analog 288
Gonorrhea 428, 429*f*
Granny's knot 367*f*
Granulosa cell tumor 462
Gynandroblastoma 462

H

Hashimoto's thyroiditis 202
Haultain procedure 263
HCG 4, 287
Hegar's
dilator 168*f*
sign 29, 30*f*
HELLP syndrome 142
Hematoma 304, 375
in parametrium 304
Hemolytic anemia 148
Hepatic necrosis 144
Herpes zoster 406
High
pelvic application 84
vaginal swab 254
Hilus cell tumor 462
Hodge pessary test 403
Homan's sign 227
Hormonal method of contraception 499
Hormone replacement therapy 297, 300, 311
HPL 5
Huntington procedure 263
Hydrops fetalis 194
Hymen 273
Hyperemesis gravidarum 120, 121, 195
Hyperprolactinemia 445
Hypertensive disorders 218
Hyperthyroidism 202, 203
Hypothyroidism 202, 203, 315, 328
Hysterectomy 321, 382, 393
Hysterosalpingography 270, 325
Hysteroscopy 315, 335

I

Iliococcygeal muscles 398*f*
Iliopectineal ligaments 493*f*
Imperforate hymen 444
Incisional hernia 386
Incomplete
abortion 164, 310, 315
Indications for pelvic lymphadenectomy 338*t*
Inevitable abortion 164
Infant chest compression 252*f*
Infertility 305, 308, 319, 403, 442, 444, 449
Injectable contraceptives 502, 503*t*
Injuries of female genital tract 302
Internal
ballottement 7
genital organs 276*f*
iliac artery ligation 257*f*
radiation therapy 354
vaginal examination 131
Intracranial hemorrhage 80
Intractable uterine atony 214
Intrauterine
blood transfusions 192
contraceptive device 314, 497, 507
copper device 510*f*
fetal death 147
growth restriction 70, 122, 198
Invasive
cancer of cervix 347
mole 175
Inverted uterus 214
Iron
deficiency anemia 147, 148, 150*f*
metabolism during pregnancy 33
Irving technique 519

J

Jacquemier's sign 28, 30
Johnson's
maneuver 262
method 263*f*
Jones metroplasty 422*f*

K

Kallman's syndrome 445
Kleihauer-Betke test 191
Klinefelter's syndrome 451
Koilonychia 149*f*

L

Lactogenesis 37
Laparoscopic
adhesiolysis of endometriotic lesions 411*f*
assisted vaginal hysterectomy 379
cutting of fallopian tube and utero-ovarian ligaments 381
ovarian drilling 468
salpingotomy 476*f*
Latzko's partial colpocleisis procedure 485
Le Fort colpocleisis 393
Left
mentoanterior position 113
mentoposterior position 113
Leiomyomas 214, 314, 317, 414, 455
Leopold's maneuver 102
Levator ani muscle 400, 401*f*
Leydig cell tumor 462
Ligaments of pelvic floor 401*f*
Liley's chart 192, 193*f*
Linea nigra 7*f*
Lipid cell tumors 463
Lippes-loop 505*f*
Lochia 221
alba 221
rubra 221
serosa 221
Lymphadenectomy 337, 354

M

Macrosomia 133
Magnesium sulfate 141
Male

condom 512, 514
infertility 451
internal genitalia 26*f*
pseudohermaphroditism 291, 294
Malignant
ovarian tumors 405
Mammogenesis 37
Manchester operation 393, 394
Manual removal of placenta 239
Masculinizing ovarian tumors 296
Mastitis 225
Mastodynia 6
Mature cystic teratoma 463
Maylard incision 368*f*
McCune-Albright's syndrome 287
Meconium aspiration syndrome 201
Medical termination of pregnancy 166
Megaloblastic anemia 153, 154*f*
Menarche 284
Meningitis 143
Menopause and hormone replacement therapy 297
Menorrhagia 314, 318, 403
Mesodermal mixed tumors 462
Mesonephroid tumors 462
Metoclopramide 196
Metformin 468
Method of
eliciting Homan's sign 227*f*
fetal assessment 44
insertion of IUCD 508*f*
Methylene blue
dye test 484
three-swab test: 484
Metroplasty 418, 423
for bicornuate uterus 420
for septate uterus 421
Midsagittal section of female pelvis 274*f*
Miscarriage 122, 147, 159, 163, 315
Mixed epithelial tumors 462
Mobile retroversion 402
Modified Gillam's ventrosuspension 404
Molding of fetal skull 64
Moschcowitz culdoplasty 394
MRKH syndrome 418
Mucinous tumors 461
Müller Munro Kerr method 78
Müllerian agenesis 418, 420, 444
Multifetal gestation 117
Myomectomy 321, 382

N

Naegele's rule 40
Natural
family planning methods 511
nonabsorbable sutures 366
orifice transluminal surgery 386
Neisseria gonorrhoeae 469
Neonatal
asphyxia and acidosis 201
encephalopathy 201
hypoglycaemia 159
jaundice 159
resuscitation 250*t*
Neural tube defects 159
Nitrazine paper test 127
Noninvasive prenatal diagnostic tests 42
Nonstress test 44, 46, 200
No-scalpel vasectomy 523

O

Obstetric hysterectomy 213
Obstructed labor 77, 103
Oligohydramnios 70, 185, 186*f*, 201
Oophorectomy 382
Oral
contraceptive 312
pills 499
glucose tolerance test 156
Ornidazole 436
Orthopnea 161
Osiander's sign 28
Osteitis pubis 494
Osteoporosis 298, 449
O'Sullivan's method 263
Ovarian hyperstimulation syndrome 459
Ovulation pain 326
Ovulatory DUB 309
Oxytocin challenge test 46

P

Paget disease of vulva 356
Palmer's sign: 29
Pap smear 270, 310, 343, 348, 353, 358
Papanicolaou test 270
Paracervical nerve block 366*f*
Parametritis 477
Parkland technique 518
Parovarian cysts 463
Partial mole 174
Peak systolic velocity 48
Pelvic
exenteration 357
inflammatory disease 307, 315, 318, 403, 437
lymph nodes 354
nerves 275
tuberculosis 405
Pelvimetry 49
Pereyra's procedure 492
Perforation of uterus 303
Perineal body 402*f*
Peritoneal tuberculosis 340
Permanent method of contraception 517
Persistent
fetal circulation 201
vaginal bleeding 369
Pfannenstiel incision 368*f*
Placenta previa 96, 177
Placental
abruption 181*t*, 232
insufficiency 248
site trophoblastic tumor 175

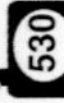

Polycystic ovarian disease 405, 466
Polyembryoma 463
Polyhydramnios 70, 120, 127, 159, 188
Pomeroy's technique 518
Posterior
colpoperineorrhaphy 393
cul-de-sac obliteration 412
Postmaturity syndrome 130
Postmenopausal
bleeding 330, 332*f*, 338
Postpartum hemorrhage 76, 115, 121, 148, 214, 252
Post-pill amenorrhea 444
Post-term pregnancy 130, 186
Post-thrombotic syndrome 227
Post-tubal ligation syndrome 521
Postvasectomy pain syndrome 524
Precocious
breast development 286*f*
puberty 285, 286
Premature
birth 181
menopause 297
ovarian failure 444
rupture of membranes 126
Premenstrual syndrome 326
Previous cesarean delivery 207
Procedure of
in vitro fertilization 458*f*
manual removal of placenta 242*f*
vasectomy 523*f*
Progestin only pill 497
Protraction disorders 74
Pseudocyesis 9
Pseudomeigs syndrome 321
Pubarche 284
Puberty 283
Pudendal nerve block 366*f*
Puerperal
pyrexia 223
sepsis 76, 224
Pulsatility index 48
Pyometra 338
Pyosalpinx 360
Pyridoxine 196

Q

Quickening 6

R

Radioimmunoassay 8
Rape 302, 304
Rectocele 392*f*
Rectovaginal
fistula 304, 432
Recurrent pregnancy losses 418
Red degeneration of fibroid 147
Repair of
anal sphincters 238*f*
episiotomy incision 235*f*
Respiratory
distress 133
syndrome 130, 201
Retained tampon or condom 432
Retropubic bladder neck suspension procedures 492
Retroverted uterus 403*f*
Rh negative pregnancy 190
Right
mentoanterior position 113
mentoposterior position 112
sacroiliac joint 50
Rupture of uterus 232

S

Salpingitis 469
Sarcoma of cervix 349
Screening for congenital malformations 158
Secondary postpartum hemorrhage 223
Semen analysis 452
Septate uterus 420
Serous tumors 461
Sertoli-Leydig cell tumor 462
Serum
iron concentration 151
testosterone 446
Sex
cord stromal tumors 462
education 285
steroid levels 287
Sexual
assault 302
dysfunctions 451
intercourse 42, 433
Sexually transmitted diseases 424
Sheehan's syndrome 80, 448
Shoulder dystocia 88, 159
Signs of
androgen excess 446
virilization 446
Simple cysts 463
Sinovaginal bulbs 27*f*
Spermicides 514
Spontaneous abortion 121, 163
Squamous
cell cancer 353*f*
papillomas 345
Square knot 367*f*
Steps of
laparoscopic myomectomy 322*f*
Latzko's partial colpocleisis 485*f*
procedure of vacuum aspiration 168*f*
Strassman metroplasty 421*f*
Stress urinary incontinence 490
Stria gravidarum 7*f*
Struma ovarii 463
Subdermal implants 504
Superficial
muscles of pelvic floor 400*f*
transverse perineal muscle 400*f*
Surgical
knots 363
needles 363

Symptothermal method 511
Synthetic nonabsorbable sutures 366
Syphilis 430

T

Tanner staging for
- breast development 447*f*
- development of pubic hair in females 447*f*

Teratomas 463
Thecoma 462
Thelarche 284
Theory of coelomic metaplasia 408
Threatened abortion 164, 173, 310, 315
Thyroxine binding globulin 202
Tibolone 301
Tobacco pouch appearance 307
Tocolytic therapy 125
Tompkins metroplasty 422*f*
TORCH test 211
Toxic shock syndrome 321
Transabdominal sonography 348*f*
TCRE 313*f*
Transdermal skin patches 301
Transvaginal urethropexies 492
Transverse
- lie 77, 100, 135
- perineal muscle 400

Trichomonas vaginalis 432
Tubal
- ectopic pregnancy 476*f*
- ligation 518
- sterilization 382, 517

Tuberculosis of genital tract 305
Turner's syndrome 444
Twin transfusion syndrome 189

U

Uchida technique 518
Ultrasound measurement of
- abdominal circumference 200*f*
- femur length 200*f*

Umbilical artery Doppler analysis 143
Unclassified
- epithelial tumors 462
- tumors 463

Undescended testes 451
Urethrovaginal fistula 482*f*
Urge incontinence 488*f*, 495
Urinary
- incontinence 398, 488
- retention and bladder dysfunction 86

Urogenital fistula 494
Use of oral contraceptive pills 329
Uterine
- artery
  - Doppler 47*f*
  - ligation 257*f*
- inversion 260
- malformations 416
- perforation 169, 338, 509
- retroversion 402
- rupture 258, 390
- subinvolution 223

Uteroplacental apoplexy 185
Uterovesical fistula 482*f*
Uterus 28, 273, 274, 299, 348
- didelphys 418

V

Vagina 28, 273, 299, 354
Vaginal
- assisted delivery 82
- atrophy 303
- birth after cesarean 208
- bleeding 183
- breech delivery 96
- cancer 352, 353*t*
- delivery of uterus 381*f*
- discharge 285, 305, 431
- dryness 298
- endometriosis 353
- hysterectomy 376, 379, 394
- inflammation 353
- introitus 52*f*
- prosthetic devices 496
- rings 497
- trauma 315
- trichomoniasis 436

Vaginectomy 354
Vaginitis 353
Vaginoplasty 418, 421
Vasa previa 121
Vasectomy 497, 521
Ventilation perfusion scanning 231
Vesical fistula 482
Vesicovaginal fistula 432, 482, 486*f*
Vessels of abdominal wall 277
von Willebrand's disease 253
Vulvar
- cancer 355, 355*f*, 357
- intraepithelial neoplasia 356

Vulvovaginal candidiasis 432

W

Whiff test 433
Wolffian ducts 26*f*

Z

Zipper injury 303

Also available...

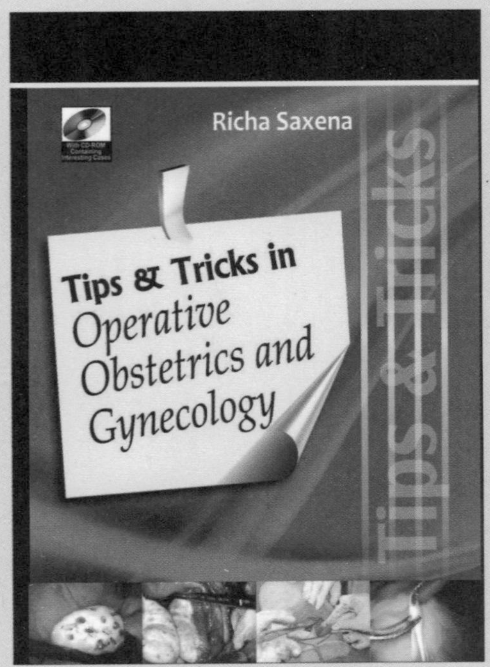